Leeds Metropolitan University

17 0177855 5

NUTRIENTS
and FOODS
in AIDS

Edited by

Ronald R. Watson

CRC Press

Boca Raton Boston London New York Washington, D.C.

Acquiring Editor:	Harvey Kane
Project Editor:	Carol Whitehead
Marketing Manager:	Becky McEldowney
Cover design:	Dawn Boyd
PrePress:	Walt Cerny
Manufacturing:	Carol Royal

Library of Congress Cataloging-in-Publication Data

Nutrients and foods in AIDS / edited by Ronald R. Watson.
     p. cm. -- (CRC series in modern nutrition)
    Includes bibliographical references and index.
    ISBN 0-8493-8561-X (alk. paper)
    1. AIDS (Disease)--Diet therapy. 2. AIDS (Disease)--Nutritional
aspects. I. Watson, Ronald R. (Ronald Ross) II. Series: Modern
nutrition (Boca Raton, Fla.)
    [DNLM: 1. Acquired Immunodeficiency Syndrome--diet therapy.
2. Acquired Immunodeficiency Syndrome--metabolism. 3. Nutrition.
WC 503.2 N976 1998]
RC607.A26N883   1998
616.97'920654--dc21
DNLM/DLC
for Library of Congress   97-48635
                                                  CIP

© 1998 by CRC Press LLC

No claim to original U.S. Government works
International Standard Book Number 0-8493-8561-X
Library of Congress Card Number 97-48635
Printed in the United States of America 1 2 3 4 5 6 7 8 9 0
Printed on acid-free paper

Series Preface

The CRC Series in Modern Nutrition is dedicated to providing the widest possible coverage to topics in nutrition. Nutrition is an interdisciplinary, interprofessional field par excellence. It is noted for its broad range and diversity. We trust that the titles and authorship in this series will reflect that range and diversity.

Published for a broad audience, the volumes of the CRC Series in Modern Nutrition are designed to explain, review, and explore present knowledge and recent trends, developments, and advances in nutrition. As such, they appeal to professionals as well as to educated laymen. The format for the series will vary with the needs of the author and the topic, including, but not limited to, edited volumes, monographs, handbooks, and texts.

Contributors from any bona fide area of nutrition, including the controversial, are welcome.

We welcome the significant contribution, *Nutrients and Foods in AIDS*, edited by Ronald R. Watson. This volume follows *Nutrition and AIDS*, also edited by Dr. Watson, published in this series by CRC Press in 1994. That volume has been well received by life scientists and caregivers concerned with AIDS. As the survival rate increases and as we learn more about AIDS and how to control or manage it, our attention increasingly focuses on factors such as nutrition and its possible impacts on the etiology and management of the disease.

This volume was designed to enlarge and expand, without overlap, our knowledge of nutrition and AIDS. As such, both volumes taken together constitute a splendid resource for all those interested in nutrition and AIDS.

Ira Wolinsky, Ph.D.
University of Houston
Houston, Texas
Series Editor

CRC SERIES IN MODERN NUTRITION

Edited by Ira Wolinsky

Published Titles

Handbook of Nutrition in the Aged, Ronald R. Watson
Manganese in Health and Disease, Dorothy Klimis-Tavantzis
Nutrition and AIDS, Ronald R. Watson
Nutrition Care for HIV Positive Persons: A Manual for Individuals and Their Caregivers, Saroj M. Bahl and James F. Hickson, Jr.
Calcium and Phosphorus in Health and Disease, John J. B. Anderson and Sanford C. Garner
Practical Handbook of Nutrition in Clinical Practice, Donald F. Kirby and Stanley J. Dudrick
Handbook of Dairy Foods and Nutrition, Gregory D. Miller, Judith K. Jarvis, and Lois D. McBean
Advanced Nutrition: Macronutrients, Carolyn D. Berdanier
Childhood Nutrition, Fima Lifshitz
Antioxidants and Disease Prevention, Harinder S. Garewal
Nutrition and Cancer Prevention, Ronald R. Watson and Siraj I. Mufti
Nutrition and Health: Topics and Controversies, Felix Bronner
Nutritional Concerns of Women, Ira Wolinsky and Dorothy Klimis-Tavantzis
Nutrients and Gene Expression: Clinical Aspects, Carolyn D. Berdanier
Advanced Nutrition: Micronutrients, Carolyn D. Berdanier
Nutrition and Women's Cancer, Barbara C. Pence and Dale M. Dunn
Nutrients and Foods in AIDS, Ronald R. Watson

Forthcoming Titles

Laboratory Tests for the Assessment of Nutritional Status, 2nd Edition, H. E. Sauberlich
Nutrition: Chemistry and Biology, 2nd Edition, Julian E. Spallholz, L. Mallory Boylan, and Judy A. Driskell
Child Nutrition: An International Perspective, Noel W. Solomons
Handbook of Nutrition for Vegetarians, Rosemary A. Ratzin
Melatonin in the Promotion of Health, Ronald R. Watson
Nutrition and the Eye, Allen Taylor
Advanced Human Nutrition, Denis Medeiros and Robert E. C. Wildman
Nutrition in Space Flight and Weightlessness Models, Helen W. Lane and Dale A. Schoeller

Preface

As HIV infection progresses to AIDS and eventual death, a significant component is undernutrition producing the added effects of starvation, a potent immunosuppressant. Nutritional supports could thus help maintain health in the HIV+ patient by repleting lost nutrients, compensating for nutritional damage done by the retrovirus-induced immunodeficiency, and stimulating the remaining immune system and cells for better host defenses. Unconventional dietary therapies are being used by AIDS patients. The goal of this book is to define recent advances in understanding the nutritional deficiencies of AIDS and HIV+ patients, as well as to explore the scientific knowledge of how nutritional and dietary changes and herbal medicines benefit or harm them. There are a large variety of alternative herbal and dietary remedies that have been suggested, and some have been tested in animals and people to stimulate immune defenses or compensate for changes induced by HIV infection. Animal models are clearly useful and helpful in testing novel remedies. There are a number of drugs and dietary materials such as cocaine, alcohol, and other immunosuppressive materials that could adversely impact damaged immune systems. The overall goal is to provide the most current, concise scientific appraisal of the status of nutrients, foods, and herbal (alternative) medicines in preventing or treating AIDS and its symptoms for improved quality of life.

Ronald R. Watson

About the Editor

Ronald R. Watson, Ph.D., initiated and directed the Specialized Alcohol Research Center at the University of Arizona College of Medicine until 1994. A theme of this National Institute of Alcohol Abuse and Alcoholism (NIAAA) Center Grant is to understand the role of ethanol-induced immuno-suppression on murine AIDS, including the use of nutrition to normalize immune dysfunction. This has led to use of antioxidants (DHEA, melatonin, and vitamin E) as treatments as well as T cell receptor peptides. Dr. Watson currently directs an NIH grant and study of oxidation and its immune enhancement of cardiotoxicity in murine AIDS.

Dr. Watson attended the University of Idaho, and graduated from Brigham Young University in Provo, Utah with a degree in chemistry in 1966. He completed his Ph.D. degree in biochemistry in 1971 at Michigan State University. His postdoctoral schooling was completed at the Harvard School of Public Health in nutrition and microbiology, including two years of postdoctoral research in immunology. He was Assistant Professor of Immunology and did research at the University of Mississippi Medical Center in Jackson from 1973 to 1974. He was an Assistant Professor of Microbiology and Immunology at the Indiana University Medical School from 1974 to 1978, and an Associate Professor at Purdue University in the Department of Food and Nutrition from 1978 to 1982. In 1982 he joined the faculty of the University of Arizona in the Department of Family and Community Medicine, Nutrition Section, and is a Research Professor in the Arizona Prevention Center. He has published 450 research papers and review chapters and edited 42 books.

Dr. Watson is a member of several national and international nutrition, immunology, and AIDS research societies. He directed the first symposium on nutrition and AIDS at FASEB and also at the International Congress on Nutrition in Australia in 1993. In 1997, he addressed the International Congress on Nutrition in Montreal on the subject of hormones and AIDS.

Contributors

P. Aukrust
Section of Clinical Immunology
  and Infectious Diseases
Medical Department A and
  Research Institute for Internal
  Medicine
University of Oslo
The National Hospital
Rikshospitalet
Oslo, Norway

Marianna K. Baum
Psychiatry and Behavioral
  Sciences
Division of Metabolism and
  Disease Prevention
University of Miami
  School of Medicine
Miami, Florida

Francine Belleville, Ph.D.
Department of Biochemistry
Central Hospital
Nancy, France

R. K. Berge
Division of Clinical
  Biochemistry
University of Bergen
Haukeland Hospital
Bergen, Norway

Lawrence A. Cone, M.D., D.Sc.
Section of Infectious Diseases
Eisenhower Medical Center
Rancho Mirage, California and
  Harbor-UCLA Medical Center
Torrence, California

Joël Constans
Service de Médecine Interne et
  Maladies Vasculaires
Hopital Saint-Andre
Bordeaux, France

Brigitte Dousset, M.D., Ph.D.
Department of Biochemistry
Central Hospital
Nancy, France

Mary G. Enig, Ph.D., F.A.C.N.
Nutritional Sciences Division
Enig Associates, Inc.
Silver Spring, Maryland

S. S. Frøland
Section of Clinical Immunology and
  Infectious Diseases
Medical Department A and Research
  Institute for Internal Medicine
University of Oslo
The National Hospital
Rikshospitalet
Oslo, Norway

Dorothy C. Humm, M.B.A., R.D., C.D.E., C.D.N.
The Preferred Nutritionist Organization
Brockport, New York

François Hussenet, M.D.
Department of Biochemistry
Central Hospital
Nancy, France

Paula Inserra
Arizona Prevention Center
University of Arizona
Tucson, Arizona

Raxit J. Jariwalla, Ph.D.
Viral, Immune and Metabolic Diseases
California Institute for Medical Research
San Jose, California

Jeongmin Lee
Arizona Prevention Center
University of Arizona Medical Center
Tucson, Arizona

Bernhard Lembcke
Division of Gastroenterology
University Hospital
J.W. Goethe University
Frankfurt, Germany

Bailin Liang, Ph.D.
Section of Rheumatology
Department of Internal Medicine
Yale University School of Medicine
New Haven, Connecticut

F. Müller
Section of Clinical Immunology and Infectious Diseases
Medical Department A and Research Institute for Internal Medicine
University of Oslo
The National Hospital
Rikshospitalet
Oslo, Norway

Bruce C. Oliver, R.D., C.D.N.
Community Health Network
Rochester, New York

Michael Ott
Division of Gastroenterology
University Hospital
J.W. Goethe University
Frankfurt, Germany

Gail Shor-Posner
Department of Psychiatry and Behavioral Sciences
Division of Metabolism and Disease Prevention
University of Miami School of Medicine
Miami, Florida

Carolyn D. Summerbell, SRD. Ph.D.
Department of Primary Care and Population Sciences
Royal Free Hospital School of Medicine
London, U.K.

A. M. Svardal
Department of Clinical Biology
Division of Pharmacology
University of Bergen
Haukeland Hospital
Bergen, Norway

P. M. Ueland
Department of Clinical Biology
Division of Pharmacology
University of Bergen
Haukeland Hospital
Bergen, Norway

James Y. Wang, Ph.D.
Division of Gastroenterology and
  Nutrition
Department of Pediatrics
University of Minnesota Medical
  School
Minneapolis, Minnesota

Ronald R. Watson, Ph.D.
Arizona Prevention Center
University of Arizona
Tucson, Arizona

Zhen Zhang
Arizona Prevention Center
University of Arizona
Tucson, Arizona

Contents

Nutrition and AIDS

chapter one

Trace elements, free radicals, and HIV progression

Brigitte Dousset, François Hussenet, and Francine Belleville

In recent years a considerable amount of information on the spectrum of clinical consequences of HIV infection has been accumulated. The most striking characteristics of this disease include severe malnutrition and wasting syndrome.[1-3] Such malnutrition involves both changes in overall body composition as well as deficiencies of specific nutrients. Since, as yet, there is only available palliative antiviral chemotherapy, alternative interventions are sought in order to prevent or alter the course and/or the progression of the disease. It has been shown that the course of infection is influenced by different factors including genetic susceptibility, age, environmental conditions, opportunistic infections, biological properties of HIV itself, therapy, metabolic changes, and nutritional status.[4-7] Among these latter, there is considerable evidence to suggest important links between trace minerals, oxidative stress, and HIV infection.[8] Indeed, alterations in trace element metabolism and increased oxidative stress associated with inadequate antioxidant capacities have been observed in HIV-infected subjects. As they constitute some of the factors which may influence immunological functions, viral replication, carcinogenesis, development of cardiomyopathy, and resistance to infections, they are, therefore, of considerable interest. Although the role of trace elements and free radicals in clinical manifestations of the disease is only partially elucidated, different observations have focused on their potential effects on the morbidity and mortality of the retrovirus infection. These substances represent a growing area of investigation in HIV infection. This review summarizes the current knowledge on trace element status and oxidative stress in HIV infection, their potential implication on pathogenesis and disease progression as well as the effects of various supplementations.

Trace element status in HIV infection

The impairment of trace element status during HIV infection was prelimi-
narily suggested in two studies describing low serum thymic hormone and
serum zinc levels in patients with AIDS.[9,10] By 1986, Dworkin et al.[11] observed
a deficit in plasma, whole blood, and red blood selenium levels in AIDS,
and subsequent studies on trace elements in clinical settings assessed — by
biochemical measurements of the baseline status — the prevalence of specific
abnormalities and the relationship between temporal alterations and disease
progression. However, the reported prevalence and incidence of trace element alterations has varied widely in all observations. These disparities may
reflect the sample sizes, different populations (risk factors, presence or
absence of treatment by antiretroviral chemotherapeutic agents), the calcu-
lation of supplemental dietary intake and specific nutrient intake, and socio-
economic status.

Selenium

There is extensive literature documenting a frequent occurrence of selenium
(Se) deficiency in HIV infection in agreement with the preliminary report of
Dworkin.[11] Thus, diminished plasma level of this trace element is common
in adult and children HIV 1-seropositive[11-20] with a global prevalence from
17 to 66%.[13,17] This deficit may exist at the early stage of the disease.[18,19]
Moreover, plasma Se concentrations are lower in patients with persistent
lymphadenopathy or AIDS related complex (ARC)[12,14] and the decline tends
to be most marked in adults with AIDS[11,12,19,21,22] rather than children.[20,23] Se
deficiency is also documented by reduced whole blood and red blood cell
concentrations in patients with ARC or AIDS without difference between
the groups.[12,15,18] Moreover, a low Se status is frequently associated with an
impairment in glutathione peroxidase (GSH-Px) function. The diminished
erythrocyte GSH-Px activity found in most[11,12,18] but not all cases[21] is further
evidence of a true Se depletion. This decline tends to be more frequent in
patients with AIDS (45%) than with ARC (27%) and correlates to plasma
selenium concentrations, hematocrit values, and total lymphocyte counts.[12,18]
The impact of Se deficiency on HIV1-infected subjects may be modulated or
amplified by the interactions of trace minerals with other related nutrients
such as vitamin E or by overlapping biochemical functions such as vitamin
A and zinc.

Zinc

By 1983, Dardenne et al. described undetectable levels of thymuline-like
activity in a patient with ARC,[10] and this finding was interpreted as showing
HIV-induced injury of the thymic epithelial cells that synthesize and release
hormones. However, this observation raised the question of whether alterations

in zinc (Zn) homeostasis might occur in HIV-1 infection. Multiple investigations regarding the Zn status in HIV-1 infection have focused mainly on the plasma/serum concentrations although variations in the values may occur rapidly within hours and do not necessarily reflect corresponding changes in tissue and cellular zinc concentrations.[24,25] Some reports describe significant biological impairment of plasma/serum Zn levels at various stages of the disease in adults[4,5,14,19,20,26,27,28] and children[20,23] while other observations provide a detailed and consistent characterization of a deficiency.[13,21,24,29-35] Thus, a marginal or clear hypozincemia is common and occurs with a total prevalence from 3 to 50% in study populations consisting of subjects with different risk factors and at various stages of the disease.[13,17,24,26,36,37] Hypozincemia is more frequent in patients undergoing azidothymidine (AZT) therapy[37] and may be, at least in part, due to AZT that decreases the concentrations of Zn in plasma despite adequate intake.[38] Asymptomatic HIV-infected children exhibit normal plasma/serum Zn values[18,23] whereas HIV-infected adults have either depressed[21,22] or normal levels.[29,33,39] The prevalence of low serum Zn concentrations is accentuated in late stages of infection: 48% and 27% of values, respectively, below 0.85 µg/l and 0.75 µg/l in CDC group III[32] and 38% in CDC group IV. The magnitude of the decline may also be progressively enhanced by the severity of the infection as characterized by a significant lowering of concentrations from asymptomatic subjects and patients with lymphadenopathy to patients with AIDS,[9,22,29,30,31,34,39] which is nevertheless not systematically related to clinical progression in adults[21,25,30] as in children.[20] Some authors carried out studies on Zn concentrations in blood cells, but no abnormality was identified in polymorphonuclear and mononuclear cells,[27] platelets,[4] or erythrocytes[4,20,26] although low level in the red blood cells (RBC) was noted in some cases.[4] The activity of Cu/Zn superoxide dismutase in RBC, considered as a more reliable marker of the Zn status, is not modified regardless of the stage of the infection.[4] In addition, Zn concentrations in urine[4,19] as well as in toenails[39] do not differ statistically between HIV-seropositive and seronegative subjects.

Copper

Abnormalities in copper (Cu) are still less clearly identified than those of Se or Zn. The serum Cu values noted in the different reports are within the normal range,[26,40] decreased,[19] or increased.[4,13,20,24,32,39] Moreover, the concentrations of Cu are subject to a significant decrease as a result of AZT treatment.[38] The variations appear to be linked to the severity of the disease,[4,19,24] and they are found more important in patients with AIDS than those who are asymptomatic or with lymphadenopathy while both latter groups exhibit similar values.[4] In children, the rise observed in the serum of non-AIDS stage is not confirmed in the AIDS group.[20] The urinary excretion[19] and the amount in toenails[39] of Cu is not altered by HIV infection.

Magnesium

Although few investigators have examined the magnesium (Mg) status in HIV infection, the observations indicate that serum Mg levels in HIV-infected subjects are either normal[19,26] or modified as characterized by hypomagnesemia demonstrated in 30 to 64.7% of cases.[13,24,41] Serum Mg values appear independent of the stage of infection.[19,24] In HIV-infected individuals with normal serum concentrations, the urinary concentrations are not statistically different from those found for uninfected[19] while hypomagnesemia is associated with renal Mg wasting.[41]

Manganese

The characterization of trace element status in HIV infection is also extended to manganese (Mn). Serum Mn concentrations are similar in asymptomatic HIV-individuals and healthy controls but significantly higher than in patients with AIDS.[19] No differences in urinary Mn levels are found between HIV-infected patients and controls.[19]

Oxidative stress in HIV-infection

Free radicals such as superoxide, O_2^-, nitric oxide, NO, and hydroxyl, OH, as well as other oxygen-derived species (ROS) such as hydrogen peroxide (H_2O_2) and hypochlorous (HOCl) are formed constantly in the human body.[42] Early after HIV infection, radical oxygenated species (ROS) increase. Several mechanisms are implicated that result in enhancement of ROS production and decrease of antioxidant defenses. The modification of intracellular ROS levels influences the immunity status of HIV-positive patients and virus replication.

Increase of ROS and free radicals

Modifications of phagocytosis cell functions has been observed *in vitro* and *in vivo* after HIV infection. The level of O_2^- generation in HL 60 cells after HIV infection is significantly higher than that of steady-state although no activation of NADPH oxidase is observed. It has also been hypothesized that cytosolic factor(s) due to virus infection might be responsible for the amplification of O_2^- generation.[43] A similar phenomenon is observed *in vivo*; ROS released by neutrophils of HIV-infected patients is increased in CDC group III whereas they are diminished in CDC group IV. This rise may be due to cytokine stimulation, mainly $TNF\alpha$[44] which increases with disease progression and degree of immunodeficiency.[45] The results of Bandes et al.[46] also suggest that in early infection, neutrophil functions or phagocytosis are more vigorous than those in uninfected donors. On the contrary, several studies *in vitro* and *in vivo* report that such activities are depressed in HIV-infected patients. So Spaer et al.[47] observed in asymptomatic subjects that the oxidation burst of isolated peripheral blood mononuclear cells was depressed following with stimulation with PHA. In the course of the disease, the opportunistic infections may contribute to the production of O_2^- and NO.[48]

Mitochondria are another source of free radical generation. Macho et al.[49] demonstrate that HIV-infected lymphocytes exhibit a reduction of mitochondrial transmembrane potential and an elevated O_2^- production, which may be important for lymphocyte depletion. However, no correlation between the clinical status of HIV carriers and mitochondrial modification was observed.

Decrease of antioxidant defenses

HIV infection is associated with an altered protection of cells from oxidative stress. A reduction of glutathione peroxidase activity is observed.[50] Cells acutely infected with HIV present a tat-mediated transcriptional decrease of Mn superoxide dismutase (Mn SOD) expression[51] and lose their ability to induce this antioxidant enzyme in response to TNFα and interleukin-1.[51,52,53] In addition, the serum catalase activity increases progressively in advancing HIV infection and is certainly due to tissue damage since a correlation exists between serum catalase and lacticodeshydrogenase.[54]

Furthermore, HIV-seropositive patients often have a specific deficiency in one or more antioxidant trace elements (see above) or vitamins. However, the prevalence of patients with at least one abnormal antioxidant value is 22% in asymptomatic subjects and 46% in symptomatic subjects with AIDS.[55] Deficiency in micronutrients may be related to malabsorption which can occur early in HIV infection. Indeed, HIV infection of small intestine cells resulted in early impairment of the function of the small bowel mucosa.[56] Moreover, metabolic changes caused by HIV activity and cytokine production contribute to this deficiency.[57]

A progressive decrease in plasma vitamin A levels is often observed[5,20,25,38] with concentrations below normal at various stages of the infection.[20,24,55] Development of vitamin A (B_6 and B_{12}) deficiency is associated with faster disease progression.[36]

Total serum carotene concentrations are reduced in HIV-infected individuals without difference between asymptomatic and AIDS patients although the levels are correlated to CD4 count or CD4/CD8 ratio.[58] Other studies reported normal plasma β carotene concentrations and a significant decrease of total carotene in HIV-seropositive patients compared to control group.[55] Total carotene levels are lower in stage IV than in stage II.[21] The normal plasma values of β carotene suggest that decline in total carotene may be due to changes in lycopene concentrations as observed in HIV-infected children.[20]

Vitamin E plasma levels are less often decreased than those of vitamin A or total carotene. Vitamin E deficiency was not found in patients with wasting syndrome.[24,25] Skurnick et al.[55] noted that vitamin E tended to be lower in HIV-infected subjects than in controls, but the difference was not significant. In contrast, circulating vitamin E is considerably reduced in HIV-seropositive patients (children or adults) with an increase of the prevalence from non-AIDS to AIDS stages.[20,23] Vitamin E is the main antioxidant of cell membranes and plasma lipoprotein and its decrease is related to the increase of lipid peroxidation evaluated by plasma malondialdehyde levels although, paradoxically, lipid peroxidation is more important in asymptomatic HIV-subjects than in the AIDS group.[22]

Ascorbic acid has been shown to inactivate, *in vitro*, a broad spectrum of viruses including HIV by inhibiting reverse transcriptase activity. In studies this inhibition persisted as long as vitamin supplementation was maintained in culture medium whereas the removal of ascorbic acid resulted in the resumption of virus replication.[59,60] There is little information about vitamin C in HIV infection, and the prevalence of deficiency varies from 0 to 27%[24] without significant difference according to the severity of the disease in adults[24,25] as well as in children.[20]

Nutrient deficiency may play a contributory role in immune function impairment in HIV-infected individuals. The results of numerous studies provide evidence that micronutrient status may be, at least partially, corrected among HIV-infected patients by use of micronutrient supplementation. An effective program of nutritional supplementation may be beneficial for these patients.[5]

Glutathione (GSH) is the main defense against intracellular oxidants acting as a cofactor in enzymatic reactions such as glutathione peroxidase, the major enzyme for H_2O_2 removal. It is also a regulator of cellular redox potential maintaining protein sulphydryl redox status, and during these reactions, the reduced form (GSH) is transformed in oxidized glutathione (GSSG) and quickly eliminated from the cells. A deficiency of GSH is found in plasma[61-64] and the decrease occurs rapidly upon infection and becomes greater as the disease progresses.[62] Contradictory results are noted in peripheral blood mononuclear cells (PBMC) including normal[45,65] or decreased,[61-63,66-69] values, which might be explained by different concentrations of GSH in subpopulations of lymphocytes and monocytes in mixed populations of PBMC.[63] Roederer et al.[66] and Staal et al.[67] have observed low and high intracellular GSH levels in the CD4+ T cell and CD8+ T cell subsets of healthy individuals and demonstrated a selective depletion of cells with high intracellular GSH values in virtually all HIV-positive individuals. This loss occurs even in asymptomatic patients with a nearly normal number of CD4+ T cells and is greatest in the later stages of the disease, likely in response to changes of cytokine concentrations.[70] Furthermore, early in the course of HIV-1 infection, the plasma glutamate level increases and aggravates the cysteine deficiency by inhibiting the membrane transport of cysteine. Clinical studies have revealed that individual cysteine and glutamate levels are correlated with the lymphocyte reactivity and CD4+ cell counts.[71]

Trace elements, immunity, and HIV replication

Existing studies suggest a complex set of multidirectional relationships among nutrition, gastrointestinal function, immunity, and HIV-replication. However, it is difficult to determine the precise role of trace element status since it is, as yet, unclear whether the observed abnormalities are merely a consequence of the disease or have a role in the pathogenesis of it. On one hand, the causes for abnormal trace element status remain unelucidated and are more likely multifactorial in origin. Thus, trace element alterations appear to be influenced by the course of infection as characterized by the rise in their prevalence over the course of the disease which may reflect the progression of the HIV infection and/or be related to antiretroviral chemo-therapeutic agents (AZT)-induced effect and/or acute phase response. On the other hand, different findings[5,12,14,25,29,32,36,72-74] raise the possibility that altered nutritional status may affect the progression by exacerbating immu-nologic, hematologic, and neurologic deficits that are common during HIV infection, contributing to the development of cardiomyopathy or carcino-genesis, modulating viral replication as well as the effectiveness of antiret-roviral therapy with medications such as AZT,[38] reducing, to some degree, appetite and increasing weight loss,[27] and impairing hormonal regulation. Although a variable degree of correlation was noted between total dietary intake and biochemical measurements taken to assess nutrition status, some micronutrient abnormalities are found in HIV-infected individuals at an early stage of the disease and in the absence of gastrointestinal malabsorp-tion, opportunistic infections, antiretroviral treatment, with daily intake within or above recommended dietary allowance level. Furthermore, differ-ent studies have shown that serum levels of Se, Zn, and Cu may predict progression to AIDS[22,39] independently of percent of CD4+ count and inde-pendently of intake.

Zinc

Zinc (Zn) is necessary for the normal functioning of all living systems.[75-77] This trace element is known to play an essential role in immune functions and others which have an impact on immune functions. Moreover, a number of immunological abnormalities in HIV-1 infection are similar to the defects observed in both experimental animals and humans with Zn deficiency. This latter is, *in vivo*, associated with a decrease in many immune functions, primarily of the T cell system. Thus, in severely Zn-deficient subjects such as patients with acrodermatitis enteropathica, a childhood disease caused by an inborn error of metabolism resulting in malabsorption of dietary zinc, a T cell lymphopenia, cutaneous anergy, a depressed responsiveness of lym-phocytes to the mitogen phytahaemagglutinin, a selective decrease in T4+ helper cells, a decreased NK cell lytic activity, and deficient thymic hormone activity were observed.[78,79] Elsewhere, Zn depletion may also contribute to the immunological aberrations of HIV-infected patients. A close correlation between immune response evaluated by proliferative response to T cell mitogens and serum Zn levels was reported in seropositive HIV patients.[33,38] Likewise, Harrer et al.[34] examined the influence of Zn on the *in vitro* proliferation of peripheral mononuclear cells from HIV-1 infected patients and showed that lymphocyte proliferation correlated clearly with the stages of the WR classification, and all patients (WR stages 4 to 6) exhibited a depressed cell proliferation. The precise mechanism for Zn-dependent immunodeficiency, in particular dysfunctions of T cells, is not clear.[78,80] Several mechanisms are probable, and it is likely that one of the major actions is on lymphocyte proliferation.[78] The other significant effect of Zn on immune activity is the decline in the thymic secretory function. A considerable body of evidence now exists that shows that serum level of thymulin is significantly decreased in zinc deficiency in the human model as well as in patients with AIDS.[10,30,81] This nonapeptide hormone is active and measurable in bioassay when it is bound to Zn.[82] Diminished values of active thymulin without changes in those of total hormone are observed in the absence or presence of low serum Zn concentration in patients with either ARC or AIDS,[10,30] and it has been suggested that the evaluation of the ratio of total/active thymulin may represent a better measurement of Zn bioavailability.[30] This hormone produced by the thymic epithelium exhibits potent immunoregulating effects including the inducement of several T cell markers, the promotion of T cell function such as allogenic cytotoxicity, suppressor function, and IL2 production.[83] The effects of Zn depletion are not restricted to T cells. This trace element activates B cells[84] to secrete immunoglobulins (polyclonal activation) and can also interact synergistically with their activators to enhance the activation and differentiation process *in vitro*. In addition, subjects with Zn deficiency induced experimentally exhibited decreased natural killer activity,[85] and an experiment has shown that this function was twice as high in Zn-supplemented mice as in pair-fed, Zn-deficient mice. Consequently, Zn deficiency favors opportunistic infections to which HIV-infected patients are susceptible.

Apoptosis may be enhanced by different mechanisms in HIV infection and a Zn deficit may contribute to this phenomenon since this trace element is an inhibitor of endonuclease activated by the loss of Ca^{++} homeostasis.[86]

Zn also plays a critical role in the virus replication because certain retroviral proteins contain peptide segments that chelate Zn ions. Each of these segments forming a three-looped structure is referred to as a Zn-finger that has been found in HIV-1 and HIV-2. The Zn finger-like domain in the gag precursor polyprotein is involved in RNA selection and packaging, and that of the mature nucleocapsid protein is required for the function of this protein in early stages of the infection.[87,88] There are also Zn-finger proteins in the structure of HIV-EP1[89] and tat.[90] Zn depletion may also diminish the effectiveness of AZT because the pathway of intracellular AZT metabolism requires the Zn-dependent enzyme thymidine kinase for conversion to its active triphosphate form.[38] On the other hand, Zn ions can also bind stably with the aspartate residues of the catalytic site of the HIV-1 protease leading to the inhibition of this enzyme that mediates the proteolytic cleavage of the viral gag and gag-pol fusion polyproteins into their functional forms.[91-93]

Zn depletion may also be one of several factors contributing to many manifestations observed in HIV-infected patients such as anorexia or impaired taste acuity by acting on the secretion and/or release of opiate and/or hypothalamic peptides, gastrointestinal manifestations such as diarrhea, and central nervous system malfunction.[94]

Zn is a modulator of several endocrinological processes — mainly growth, glucose homeostasis, gonadal function, thyroid function, adrenal hormones, prolactin and calcium-phosphorus metabolism — that can be considerably perturbed by a deficiency.[95] Thereby, Zn might be at least partially implicated in hormonal dysfunction observed during the infection to which the connection with the wasting syndrome is still ill-defined.[2,3]

Several findings argue in favor of the serum Zn level being a risk marker of progression.[17,39] Subjects who progressed to AIDS in succeeding years had significantly lower Zn levels than nonprogressors[39] and Zn deficiency may predict progression to AIDS independently of the percentage of CD4 cells and independently of intake. Beck et al.[13] found a positive correlation between Zn and Se values and suggested that both trace elements could affect viral replication in a competitive modulatory fashion. A similar relationship as well as inverse correlations between Zn and β2 microglobulin concentrations is reported by Allavena.[17]

It has been, therefore, hypothesized that Zn supplementation might be useful in retarding progression of the immune deficiency in HIV-1 infection[31] although the relationship between dietary Zn intake and level measured in the serum[32,36] is not reported in some observations.[39,58] So, normalization of plasma Zn levels is linked to slower disease progression in both AZT-treated as well as non-AZT-treated individuals and to a significant increase in the level of CD4+ cells in this latter group.[36] In response to supplementation, patients with AIDS (children: 2 mg Zn/d for 3 weeks; adults: 1 mg Zn/d for 10 weeks) exhibit an elevation in serum Zn baseline levels,[9,27] CD4/CD8 ratios,[9,96] CD4 counts,[27] and a concomitant weight gain.[27] An increment in the lymphocyte response to mitogens occurs in asymptomatic patients treated by 125 mg of Zn for 3 weeks.[97] Nevertheless, high intakes of Zn from food alone and from total intake (food and supplementation) are associated with an increased hazard of developing AIDS, and the proportion of surviving AIDS-free is 70.4, 61.4, and 52.9% in groups with Zn intake ≤14.1mg/day, 14.1–20 mg/day, and >20 mg/day, respectively.[98]

Selenium

Diverse clinical manifestations have been related to selenium (Se) deficiency. It was reported to promote congestive cardiomyopathy known as Keshan disease.[99] Cardiomyopathy is also noted in patients who have suboptimal intake of Se[100,101] as in children or adults with AIDS.[16,102-109] Further, Se deficiency has been found to be implicated in the pathogenesis of human myopathy and is considered as a possible cofactor in muscle involvement in HIV-infected patients because of its clear correlation with the existence of muscle symptoms.[110]

The immune response is also susceptible to an alteration in Se status,[111,112] but whether this impairment could have any secondary effect on immune function in AIDS is unknown. The biological roles of Se are closely linked to the requirement of seleno-cysteine for activity of GSH-Px and phospho-lipidhydroperoxide glutathione peroxydase (PLGSH-Px), both of which catalyze the reduction of the substrates H_2O_2, organic peroxides using reduced gluthatione as a hydrogen donor. GSH-Px and/or PLGSH-Px tissues, platelets, and other lymphoid cells are responsible for the reduction of prostaglandin G_2 in the arachidonic acid cascade leading to the synthesis of thromboxane A_2, prostacyclin, and prostaglandins. One or both of the Se-enzymes in cells are responsible for the reduction of 5-HPTE, 12-HPTE, and 15-HPTE in the synthesis of leucotrienes and lipoxins. Numerous investigations have demonstrated a reduction of eicosanoid biosynthesis in the absence of Se and GSH-Px.[113,114] The decreased production of chemotatic factors such as leucotriene B_4 by neutrophils may reduce the ability of circulating phagocytes to migrate to sites of infection and inflammation. It is likely that the antiinflammatory activity and immune functions of Se are mediated in part by the Se-containing peroxydases owing to both the reduction of hydroperoxides and the synthesis of eicosonoids.[115]

Diverse abnormalities of the development and function of the immune system with low Se status have been described.[112] Thus, Se deficiency was reported to be associated with impaired responses to vaccines, lowered helper T cell numbers, decreased immune cytotoxicity, and impaired phagocytic function.[116,117] The ability of phagocytes to ingest microbial pathogens seems not significantly altered by Se status, but post-phagocytic killing could be depressed by a deficiency. Several different types of observations suggest that Se and GSH-Px are important modulators of the oxidative products of the respiratory burst of phagocytic cells. Although hydrogen peroxide is a constituent of the respiratory burst, release of increased amounts of this molecule leads to damage of lysosomial membranes. Thus, in turn, Se may affect the ability of the host to resist infection by microbial pathogens. In animals, Se depletion results in impaired fungicidal activity by neutrophils leading to yeast infections.[112]

Se deficiency as well as GSH-Px depletion produce an oxidative stress damaging the cell membranes and, consequently, the functions of the cells of the immune system which are membrane-dependent processes such as the secretion of lymphokins and antibodies, antigen reception, lymphocyte transformation, and contact cell lysis.[15]

AIDS is also associated with a striking risk of carcinoma. Experimental and epidemiological links exist between Se and a variety of tumor types, but very little is known about the role of nutritional elements in carcinogenesis in HIV infection.[18]

A new hypothesis for the regulation of HIV expression by Se has been proposed by Taylor et al. suggesting a mechanism whereby the depletion could accelerate the virus transcription. Indeed, Taylor et al.[118,119] found potential selenocysteine insertion sequences in the RNA of HIV structures that are known to be necessary and sufficient for the incorporation of selenocysteine at UGA «stop» codon. The insertion of seleno-cysteine at the UGA «stop» codons during the process called termination suppression permits reading through the «stop» codon and extending the protein sequence.[120] The potential selenocysteine-containing gene products had similarities to a number of DNA-binding proteins of papillomavirus, which bound to DNA act as transcriptional activators or repressors depending on how the gene is spliced. Taylor had suggested that one form of the proposed DNA-binding protein could act as a repressor of HIV transcription and that Se deficiency within an infected cell could be a signal for unrestrained expression of viral genes and a trigger for release from latency.

It would be possible that the depletion in Se might have a further direct or indirect negative impact on the progression of the disease although it is clear that it is not the main etiology of immune defects occurring in HIV infection. By reflecting in part the HIV activity and contributing to the development of AIDS, the blood levels of Se seem to be, like those of Zn and Cu, prognostic biological markers of progression.[17,40]

The relationship between adjuvant Se supplementation and the reversal of Se deficiency was assessed. Se in the forms normally contained in foods appear to be absorbed by most HIV-infected subjects, and with 400 µg of selenium yeast or 80 µg/d of sodium selenite, the blood Se levels increase without parallel change in immunological parameters (CD4 count, CD4/CD8 ratio, red and white cell counts).[14,15] Upon Se repletion, an increase to normal value of the left ventricle shortening fraction reflecting an improvement of cardiac function was noted.[106] In response to oral daily supplementation, diminished recurrent illness, improvement of gastrointestinal functions and appetite, and positive neurologic and psychologic changes have also been described.[121] It has been suggested that the determination of phosphoprotein CD20 may be a parameter of interest in the supplementation follow-up. Its expression occurs on peripheral B cells but not on T cells, NK cells, or monocytes and is related to intracellular B cell level in HIV-infected patients.[121] Indeed, Se modulates intracellular and extracellular levels by various mechanisms although the decrease in total intracellular GSH in PBMC subsets is due in part to the constant loss of T cells — especially those with high levels — while a great disparity characterizes the amount of the other cells.[67]

Oxidative stress, immunity, and HIV replication

A wide variety of research supports the theory that oxidative stress may contribute to several aspects of HIV disease pathogenesis and is involved in the progression of HIV disease by enhancing viral replication and inflammatory response, decreasing immune cell proliferation, loss of immune function, apoptosis, chronic weight loss, and exacerbating the sensitivity to drugs. However, these phenomena are also influenced by other metabolic events that are not related directly to oxidant overproduction.

Immune functions are strongly influenced by redox potentials,[122-124] and the constitutive difference in endogenous antioxidants[66,67] may contribute to the various sensitivities to oxidizing stress among lymphocyte sub-populations.[22] Indeed, GSH is an important factor for T cell proliferation, T and B cell differentiation, cytotoxic T cell activity, and NK activity.[125-129] Leukocytes contain a high concentration of ascorbate, which is expended during infection, and phagocytosis.[130] and deficiency in vitamin C lead to diminished delayed cutaneous hypersensitivity reactions and phagocytic cell function.[131] Vitamin E stimulates the mitogenesis and the helper functions of T cells and perhaps cooperation of T and B cells.[132] Deficiency in vitamin A is associated with a decrease of lymphocyte counts, a suppression of antibody production after immunization, a reduction of peripheral macrophages, and lymphocyte response to mitogenesis.[133] *In vitro*, the recognition of antigen by T cells, but not antigen uptake or processing by antigen-presenting cells, is inhibited by low concentrations of aldehydes and amines,[134] and the direct as well as antibody-dependent cytotoxicity of lymphocytes is decreased by oxidative stress.[135,136] Lipid peroxidation and/or cytotoxic aldehydes can block macrophage action, inhibit protein synthesis, kill bacteria and act as chemotaxis for phagocytosis.[134,137] Oxidative stress and depressed GSH levels lead to abnormal production of certain cytokines such as TNFα or that of interleukin receptor (IL-2). Then, the release of cytokines resulting in activation of the immune system encourages cell lysis, lysosoma enzyme release, free radical generation, and re-initiation of the cycle.

Apoptosis, or programmed cell death (PCB), may be induced by oxidative stress[132,138,139] and be partially responsible for the progressive loss of CD4 lymphocytes occurring in HIV infection.[140-143] It has been proposed that an oxidative signal for T cell apoptosis can originate both extracellularly and intracellularly,[139] and the mechanisms of oxidant-mediated cell injury include membrane lipid peroxidation and loss of Ca++ homeostasis, DNA damage, and metabolic pathways.[143]

Elsewhere redox status of cells as well as intracellular glutathione level regulate HIV-virus replication, and an inverse relationship between intracellular CD4 antioxidant capacity and replication of HIV has been reported. Different findings argue in favor of an enhancement of HIV replication by oxidative stress. Reactive oxygen intermediates like hydrogen peroxide have been shown to serve as messagers in the induction of the nuclear factor κB (NFκB).[144] This latter is a pleiotropic cellular transcription factor that regulates a wide variety of cellular (IL-2, IL-2 receptor, IL-6, TNFα) and viral genes. Its activation can be brought about by a variety of pathogenic or pathogen-elicited stimuli including cytokines, mitogens, bacteria and related products, virus and viral products, physical stress, oxidants such as H_2O_2, and a variety of chemical agents such as phorbol esters, and certain phosphatase inhibitors. NFκB activation is involved in HIV gene expression and then may be crucial in regulating AIDS latency.[145] The long terminal repeat (LTR) region of HIV proviral DNA contains two juxtaposed κB enhancer elements. In cells, as long as HIV is in its latent state, NFκB remains within the cytosol in an inactive form bound to the inhibitory IκB protein. The production of excessive and unquenched levels of free radicals leads to the dissociation of IκB from the NFκB in the cytoplasm, the subsequent translocation of active NFκB into the nucleus, and the transcriptional activation of the proviral DNA and of many cytokines.[146,147] The nuclear translocation of NFκB requires a certain amount of GSSG while an excess of GSSG inhibits binding of NFκB at the level of DNA.[148] On the contrary, agents that interfere directly or indirectly with the activation of NFκB inhibit *in vitro* HIV replication. Then, substances such as L-cysteine, L- and D-N-acetylcysteine, glutathione, SOD, dithiocarbamates, pentoxifylline, vitamin E succinate and vitamin C reduce NFκB activation in HIV-1-infected T cells.[59,149-155] Ascorbic acid also reduces the stability of virion-associated reverse transcriptase.[60] In addition, the effectiveness of antiretroviral therapy with medications such as AZT is modulated by the nutritional status. The addition of vitamin E acts *in vitro* in combination with AZT synergistic effects to inhibit the HIV-1 virus by modulating glycosylation of viral proteins.[156]

Oxidative stress involved in the progression may also implicate HIV transmission from cell to cell by syncytia formation. Kamekoa et al. (1993)[157] showed that HIV-spread is amplified during cell-cell transmission by superoxide. This effect through an enhancement of HIV-induced syncytia formation is specific and reduced by SOD and ceruloplasmin. It is also mediated by CD4 that is the region present on the surface of helper T lymphocytes and mononuclear phagocytes and reactive with gp120.

Interactive effects of oxidative stress and disturbed production of cytokines and hormones may constitute a possible mechanism contributing to the elevated resting energy expenditure (REE) and hypermetabolism. It has also been suggested that certain complications such as renal and hepatic dysfunction or sensitivity to drugs such as sulfamethoxazole and acetaminophen could be related to oxidative stress.[158-161]

Several investigations regarding the status in vitamins, glutathione, peroxidase, glutathione and cysteine have demonstrated that deficiencies in these substances occur early in the HIV infection and suggested they tend to complicate the progression of infection although they are themselves influenced by the course of the disease. Indeed, regardless of the treatment by AZT, biochemical measurements are related to dietary intake of vitamins A, E, B_6, B_{12} but unrelated to intake of retinol and vitamin C.[32,38,98] Recommended dietary allowance intake levels are generally associated with normal plasma nutrient levels in HIV-seronegative but not HIV-seropositive subjects[5] and do not appear adequate for HIV-infected individuals since significantly higher nutrient intake is necessary to achieve normal plasma nutrient values in HIV-seropositive patients.[5] Furthermore, daily intake of vitamin A from 9.06 to 20.6 IU/d and vitamin C >715 mg may slow progression to AIDS.[98] Interestingly, the risk of AIDS is more clearly related to the total intake levels in these vitamins than intake from food only and is not correlated with supplements.[131] The decreased serum retinol concentrations, indicative of vitamin A deficiency, appear also to be independently associated with mortality, but not with the development of infections such as tuberculosis.[162] On the contrary, another recent report shows negative results for the effect of vitamin A intake on disease progression.[163]

These findings on the role of oxidative stress[164] raised the question whether micronutrient supplementation might be beneficial in HIV infection. Indeed, total daily intake of vitamins C and A, like that of Zn, is an independent predictor of AIDS.[98] Changes in vitamin A from biochemical deficiency to adequacy were positively associated with an estimated increase on the level of CD4+ and linked to slower disease progression in both AZT-treated as well as untreated individuals.[5,165] The relation between vitamin A intake and AIDS progression appears to have a U-shaped form with the middle two quartiles of intake having the most benefit.[98] With high doses of ascorbate (50–200 g/day), Cathcart[166] has reported clinical improvement and decreased symptoms despite a lack of change in their CD4/CD8 ratios. The lesions of oral hairy leucoplakia in HIV-infected patients were completely resolved after a local application of 0.1% vitamin A, twice daily, but recurred when the treatment was stopped.[167] Because oral supplementation in β carotene provokes an increase of approximately 30% in circulating CD4 lymphocytes in healthy subjects,[168] the potential benefit of this provitamin A was also considered. Following a treatment with 60 mg/d over a 4-month period, Garewal et al.[169] observed an increase in the number of cells with NK markers only, while Coodley[170] noted an improvement in total white blood cell count and in mean percent changes in CD4 counts and CD4/CD8 ratios after 180mg/d for 1 month. Oral administration of N-acetylcysteine (NAC) has been proposed in order to correct the deficiency of cysteine and glutathione in plasma and mononuclear cells of HIV-infected subjects, but contradictory results of subsequent replenishment of plasma or PBMC GSH have been reported.[63,171] Unexpectedly, in response to supplementation by vitamin E the plasma levels of MDA are increased while neither the values of GSH nor CD4+ counts are modified.[172]

In conclusion, nutrition may be considered among the cofactors that influence the development of AIDS in HIV-infected patients. Although a variety of nutritional imbalances occur during the HIV infection, the degree to which they alter the immune functions and/or response to infections is generally not well quantified. In addition, their role in specific aspects of disease progression is not clearly established. Nutritional therapy can to some extent improve different parameters and need, therefore, to be considered in effective programs. Strategies of intervention must be defined with a principal goal: to maintain optimal nutritional status. However, because of the limited nature of the data, clinical recommendations are difficult to establish since such treatments may carry a risk of excess dietary provision in some factors that may have adverse effects on immune status, resistance to infections, and susceptibility to or progression of cancer.

References

1. Keusch, G.T. and Farthing, M.J.G., Nutritional aspects of AIDS, *Annu. Rev. Nutr.*, 10, 475, 1990.
2. Coodley, G.O., et al., The HIV wasting syndrome: a review, *J. Acquir. Immune Defic. Syndr.*, 7, 681, 1991.
3. Weinroth, S.E., et al., Wasting syndrome in AIDS: pathophysiologic mechanisms and therapeutic approaches, *Infect. Agents Dis.*, 4, 76, 1995.
4. Walter, R.M., et al., Zinc status in human immunodefiency virus infection, *Life Sci.*, 46, 1597, 1990.
5. Baum, M.K., et al., Inadequate dietary intake and altered nutrition status in early HIV-1 infection, *Nutrition*, 10, 16, 1994.
6. Cheng-Meyer, C., et al., Biological features of HIV-1 that correlate virulence in the host, *Science*, 240, 80, 1988.
7. Blaxhult, A., et al., The influence of age on the latency period to AIDS in people infected by HIV through blood transfusion, *AIDS*, 4, 125, 1990.
8. Michael, S., HIV, AIDS, cancer and immune system: the domino effect of trace elements and vitamins, *Proceedings of the 10th International Conference on AIDS*, Abstract PBO300, Yokohama, 1994.
9. Caselli, M. and Bicocchi, R., 1986 Taux seriques du zinc chez les malades atteints du syndrome d'immunodeficit acquis, *La Presse Med.*, 15, 1877, 1986.
10. Dardenne, M., et al., Low serum thymic hormone levels in patients with acquired immunodeficiency syndrome, *N. Engl. J. Med.*, 1, 48, 1983.
11. Dworkin, B.M., et al., Selenium deficiency in the acquired immunodeficiency syndrome, *J. Parenteral Enteral Nutr.*, 10, 405, 1986.
12. Dworkin, B.M., et al., Abnormalities of blood selenium and glutathione peroxydase activity in patients with acquired immunodeficiency syndrome and AIDS-related complex, *Biol. Trace Elem. Res.*, 5, 167, 1988.
13. Beck, K.W., et al., Serum trace element levels in HIV-infected subjects, *Biol. Trace Elem. Res.*, 25, 89, 1990.
14. Cirelli, A., et al., Serum selenium concentration and disease progress in patients with HIV infection, *Clin. Biochem.*, 24, 211, 1991.
15. Olmsted, L., et al., Selenium supplementation of symptomatic human immunodeficiency virus infected patients, *Biol. Trace Elem. Res.*, 20, 59, 1989.
16. Mantero-Atienza, E., et al., Selenium status of HIV-1 infected individuals, *J. Parenteral Enteral Nutr.*, 15, 693, 1991.
17. Allavena, C., et al., Zinc and selenium blood values: other prognostic biological parameters in the progression of human immunodeficiency virus infection, in *Biologie prospective, Comptes rendus du 8e Colloque de Pont-à-Mousson.*, Galteau, M.M., Siest, G., Henny, J., Eds., John Libbey Eurotext, Paris, 1993.
18. Dworkin, B.M., Selenium defiency in HIV infection and the acquired immunodeficiency syndrome (AIDS), *Chem. Biol. Interact.*, 91, 181, 1994.
19. Schuhmacher, M., et al., Trace elements in patients with HV-1 infection, *Trace Elem. Electr.*, 11, 130, 1994.

20. Perriquet, B.A., et al., Micronutrient levels in HIV-1-infected children, *AIDS*, 9, 887, 1995.
21. Sappey, C., et al., Vitamin, trace element and peroxyde status in HIV seropositive patients: asymptomatic patients present a severe β-carotene deficiency, *Clin. Chim. Acta*, 230, 35, 1994.
22. Favier, A., et al., Antioxydant status and lipid peroxydation in patients infected with HIV, *Chem. Biol. Interact.*, 91, 165, 1994.
23. Malvy, D. J-M., et al., Relationship of plasma malondialdehyde, vitamin E and antioxydant micronutrients to human immunodeficiency virus-1 seropositivity, *Clin. Chim. Acta*, 224, 89, 1994.
24. Bogden, J.D., et al., Micronutrient status and human immunodeficiency virus (HIV) infection, *Ann. N. Y. Acad. Sci.*, 587, 189,1990.
25. Coodley, G.O., et al., Micronutrient concentrations in the HIV wasting syndrome, *AIDS*, 7, 1595, 1993.
26. Heise, W., et al., Concentrations of magnesium, zinc and copper in serum of patients with acquired immuno-deficiency syndrome, *J. Clin. Chem. Clin. Biochem.*, 27, 515,1989.
27. Isa, L., et al., Blood zinc status and zinc treatment in human immunodeficiency virus-infected patients, *Int. J. Clin. Lab. Res.*, 22, 45, 1992.
28. Buhl, M., et al., Serum zinc in homosexual men with antibodies against human immunodeficiency virus, *Clin. Chem.*, 34, 1929, 1988.
29. Falutz, J., et al., Zinc as a cofactor in human immunodeficiency virus-induced immunosuppression, *JAMA*, 259, 2850, 1988.
30. Mocchegiani, E., et al., Zinc-dependent thymic hormone failure in AIDS, *Ann. N. Y. Acad. Sci.*, 650, 94, 1992.
31. Fabris, N. and Mocchegiani, E., AIDS, zinc deficiency, and thymic hormone failure, *JAMA*, 259, 839, 1988.
32. Beach, R.S., et al., Specific nutrient abnormalities in asymptomatic HIV-1 infection, *AIDS*, 6, 701,1992.
33. Falutz, J., The role of zinc in HIV-induced immunosuppression, *Ann. N. Y. Acad. Sci.*, 587, 286, 1990.
34. Harrer, T., et al., *In vitro* activation of peripheral mononuclear cells by zinc in HIV-infected patients and healthy controls, *Clin. Exp. Immunol.*, 89, 285, 1992.
35. Lebanore, M., et al., Zinc and lymphocyte subsets in patients with HIV infection, *Minerva Med.*, 78, 1805, 1987.
36. Baum, M.K., et al., Micronutrients and HIV-1 disease progression, *AIDS*, 9, 1051, 1995.
37. Shoemaker, J.D., et al., Zinc in human immunodeficiency virus infection, *JAMA*, 260, 1881, 1988.
38. Baum, M.K., et al., Zidovudine-associated adverse reactions in a longitudinal study of asymptomatic HIV-1-infected homosexual males, *J. Acquir. Immune Defic. Syndr.*, 4, 1218, 1991.
39. Graham, N.M.H., et al., Relationship of copper and zinc levels to HIV-1 seropositivity and progression to AIDS, *J. Acquir. Immune Defic. Syndr.*, 4, 976, 1991.
40. Dousset, B., et al., Relations of trace element status to immunological activity markers and progression of human deficiency virus infection, *Proceedings of the 10th International Conference on AIDS*, Abstract PBO063, Yokohama, 1994.
41. Brod-Miller, C., et al., Hypomagnesemia (HMg) in acquired immune defiency syndrome (AIDS), *J. Am. Soc. Nephrol.*, 1, 329, 1990.

42. Gutteridge, J.M.C., Biological origin of free radicals, and mechanisms of antioxidant protection, *Chem. Biol. Interact.*, 91, 133, 1994.

43. Kimura, T., et al., Amplification of superoxide anion generation in phagocytic cells by HIV-1 infection, *FEBS Lett.*, 326, 232, 1993.

44. Jarstrand, C. and Akerlund, B., Oxygen radical release by neutrophils of HIV-1 infected patients, *Chem. Biol. Interact.*, 91, 141, 1994.

45. Aukrust, P., et al., Increased levels of oxydized glutathione in CD4+ lymphocytes associated with disturbed intracellular redox balance in human immunodeficiency virus type 1 infection, *Blood*, 86, 258, 1995.

46. Bandes, J.C., et al., Increased phagocytosis and generation of reactive oxygen products by neutrophils and monocytes of men with stage 1 human immunodeficiency virus infection, *J. Infect. Dis.*, 168, 75, 1993.

47. Spear, G.T., et al., Decreased oxidative burst activity of monocytes from asymptomatic HIV-infected individuals, *Clin. Immunol. Immunopathol.*, 54, 184, 1990.

48. Baldeweg, T., et al., Serum nitrite concentration suggests a role for nitric oxide in AIDS, *AIDS*, 10, 451, 1996.

49. Macho, A., et al., Mitochondrial dysfunctions in circulating T lymphocytes from human immunodeficiency virus-1 carriers, *Blood*, 86, 2481, 1995.

50. Sandstrom, P.A., et al., Lipid hydroperoxides induce apoptosis in T cells displaying a HIV-associated glutathione peroxydase deficiency, *J. Biol. Chem.*, 269, 798, 1994.

51. Flores, S.C., et al., Tat protein of human deficiency virus type 1 represses expression of manganese superoxide dismutase in HeLa cells, *Proc. Natl. Acad. Sci. U.S.A.*, 90, 7632, 1993.

52. Greenspan, H.C., The role of reactive oxygen species, antioxidants and phytopharmaceuticals in human immunodeficiency virus activity, *Med. Hypotheses*, 40, 85, 1993.

53. Wong, G.H., et al., Manganous superoxide dismutase is essential for cellular resistance to cytotoxicity of tumor necrosis factor, *Cell*, 58, 923, 1989.

54. Leff, J.A., et al., Progressive increases in serum catalase activity in advancing human immunodeficiency virus infection, *Free Rad. Biol. Med.*, 13, 148, 1992.

55. Skurnick, J.H., et al., Micronutrient profile in HIV-1 infected heterosexual adults, *J. Acquir. Immune Defic. Syndr.*, 12, 75, 1996.

56. Stone, J.D., et al., Development of malabsorption and nutritional complications in simian immunodeficiency virus infected rhesus macaques, *AIDS*, 8, 1245, 1994.

57. Hommes, M.J.T., et al., Resting energy expenditure and substrate oxidation in human immunodeficiency virus (HIV-1) infected asymptomatic men: HIV affects host metabolism in the early asymptomatic stage, *Am. J. Clin. Nutr.*, 54, 311, 1991.

58. Ulrich, R., et al., Serum carotene deficiency in HIV-infected patients, *AIDS*, 8, 661, 1994.

59. Harakeh, S. and Jariwalla, R.J., Comparative study of the anti-HIV activities of ascorbate and thiol-containing reducing agents in chronically HIV-infected cells, *Am. J. Clin. Nutr.*, 54, 1231S, 1991.

60. Harakeh, S. et al., Mechanistic aspects of ascorbate inhibition of human immunodeficiency virus, *Chem. Biol. Interact.*, 91, 207, 1994.

61. Buhl, R., et al., Systemic glutathione deficiency in symptom-free HIV-seropositive individuals, *Lancet*, ii, 1294, 1989.

62. Eck, H-P., et al., Low concentrations of acid-soluble thiol (cysteine) in the blood plasma of HIV-1 infected patients, *Biol. Chem. Hoppe-Seyler*, 370, 101, 1989.

63. De Quay, B., et al., Glutathione depletion in HIV-infected patients: role of cysteine deficiency and effect of oral N-acetylcysteine, *AIDS*, 6, 815, 1992.

64. Helbling, B., et al., Decreased release of glutathione into the systemic circulation of patients with HIV infection, *Eur. J. Clin. Invest.*, 26, 38, 1996.

65. Pirmohamed, M., et al., Intracellular glutathione in the peripheral blood cells of HIV-infected patients: failure to show a deficiency, *AIDS*, 10, 501, 1996.

66. Roederer, M., et al., CD4 and CD8 T cells with high intracellular glutathione levels are selectively lost as the HIV infection progresses, *Int. Immunol.*, 3, 933, 1991.

67. Staal, F.J.T., et al., Intracellular glutathione levels in T-cell subsets decrease in HIV-infected individuals, *AIDS Res. Hum. Retroviruses*, 8, 305, 1992.

68. Staal, F.J.T., et al., Glutathione deficiency and human immunodeficiency virus infection, *Lancet*, 339, 909, 1992.

69. Staal, F.J.T., et al., Glutathione and immunophenotypes of T and B lymphocytes in HIV-infected individuals, *Ann. N. Y. Acad. Sci.*, 651, 453, 1992.

70. Hortin, G.L., et al., Changes in plasma amino-acid concentrations in response to HIV-1 infection, *Clin. Chem.*, 40, 785, 1994.

71. Droge, W., Cysteine and glutathione deficiency in AIDS patients: a rationale for the treatment with N-acetyl-cysteine, *Pharmacology*, 46, 61, 1993.

72. Odeh, M., The role of zinc in acquired immunodeficiency syndrome, *J. Intern. Med.*, 231, 463, 1992.

73. Moseson, M., et al., The potential role of nutritional factors in the induction of immunologic abnormalities in HIV-positive homosexual men, *J. Acquir. Immune Defic. Syndr.*, 2, 235, 1989.

74. Beach, R.S. and Laura, P.F., Nutrition and the acquired immunodeficiency syndrome, *Ann. Intern. Med.*, 99, 565, 1983.

75. McClain, C.J., et al., Clinical spectrum and diagnosis aspects of human zinc deficiency, in *Essential and Toxic Trace Elements in Human Health and Disease*, Prasad, A.S., Ed., Alan R Liss, New York, 1988.

76. Klug, A. and Rhodes A., 'Zinc-fingers'. A novel protein motif for nucleic acid recognition, *Trends Biochem. Sci.*, 12, 461, 1987.

77. Falchuk, R.H., Zinc in developmental biology: the role of metal dependent transcription regulation, in *Essential and Toxic Trace Elements in Human Health and Disease: An Uptake*, Prasad, A.S., Ed., Wiley-Liss, New York, 1993.

78. Prasad, A.S., Marginal deficiency of zinc and immunological effects, in *Essential and Toxic Trace Elements in Human Health and Disease: An Uptake*, Prasad, A.S., Ed., Wiley-Liss, New York, 1993.

79. Moynahan, E.J., Acrodermatitis enteropathica: a lethal inherited human zinc deficiency disorder, *Lancet*, ii, 399, 1974.

80. Ohsawa, M., Nutritional and toxicological implication of trace elements in the immune response, in *Essential and Toxic Trace Elements in Human Health and Disease: An Uptake*, Prasad, A.S., Ed., Wiley-Liss, New York, 1993.

81. Incefy, G.S., et al., Low circulating thymulin-like activity in children with AIDS and AIDS-related complex, *AIDS Res. Hum. Retroviruses*, 2, 109, 1983.

82. Dardenne, M., et al., Biochemical and biological aspects of the interaction between thymulin and zinc, in *Essential and Toxic Trace Elements in Human Health and Disease: An Uptake*, Prasad, A.S., Ed., Wiley-Liss, New York, 1993.

83. Pleau, J.M., et al., Specific receptor for the serum thymic factor (FTS) in lymphoblastoid cultured cell lines, *Proc. Natl. Acad. Sci. U.S.A.*, 77, 2861, 1980.
84. Cunningham-Rundles, S., et al., Physiological and pharmacological effects of zinc on immune response, *Ann. N. Y. Acad. Sci.*, 587, 113, 1990.
85. Tapazoglou, E., et al., Decreased natural killer cell activity in zinc deficient subjects with sickle cell disease, *J. Lab. Clin. Med.*, 105, 19, 1985.
86. Duvall, E. and Wyllie, A.H., Death and the cell, *Immunol. Today*, 7, 115, 1986.
87. South, T.L., et al., Zinc fingers and molecular recognition. Structure and nucleic acid binding studies of an HIV zinc finger-like domain, *Biochem. Pharmacol.*, 40, 123, 1990.
88. Gorelick, R.J., et al., The two zinc fingers in the human immunodeficiency virus type 1 nucleocapsid protein are not functionally equivalent, *J.Virol.*, 67, 4027, 1993.
89. Maekawa, T., et al., Putative metal finger structure of the human immunodeficiency virus type 1 enhancer binding protein HIV-EP1, *J. Biol. Chem.*, 64, 14591, 1989.
90. Frankel, A.D., et al., Tat protein from human immunodeficiency virus forms a metal-linked dimer, *Science*, 240, 70, 1988.
91. Zhang, Z., et al., Zinc inhibition of renin and the protease from human immunodeficiency virus type 1, *Biochemistry*, 36, 8717, 1991.
92. York, D.M., et al., Molecular modeling studies suggest that zinc ions inhibit HIV-1 protease by binding at catalytic aspartates, *Environ. Health Perspect.*, 101, 246,1993.
93. York, D.M., et al., Simulations of the solution structure of HIV-1 protease in the presence and absence of bound zinc, *J. Comp. Chem.*, 15, 61, 1994.
94. Naveh, Y., Zinc in clinical medicine. I. Biochemical and clinical aspects, *Harefuah*, 117, 145, 1989.
95. Neve, J., Clinical implications of trace elements in endocrinology, *Biol. Trace Elem. Res.*, 32, 173, 1992.
96. Mathe, G., et al., Experimental to clinical attempts in immunorestoration with bestatin and zinc, *Comp. Immun. Microbiol. Infect. Dis.*, 9, 241, 1986.
97. Zazzo, J.F., et al., Effect of zinc on immune status of zinc depleted ARC patients, *Clin. Nutr.*, 8, 259, 1989.
98. Tang, A.M., et al., Dietary micronutrient intake and risk of progression to acquired immunodeficiency syndrome (AIDS) in human immunodeficiency virus type 1 (HIV-1)-infected homosexual men, *Am. J. Epidemiol.*, 138, 937, 1993.
99. Keshan Disease Research Group of the Chinese Academy of Medical Sciences, Observations on effect of sodium selenite in prevention of Keshan disease, *Chin. Med. J.*, 92, 471, 1979.
100. Johnson, R.A., et al., An occidental case of cardiomyopathy and selenium deficiency, *N. Engl. J. Med.*, 304, 1210, 1981.
101. Reeves, W.C., et al., Reversible cardiomyopathy due to selenium deficiency, *J. Parenteral Enteral Nutr.*, 13, 663, 1989.
102. Fink, L., et al., Cardiac abnormalities in acquired immune deficiency syndrome, *Am. J. Cardiol.*, 54, 1161, 1984.
103. Cammarosano, C. and Lewis, W., Cardiac lesions in acquired immune deficiency syndrome (AIDS), *J. Am. Coll. Cardiol.*, 5, 703, 1985.
104. Cohen, I.S., et al., Congestive cardiomyopathy in association with the acquired immunodeficiency syndrome, *N. Engl. J. Med.*, 315, 628, 1986.

105. Steinherz, L.J., et al., Cardiac involvement in congenital acquired immunodeficiency syndrome, *Am. J. Dis. Child.*, 140, 1241, 1986.
106. Zazzo, J.F., et al., Is nonobstructive cardiomyopathy in AIDS a selenium deficiency-related disease?, *J. Parenteral Enteral Nutr.*, 12, 537, 1988.
107. Dworkin, B., et al., Reduced cardiac selenium content in the acquired immunodeficiency syndrome, *J. Parenteral Enteral Nutr.*, 13, 644, 1989.
108. Kavanaugh-McHugh, A.L., et al., Selenium deficiency and cardiomyopathy in acquired immunodeficiency syndrome, *J. Parenteral Enteral Nutr.*, 15, 347, 1991.
109. Lipshultz, S.E., et al., Cardiac structure and function in children with human immunodeficiency virus infection treated with zidovudine, *N. Engl. J. Med.*, 327, 1260, 1992.
110. Chariot, P. and Gherardi, R., Myopathy and HIV infection, *Curr. Opin. Rheumatol.*, 7, 497, 1995.
111. Spallholz, J.E., et al., Advances in understanding selenium's role in the immune system, *Ann. N. Y. Acad. Sci.*, 587, 123, 1990.
112. Stabel, J.R. and Spears J.W., Role of selenium in immune responsiveness and disease resistance, in *Human Nutrition — A Comprehensive Treatise, Nutrition and Immunology (Vol. 8)*, Klurfeld, D.M., Ed., Plenum Press, New York, 1993.
113. Bryant, R.W. and Bailey, J.M., Altered lipoxygenase metabolism and decreased glutathione peroxydase activity in platelets from selenium-deficient rats, *Biochem. Biophys. Res. Commun.*, 92, 268, 1980.
114. Schoene, N.W., et al., Altered arachidonic acid metabolism in platelets and aortas from selenium-deficient rats, *Nutr. Res.*, 6, 75, 1986.
115. Robinson, D.R., et al., Lipid mediators of inflammatory and immune reactions, *J. Parenteral Enteral Nutr.*, 12, 37S, 1988.
116. Kiremidjian-Schumacher, L. et al., Selenium and immune cell functions. I. Effect on lymphocyte proliferation and production of interleukin 1 and interleukin 2, *Proc. Soc. Exp. Biol. Med.*, 193, 136, 1990.
117. Roy, M., et al., Selenium and immune cell functions. II. Effect on lymphocyte-mediated cytotoxicity, *Proc. Soc. Exp. Biol. Med.*, 193, 143, 1990.
118. Taylor, E.W., et al., A basic approach to the chemotherapy of AIDS: novel genes in HIV-1 potentially encode selenoproteins expressed by ribosomial frameshifting and termination suppression, *J. Med. Chem.*, 37, 2637, 1994.
119. Taylor, E.W., From pseudoknots to selenium: a new theory of HIV pathogenesis, *Int. Antiviral News*, 3, 18, 1995.
120. Zachara, B.A., Mammalian selenoproteins, *J. Trace Elem. Electrolytes Health Dis.*, 6, 137, 1992.
121. Schrauzer, G.N. and Sacher, J., Selenium in the maintenance and therapy of HIV-infected patients, *Chem. Biol. Interact.*, 91, 199, 1994.
122. Fidelus, R.K., The generation of oxygen radicals: a positive signal for lymphocyte activation, *Cell Immunol.*, 113, 175, 1990.
123. Maly, F-E., The B lymphocyte: a newly recognized source of reactive oxygen species with immunoregulatory potential, *Free Radic. Res. Commun.*, 8, 143, 1990.
124. Bilzer, M. and Lauterburg, B.H., Glutathione metabolism in activated human neutrophils: stimulation of glutathione synthesis and consumption of glutathione by reactive oxygen species, *Eur. J. Clin. Invest.*, 21, 316, 1991.
125. Meister, A., Glutathione metabolism and its selective modification, *J. Biol. Chem.*, 263, 17205, 1988.

126. Hamilos, D.L. and Wedner, H.J., The role of glutathione in lymphocyte activation. I. Comparison of inhibitory effects of buthionine sulfoximine and 2-cyclohexene-1-one by nuclear size transformation, *J. Immunol.*, 135, 2740, 1985.
127. Droge, W., et al., Glutathione augments the activation of cytotoxic T lymphocytes *in vivo*, *Immunobiology*, 172, 151, 1986.
128. Yamamauchi, A. and Bloom, E.T., Requirement of thiol compounds as reducing agents for IL-2 mediated induction of LAK activity and proliferation of human NK cells, *J. Immunol.*, 151, 5535, 1993.
129. Droge, W., et al., Functions of glutathione and glutathione disulfide in immunology and immunopathology, *FASEB J.*, 8, 1131, 1994b.
130. Thomas, W.R. and Holt, P.G., Vitamin C and immunity: an assessment of the evidence, *Clin. Exp. Immunol.*, 32, 370, 1978.
131. Cunningham-Rundles, S., Effects of nutritional status on immunological function, *Am. J. Clin. Nutr.*, 35, 1202, 1982.
132. Hollins, T.D., T4 cell receptor distortion in acquired immune deficiency syndrome, *Med. Hypotheses*, 26, 107, 1988.
133. Beisel, W.R., Single nutrients and immunity, *Am. J. Clin. Nutr.*, 35(suppl.), 417, 1982.
134. Winrow, V.R., et al., Free radicals in inflammation: second messagers and mediators of tissue destruction, *Br. Med. Bull.*, 49, 506, 1993.
135. Grever, M., et al., The effect of oxidant stress on human lymphocyte cytotoxicity, *Blood*, 56, 284, 1980.
136. Dallegri, F., et al., Down-regulation of K-cell activity by neutrophils, *Blood*, 65, 571, 1985.
137. Halliwell, B. and Gutteridge, J.M.C., Role of free radicals and catalytic metal ions in human disease: an overview, *Methods Enzymol.*, 186, 1, 1990.
138. Hockenbery, D.M., et al., Bcl-2 functions in an antioxydant pathway to prevent apoptosis, *Cell*, 75, 241,1993.
139. Buttke, T.M. and Sandstrom, P.A., Oxydative stress as a mediator of apoptosis, *Immunol. Today*, 15, 7, 1994.
140. Laurent-Crawford, A.G., et al., The cytopathic effect of HIV is associated with apoptosis, *Virology*, 185, 829, 1991.
141. Banda, N.K., et al., Crosslinking CD4 by human immunodeficiency virus gp120 primes T cells for activation-induced apoptosis, *J. Exp. Med.*, 176, 1099, 1992.
142. Ameisen, J.C., Programmed cell death and AIDS: from hypothesis to experiment, *Immunol. Today*, 13, 388, 1992.
143. Greenspan, H.C. and Arouma, O., Could oxidative stress initiate programmed cell death in HIV infection? A role for plant derived metabolites having synergistic antioxydant activity, *Chem. Biol. Interact.*, 91, 187, 1994.
144. Sen, C.K. and Packer, L., Antioxydant and redox regulation of gene transcription, *FASEB J.*, 10, 709, 1996.
145. Griffin, G.E., et al., Activation of HIV gene expression during monocyte differenciation by induction of NF-κB, *Nature*, 339, 70, 1989.
146. Brach, M.A., et al., Leukotriene B$_4$ transcriptionally activates interleukin-6 expression involving NF-κB and NF-IL6, *Eur. J. Immunol.*, 22, 2705, 1992.
147. Meyer, M., et al., Regulation of the transcription factors NF-κB and AP-1 by redox changes, *Chem. Biol. Interact.*, 91, 91, 1994.

148. Galter, D., et al., Distinct effects of glutathione disulphide on the nuclear transcription factor κB and the activator protein-1, *Eur. J. Biochem.*, 221, 639, 1994.
149. Roederer, M., et al., Cytokine-stimulated human immunodeficiency virus replication is inhibited by N-acetyl cysteine, *Proc. Natl. Acad. Sci.*, 87, 4884, 1990.
150. Mihm, S., et al., Inhibition of HIV-1 replication and NF-κB activity by cysteine and cysteine derivatives, *AIDS*, 5, 497, 1991.
151. Fazely, F., et al., Pentoxifylline (Trental) decreases the replication of the human immunodeficiency virus type 1 in human peripheral blood mononuclear cells and in cultured T cells, *Blood*, 77, 1653, 1991.
152. Schreck, R., et al., Dithiocarbamates as potent inhibitors of nuclear factor κB activation in intact cells, *J. Exp. Med.*, 175, 1181, 1992.
153. Staal, F.J.T., et al., Antioxidants inhibit stimulation of HIV transcription, *AIDS Res. Hum. Retroviruses*, 9, 299, 1993.
154. Biswas, D.K., et al., Pentoxifylline inhibits HIV-1 LTR-driven gene expression by blocking NF-κB action, *J. Acquir. Immune Defic. Syndr.*, 6, 778, 1993.
155. Navarro, J., et al., Pentoxifylline inhibits acute HIV-1 replication in human T cells by a mechanism not involving inhibition of tumor necrosis factor synthesis or nuclear factor-κB activation, *AIDS*, 10, 469, 1996.
156. Gogu, S.R., et al., Increased therapeutic efficacy of zidovudine in combination with vitamin E, *Biochem. Biophys. Res. Commun.*, 165, 401, 1989.
157. Kameoka, M., et al., Superoxide enhances the spread of HIV-1 infection by cell-to-cell transmission, *FEBS Lett.*, 331, 182, 1993.
158. Henry, J.A., Glutathione and HIV infection, *Lancet*, 335, 236, 1990.
159. Carr, A., et al., Allergic manifestations of human immunodeficiency virus (HIV) infection, *J. Clin. Immunol.*, 11, 55, 1991.
160. Shriner, K. and Goetz, M.B., Severe hepatotoxicity in a patient receiving both acetaminophen and zidovudine, *Am. J. Med.*, 93, 94, 1992.
161. Rieder, M.J., et al., Sulfonamide toxicity in HIV infection, *Clin. Pharmacol. Ther.*, 55, 181, 1994.
162. Rwangabwoba, J.M., et al., Vitamin A status and development of tuberculosis and/or mortality, *Proceedings of the 11th International Conference on AIDS*, Abstract We.B.3268, Vancouver, 1996.
163. Denotter, D.M., et al., The relationship of dietary micronutrient intake to disease progression in a cohort of HIV + gay men, *Proceedings of the 11th International Conference on AIDS*, Abstract We.B.3259, Vancouver, 1996.
164. Pace, G.W. and Leaf, C.D., The role of oxidative stress in HIV disease, *Free Radic. Biol. Med.*, 19, 523, 1995.
165. Semba, R.D., et al., Increased mortality associated with vitamin A deficiency during human immunodeficiency virus type 1 infection, *Arch. Int. Med.*, 153, 2149, 1993.
166. Cathcart, R.F., Vitamin C in the treatment of acquired immune deficiency syndrome, *Med. Hypotheses*, 18, 67, 1985.
167. Schofer, H., et al., Treatment of oral hairy leuloplakia in AIDS patients with vitamin A acid (topically) as acyclovir (systematically), *Dermatologica*, 174, 150, 1987.
168. Alexander, M., et al., Oral beta carotene can increase the number of OKT4+ cells in human blood, *Immunol. Lett.*, 9, 221, 1985.
169. Garewal, H.S., et al., A preliminary trial of beta carotene in subjects infected with the human immunodeficiency virus, *J. Nutr.*, 122, 728, 1992.

170. Coodley, G.O., et al., β carotene in HIV infection, *J. Acquir. Immune Defic. Syndr.*, 6, 272, 1993.
171. Witschi, A., et al., Supplementation of N-acetylcysteine fails to increase glutathione in lymphocytes and plasma of patients with AIDS, *AIDS Res. Hum. Retroviruses*, 11, 141, 1995.
172. Lalonde Richard, G., et al., Diet and supplements do not reduce oxidative stress in clinically stable persons with HIV infection, *Proceedings of the 11th International Conference on AIDS*, Abstract We.B.3257, Vancouver, 1996.

chapter two

Selenium and AIDS

Joël Constans

The essential role of selenium in human health has been demonstrated recently. Dietary selenium supplementation has been shown to prevent a congestive cardiomyopathy in China (Keshan disease).[1] In patients with prolonged total parenteral nutrition, selenium supplementation prevented a muscular dystrophy.[2] The biochemical function of selenium is in part related to glutathione peroxidase (GSH-Px), an intracellular enzyme that catalyzes the oxidation of reduced glutathione by peroxides to form oxidized glutathione and water. Each of the four units of GSH-Px needs seleno-cysteine, and an adequate plasma selenium concentration is requested for a correct function of GSH-Px.[3] Selenium influences the functions of the immune system in animals, and immunologic abnormalities such as impaired cytotoxicity or phagocytosis or poor response to vaccines occur in selenium-deficient animals.[4,5,6] An antiviral effect of selenium has also been suggested: addition of sodium selenite to table salt has significantly lowered the hepatitis B infection rate.[7] A deficiency in selenium is rare in healthy subjects although dietary selenium intakes vary a lot from one country to another because of differences in selenium concentration in food and soil (the highest selenium concentrations are found in fishes).[8] Selenium deficiencies may occur in pathological conditions such as malnutrition or malabsorption.[2,9,10] More than half of all AIDS patients have wasting defined as a 10% body weight loss, and malabsorption is often demonstrated in HIV-positive patients[11,12] so that several authors investigated plasma selenium concentration in HIV-positive subjects.

Plasma selenium concentration in HIV-positive patients

Most authors have reported that plasma selenium concentration is low in HIV-positive patients.[13-20] Dworkin found that 12 AIDS patients had a mean selenium concentration half lower than 27 healthy controls.[13] Cirelli measured

Table 1   Summary of the Selenium Concentrations Found
in HIV-Positive Patients (µg/l)

	AIDS	ARC	Symptom Free	Controls
Cirelli[14]	65 ± 17	68 ± 13	69 ± 9	103 ± 6
Olmsted[15]	123 ± 30	126 ± 40	—	195 ± 20
Dworkin[13]	43 ± 10	—	—	95 ± 20
Constans[17]	61 ± 20	—	71 ± 10	83 ± 20
Revillard[21]	73 ± 20	—	94 ± 18	83 ± 10
Favier[16]	44 ± 19	—	70 ± 14	72 ± 12
Beck[19]	62 ± 15	—	—	76 ± 10
Zazzo[21]	59 ± 20	—	—	87 ± 10

plasma selenium in 67 HIV+ patients divided into 4 groups: symptom-free, persistent generalized adenopathies, AIDS-related complex (ARC), and AIDS.[14] He found that selenium concentrations were lower in all these groups than in 15 healthy controls. Olmsted found lower selenium concentrations in 24 patients with AIDS and 26 with ARC than in 28 healthy controls.[15] We divided 95 HIV-positive patients into 4 groups according to CD4 cells count (>400/mm3, 200–400/mm3, 50–200/mm3, and <50/mm3), and we found low plasma selenium concentrations in all these groups when compared to 20 healthy controls.[17,18] Beck reported that 59 HIV-positive patients had lower plasma selenium than 26 controls.[19] Mantero-Atienza found that 8 out of 54 asymptomatic HIV-positive patients had demonstrated low plasma selenium concentrations (<90 µg/l), while 31 had marginally low plasma selenium (90 to 120 µg/l).[20] In only one study, plasma selenium did not differ between HIV-positive patients and controls,[21] but in a further study, the same authors also found low plasma selenium concentrations in 18 AIDS subjects.[16]

Sufficient data are now available to consider that plasma selenium concentration decreases in HIV-positive patients and that plasma selenium is lower in AIDS patients than in others. The decrease in selenium parallels the decrease in CD4 cells[17,18] and a correlation has been reported between plasma selenium and CD4 cells count or p24 antigenemia, two indicators of disease progression.[17] A correlation has also been found in HIV-positive patients between plasma selenium and two nutritional parameters: albumin concentration and body mass index.[13,17]

Mechanisms of selenium depletion during HIV infection

It is obvious that malabsorption plays some role in selenium depletion in HIV infection. AIDS patients often have intestinal infections related to Cryptosporidium, Microsporidia, Cytomegalovirus, Mycobacterium avium or Kaposi's sarcoma.[22] Malabsorption may even occur without an identified pathogen, and HIV itself might directly injure the small intestine.[23] Protein-losing enteropathy has been found in 70% of AIDS patients with hypo-albuminemia and in 33%

of the normo-albuminemic subjects.[12] A correlation has been found in two studies between selenium and albumin plasma concentrations.[13,17] Also HIV-positive patients with wasting have decreased caloric and protein intake, and decreased selenium dietary intake possibly plays a role in selenium deficiency.[24] Other mechanisms might also be implied in selenium depletion. A decrease in plasma selenium has been reported during Legionnaires' disease and in various viral and bacterial infections.[25,26] The reasons for this transient decrease in plasma selenium concentration are unknown. As in these infectious processes without malnutrition, HIV infection might also induce selenium deficiency in part regardless of nutritional status because HIV-positive patients with high CD4 cell count and no evidence of malnutrition have lower plasma selenium than controls.[17]

Effect of the decrease in plasma selenium on HIV infection progression

Low plasma selenium concentration might have a negative effect on HIV infection. HIV-positive patients have a disturbance of the free radicals/natural antioxidants balance suggesting an oxidative stress. HIV-positive patients have a decrease in plasma cysteine, T-cell glutathione and plasma vitamin A, all part of the antioxidant system.[17,27,28,29] They also have an increase in malon-dialdehyde, an end-product of lipid peroxidation and in reduced homocysteine, a pro-oxidant substance.[17,30,31] Peroxidation of fatty acids has been demonstrated in HIV-positive patients.[17] A deficiency in selenium may result in a decreased efficacy of glutathione peroxidase, a major antioxidant system. Because free radicals may able to stimulate HIV replication and CD4 lymphocytes apoptosis, a decreased selenium concentration might result in increased oxidative stress, HIV replication, and accelerated CD4 lymphocytes death.[32] Moreover, selenium deficiencies have been reported to result in alterations of the immune system, and a decrease in selenium might by itself result in immune deficiency.

We have previously studied the compared predictive values of plasma selenium and classical markers of HIV infection progression (CD4 cells, beta-2 microglobulin, and p24 antigenemia) in 95 patients with a mean follow-up of 1 year.[33] All these markers correlated with the occurrence of death or AIDS-defining opportunistic infections during the following year. In a multivariate analysis, only two markers correlated with these two endpoints: CD4 cells count and plasma selenium concentration.[33]

Selenium and cardiomyopathy in AIDS

Selenium deficiency has been shown to be implied in a congestive cardiomyopathy (namely, Keshan disease) in some areas of China. Although this disease seems to be multifactorial, selenium supplementation prevents its occurrence.[1,34] Congestive cardiomyopathy has also been reported in patients under prolonged total parenteral nutrition.[35,36,37] In HIV-positive patients, cardiomyopathy may occur, sometimes with opportunistic infectious agents and sometimes not, and a deficiency in selenium has been hypothesized to explain such cardiomyopathies.[38] Dworkin measured selenium content in the heart of 8 AIDS patients at autopsy without overt cardiac disease and in 9 age-matched HIV-negative subjects.[39] The mean cardiac selenium concentration was 0.327 µg/g ±0.082 in the AIDS patients and 0.534 µg/g ±0.184 in the others. Most of the AIDS patients had a histologically normal heart but two had foci of myocyte necrosis, fibrosis, and monocyte infiltrations. These abnormalities look like those reported in patients with Keshan disease.

Kavanaugh-McHugh reported the case of a five-year-old boy with AIDS and cardiomyopathy who had a low plasma selenium level (29 µg/ml) and whose cardiac status improved under selenium supplementation.[40] Zazzo found low plasma selenium concentrations in 8 out of 10 AIDS patients with cardiomyopathy.[41] Left ventricle function returned to normal in 6 of those under selenium supplementation. Thus, AIDS-associated cardiomyopathy might in part be related to selenium deficiency.

Supplementation of HIV-positive patients with selenium

Very few assays of selenium supplementation have been carried out in HIV-positive subjects. Cirelli supplemented 12 HIV-positive patients, 8 of which had AIDS, with 80 µg selenium (sodium selenite) and 25 mg vitamin C daily for 2 months.[14] He found a two-time increase in selenium concentration. The authors reported an evident subjective symptomatic improvement. However, in this study, CD4+ T cell count, CD4/CD8 ratio, serum albumin, hemoglobin, and erythrocyte sedimentation rate did not vary.

Olmsted supplemented 19 AIDS or ARC patients with 4 tablets daily of 100 µg selenium yeast for 70 days.[15] He observed a 2-time increase in mean whole blood selenium. However, 2 patients had a decrease in plasma selenium while supplemented although they had no sign of gastrointestinal disturbance or opportunistic disease. The authors think that these 2 patients had poor compliance to treatment. Of the 19 supplemented patients, 14 reported subjective improvement assessed from a subjective health status questionnaire. One patient felt his health deteriorated although his blood selenium concentration increased from 0.11 to 0.23 µg/ml, and 4 felt no change in their health.

We supplemented 15 patients with 100 µg selenium (sodium selenite) for 1 year and compared them to 22 unsupplemented patients.[42,43] Both groups were comparable at inclusion for clinical status and CD4 cell count. No difference was observed between selenium recipients and controls for the occurrence of death, opportunistic infections, or CD4 cell count. There was a two-fold increase in median plasma selenium concentration in the selenium recipients, while in unsupplemented patients, plasma selenium decreased. Red blood cell glutathione peroxidase rose in the supplemented patients and decreased in the others. MDA, an end-product of lipid peroxidation, decreased in the selenium recipients and increased in the controls. Moreover, beta-2 microglobulin, a marker of immune activation and negative prognosis in HIV infection, significantly decreased in the selenium recipient patients and increased in the controls. These results indicate that 100 μg selenium daily is well tolerated and absorbed in HIV-positive patients and that such selenium supplementation improves oxidative stress and decreases beta-2 microglobulin. Again, clinical status and CD4 cell count did not improve in these patients with advanced immunodepression (most patients had less than 200 CD4 cells/mm3). Supplementation with selenium should be evaluated in patients with less advanced disease. However, the lack of improvement of CD4 cell count does not necessarily indicate the lack of influence of selenium on HIV infection since the correlation of plasma selenium concentration with the outcome is independent of the CD4 cell count.[33] There is, so far, no data on the potential effect of selenium on HIV viral load.

Conclusion

There are now sufficient data that HIV-positive patients have a decrease in plasma selenium. This decrease parallels the fall in CD4 cells and worsening of the disease. The mechanisms of selenium depletion in AIDS probably include decreased intake and malabsorption, but other mechanisms might be implicated. Low plasma selenium concentration is indicative of a poor prognosis in HIV-positive patients regardless of the CD4 cell count. Moreover, selenium deficiency is one of the possible mechanisms of congestive cardiomyopathy in AIDS. Supplementation with high selenium doses might have deleterious effects[44] and a 100 μg daily selenium dosage seems to be sufficient to restore normal plasma concentrations.[42] However, the benefit of selenium supplementation has not been established so far and further investigation is needed before recommending routine selenium supplementation in HIV-positive patients. The possibility of preventing cardiomyopathy with selenium supplementation should also be considered in clinical trials.

References

1. Keshan Disease Research Group, Observation of the effect of sodium selenite in prevention of Keshan disease, *Chin. Med. J.*, 92, 471, 1979.
2. Van Riij, A.M., Thomson, C.D., McKenzie, J.M., and Robinson, M.F., Selenium deficiency in total parenteral nutrition, *Am. J. Clin. Nutr.*, 32, 2076, 1979.
3. Rotruck, J.T., Pope, A.L., Gauther, H.E. et al. Selenium: biochemical role as a component of glutathione peroxidase, *Science*, 179, 588, 1973.
4. Kiremidjian-Schumacher, L., Roy, M., Wishe, H.I. et al., Selenium and immune cell functions. I. Effect on lymphocyte proliferation and production of interleukin 1 and interleukin 2, *Proc. Soc. Exp. Biol. Med.*, 193, 136, 1990.
5. Chaudra, R.K. and Dayton, D.H., Trace-element regulation of immunity and infection, *Nutr. Res.*, 2, 721, 1982.
6. Mecker, H.C., Eskew, M.L., Schenschenzuber, W. et al., Antioxidant effects on cell mediated immunity, *J. Leukocyte Biol.*, 38, 451, 1985.

7. Yu, S.Y., Li, W.G., Zhy, Y.J., Yu, W.P., and Hou, C., Chemoprevention trials of human hepatitis with selenium supplementation in China, *Biol. Trace Elem. Res.*, 20, 15, 1989.
8. Simonoff, M., Hamon, C., Moretto, P., Llabador, Y., and Simonoff, G., Selenium in foods in France, *J. Food Comp. Anal.*, 1, 295, 1988.
9. Watson, R.D., Cannon, R.A., Kurland, G.S. et al., Selenium responsive myositis during prolonged home total parenteral nutrition in cystic fibrosis, *JPEN*, 9, 58, 1985.
10. Kien, C.L. and Ganrther, H.E., Manifestations of chronic selenium deficiency in a child receiving total parenteral nutrition, *Am. J. Clin. Nutr.*, 37, 319, 1983.
11. Coodley, G.O., Loveless, M.O., and Merrill, T.M., The HIV wasting syndrome: a review, *J. Acquir. Immune Defic. Syndr.*, 7, 681, 1994.
12. Laine, L., Garcia, F., McGilligan, K., Malinko, A., Sinatra, F., and Thomas, D.W., Protein-losing enteropathy and hypoalbuminemia in AIDS, *AIDS*, 7, 837, 1993.
13. Dworkin, B.M., Rosenthal, W., Wormser, G., and Weiss, L., Selenium deficiency in the acquired immunodeficiency syndrome, *JPEN*, 10, 405, 1986.
14. Cirelli, A., Ciardui, M., De Simone, C. et al., Serum selenium concentration and disease progress in patients with HIV infection, *Clin. Biochem.*, 24, 211, 1991.
15. Olmsted, L., Schrauzer, N., Flores-Arce, M., and Dowd, J., Selenium supplementation of symptomatic human immunodeficiency virus infected patients, *Biol. Trace Elem. Res.*, 20, 59, 1989.
16. Favier, A., Sappey, C., Leclerc, P., Faure, M., and Micoud, M., Antioxidant status and lipid peroxidation in patients infected with the HIV, *Chem. Biol. Interact.*, 91, 165, 1994.
17. Constans, J., Peuchant, E., Pellegrin, J.L. et al., Fatty acids and plasma antioxidants in HIV-positive patients, correlation with nutritional and immunological status, *Clin. Biochem.*, 28, 421, 1995.
18. Sergeant, C., Simonoff, M., Hamon, C. et al. Plasma antioxidant status (selenium, retinol and alpha-tocopherol) in HIV infection, in *Oxidative Stress, Cell Activation and Viral Infection*, Pasquier, C. et al., Ed., Birkhäuser Verlag, Basel, Switzerland, 1994, 341.
19. Beck, K., Scramel, P., Hedl, H.A., Jaeger, H., and Kaboth, W., Serum trace-element levels in HIV-infected subjects, *Biol. Trace Elem. Res.*, 25, 89, 1990.
20. Mantiero-Atienza, E., Beach, R.S., Gavancho, M.C., Morgan, R., Shor-Posner, G., and Fordyce-Baum, M.K., Selenium status of HIV-1 infected individuals, *JPEN*, 15, 69, 1991.
21. Revillard, J.P., Vincent, C.M.A., Favier, A.E., Richard, M.J., Zittoun, M., and Kazatchkine, M.D., Lipid peroxidation in human immunodeficiency virus infection, *J. Acquir. Immun. Defic. Syndr. Hum. Retrovirol.*, 5, 637, 1992.
22. Ullrich, R., Heise, W., Bergs, C., L'Age, M., Riecken, G.O., and Zeitz, M., Gastrointestinal symptoms in patients with human immunodeficiency virus: relevance of infective agents isolated from the gastrointestinal tract, *Gut*, 33, 1080, 1992.
23. Ullrich, R., Zeitz, M., Heise, W. et al., Small intestinal structure and function in patients infected with human immunodeficiency virus (HIV): evidence for HIV-induced enteropathy, *Ann. Intern. Med.*, 111, 15, 1989.
24. Macallan, D.C., Noble, C., Baldwin, C. et al., Energy expenditure and wasting in human immunodeficiency virus infection, *N. Eng. J. Med.*, 333, 83, 1995.

25. Chen, J.R. and Anderson, J.M., Legionnaire's disease: concentrations of selenium and other elements, *Science*, 206, 1426, 1979.
26. Sammalkorpi, K., Valtonen, V., Alfthon, G., Aro, A., and Huttemen, J., Serum selenium in acute infections, *Infection*, 16, 222, 1988.
27. Roederer, M., Staal, F.J.T., Anderson, M.T., and Herzenberg, L.A., Glutathione deficiency and human immunodeficiency virus infection, *Lancet*, 339, 909, 1992.
28. Dröge, W., Eck, H.P., and Mihm, S., HIV-induced cysteine deficiency and T-cell dysfunction: a rationale for treatment with N-acetyl cysteine, *Immunol. Today*, 13, 211, 1992.
29. Semba, R.D., Graham, N.H., Caiffa, W.T. et al., Increased mortality associated with vitamin A deficiency during human immunodeficiency virus type 1 infection, *Arch. Intern. Med.*, 153, 2153, 1993.
30. Müller, F., Svardal, A., Ankronst, P., Berge, R.K., Veland, P., and Froland, S.S., Elevated plasma concentration of reduced homocysteine in patients with human immunodeficiency virus infection, *Am. J. Clin. Nutr.*, 63, 242, 1996.
31. Sönnerborg, A., Carlin, G., Akerlund, B. et al., Increased production of malondialdehyde in patients with HIV infection, *Scand. J. Infect. Dis.*, 20, 287, 1988.
32. Greenspan, H.C. and Aruoma, O.I., Oxidative stress and apoptosis in HIV infection.: a role for plant-derived metabolites with synergistic antioxidant activity, *Immunol. Today*, 15, 209, 1994.
33. Constans, J., Pellegrin, J.L., Sergeant, C. et al., Serum selenium predicts outcome in HIV infection, *J. Acquir. Immun. Defic. Syndr. Hum. Retrovirol.*, 10, 392, 1995.
34. Li, G., Wang, F., Kang, D. et al., Keshan disease: an endemic cardiomyopathy in China, *Hum. Pathol.*, 16, 602, 1985.
35. Volk, D.M. and Cutliff, S.A., Selenium deficiency and cardiomyopathy in a patient with cystic fibrosis, *J. Kentucky Med. Assoc.*, 84, 222, 1986.
36. Fleming, C.R., Lie, J.T., McCall, J.T. et al., Selenium deficiency and fatal cardiomyopathy on home parenteral nutrition, *Gastroenterology*, 83, 689, 1982.
37. Johnson, R.A., Baker, S.S., Fallon, J.T. et al., An occidental case of cardiomyopathy and selenium deficiency, *N. Eng. J. Med.*, 304, 1210, 1981.
38. Cohen, I.S., Anderson, D.W., Virmani, R. et al., Congestive cardiomyopathy in association with the acquired immunodeficiency syndrome, *N. Eng. J. Med.*, 315, 628, 1986.
39. Dworkin, B.M., Antonecchia, P.P., Smith, F. et al., Reduced cardiac selenium content in the acquired immunodeficency syndrome, *JPEN*, 13, 644, 1989.
40. Kavanaugh-McHugh, A.L., Ruff, A., Perlman, A. et al., Selenium deficiency and cardiomyopathy in acquired immunodeficiency syndrome, *JPEN*, 13, 347, 1991.
41. Zazzo, J.F., Chalas, J., LaFont, A. et al., Is nonobstructive cardiomyopathy in AIDS a selenium deficiency-related disease?, *JPEN*, 12, 537, 1988.
42. Constans, J., Delmas-Beauvieux, M.C., Sergeant, C. et al., One-year antioxidant supplementation with beta-carotene or selenium for human immunodeficiency virus-positive patients: a pilot study, *Clin. Infect. Dis.* (in press).
43. Delmas-Beauvieux, M.C., Peuchant, E., Couchouron, A. et al., Blood antioxidant enzymatic system and glutathione status in HIV-infected patients: effects of selenium or beta-carotene supplementation, *Am. J. Clin. Nutr.* (in press).
44. Schrauzer, G.N. and Sacher, J., Selenium in the maintenance and therapy of HIV-infected patients, *Chem. Biol. Interact.*, 91, 199, 1994.

chapter three

The thiols glutathione, cysteine, and homocysteine in human immunodeficiency virus (HIV) infection

F. Müller, P. Aukrust, A.M. Svardal, R.K. Berge, P.M. Ueland, and S.S. Frøland

Introduction

Infection with human immunodeficiency virus type 1 (hereafter referred to as HIV) results in a progressive impairment of immune function, ultimately leading to opportunistic infections and malignancies of the acquired immunodeficiency syndrome (AIDS). The fundamental immunologic abnormality is a progressive impairment of the number and functions of CD4+ lymphocytes. Because the CD4+ lymphocytes are important immune regulatory cells, various immune functions are affected. In recent years, several reports have suggested that impaired antioxidant defense plays a role in the immunopathogenesis of HIV infection.[1-5] Several investigators have suggested that clinical trials with antioxidants, in particular with glutathione replenishing drugs, should be carried out.[6-9]

Reactive oxygen species

As an essential part of human metabolism, oxygen is required to transform different substrates for the release of energy, oxidize endogenous compounds, and detoxify xenobiotics. In these processes, most of the oxygen acts as a terminal 4-electron acceptor and is completely reduced to water. However, a small amount of oxygen is normally partially reduced, yielding various reactive oxygen species (ROS). ROS include free radicals, i.e., molecular

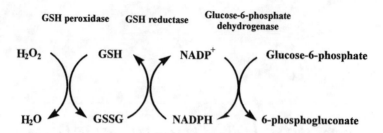

Figure 3.1   Glutathione is the substrate of glutathione peroxidase catalyzing detox-ification of hydrogen peroxide and other oxidants while glutathione reductase cata-lyzes the regeneration of reduced from oxidized glutathione. Glutathione reductase is dependent on NADPH, which in turn is generated from NADP+ by the pentose phosphate pathway.

species containing one or more unpaired electrons, such as the hydroxyl radical and superoxide anion, and species that are not, but may readily be converted to oxygen radicals, e.g., hydrogen peroxide, in the presence of, for example, iron or copper ions.[10,11]

Reactions of free radicals with other biological molecules tend to proceed as chain reactions: one radical begets another and so on[10-12] leading to oxi-dative damage of proteins, carbohydrates, lipids, and DNA.

Antioxidants

The steady state formation of ROS is normally balanced by a similar rate of consumption by antioxidants that are enzymatic and/or nonenzymatic.[11,13,14] Oxidative stress results from imbalance in this ROS-antioxidant equilibrium in favor of the ROS.[14]

Important scavenger enzymes are superoxide dismutase that catalyzes the conversion of superoxide anion to hydrogen peroxide, catalase that pro-motes the conversion of hydrogen peroxide to water and oxygen, and glu-tathione peroxidase which reduces intracellular oxidants, such as hydrogen peroxide, by the conversion of reduced glutathione (GSH) to oxidized glu-tathione (GSSG), as shown in Figure 3.1.[10,11,13,14]

There are also many structural defenses, such as compartmentalization of hydrogen peroxide-generating enzymes in peroxisomes, and chelation of free iron or copper ions in transferrin, ferritin, lactoferrin, albumin, or ceru-loplasmin, thereby preventing these metal ions from participating in ROS generation.[10-12,15,16]

In addition to the primary defenses (scavenger enzymes and metal-ion sequestration), secondary defenses are also present. Lipid-soluble α-toco-pherol, the most effective antioxidant component of vitamin E,[11] and water-soluble ascorbic acid (vitamin C) may function as chain-breaking antioxi-dants, creating new ROS which are both poorly reactive and can be recon-verted to the antioxidant compound.[10,11,15,16]

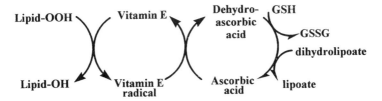

Figure 3.2   The relationship between lipophilic and hydrophilic antioxidants is shown in this figure. Vitamin E is regenerated from its radical by ascorbate which in this process is oxidized to dehydroascorbate. Dehydroascorbate can be recycled by several pathways, such as by GSH and by dihydrolipoate.

Cells also contain systems which can repair DNA damage after attack by radicals (e.g., a series of glycosylases), degrade protein damage by radicals (e.g., proteases), and metabolize lipid hydroperoxides (e.g., glutathione peroxidase and phospholipase A_2).[10,11,17] Almost all of these defenses appear to be inducible, i.e., the capacity increases in response to damage.[11]

Glutathione: the major intracellular antioxidant

Glutathione is a cysteine containing tripeptide (γ-glutamyl-cysteinyl-glycine) that is found in eukaryotic cells at millimolar concentrations and is regarded as the major intracellular redox buffering principle.[10,11] Glutathione is the substrate of selenium-dependent glutathione peroxidase catalyzing detoxification of hydrogen peroxide and other oxidants while glutathione reductase catalyzes the regeneration of reduced from oxidized glutathione (Figure 3.1). Flavin adenine dinucleotide (FAD), which is synthesized from riboflavin (vitamin B_2), is required as a cofactor for glutathione reductase. Another antioxidant enzyme, glutathione transferase, inactivates reactive electrophilic species[11] and participates in the metabolism of such endogenous compounds as steroids and leukotrienes.[10,11] Moreover, glutathione itself has antioxidant properties.[18] Finally, GSH provides reducing power for the maintenance of other antioxidants, e.g., ascorbic acid (vitamin C), vitamin E, and β-carotene.[10,11]

Ascorbic acid is a powerful antioxidant that reacts with superoxide, peroxide, and hydroxyl radicals causing the formation of dehydroascorbic acid. Dehydroascorbic acid is converted back to the reduced form, ascorbic acid, by GSH.[19] Ascorbic acid and glutathione act together as antioxidants (Figure 3.2), and there is evidence to suggest that GSH can spare ascorbic acid and vice versa.[20,22]

Vitamin E, the major lipophilic antioxidant protecting cell membranes against lipid peroxidation, is coupled to the hydrophilic antioxidants glutathione and ascorbic acid as indicated in Figure 3.2.[23] Also, as shown in Figure 3.2, the alpha-lipoic acid/dihydrolipoic acid couple contributes in the network of interlinked antioxidant systems.[23,24] Dihydrolipoic acid reacts with various ROS in addition to its interaction with ascorbic acid[24] and GSH.[25]

Reduced glutathione not only protects cells against oxidative damage induced by enhanced ROS generation. It is now recognized that glutathione is an important component of the pathway that uses NADPH to provide cells with their reducing equivalents.[20,26] Such reducing power is used for the conversion of ribonucleotides to deoxyribonucleotides and for a variety of thiol-disulfides interconversions.[11,12,26] Glutathione is, therefore, important both for the synthesis and repair of DNA and the folding of newly synthesized proteins, thus influencing the cell cycle regulation and the function of several enzymes. The glutathione redox balance is also of importance for maintenance of the thiol groups of intracellular proteins and other molecules, e.g., cysteine and coenzyme A.[26]

Figure 3.3 summarizes the reactions involved in the synthesis of glutathione. Reduced glutathione is synthesized intracellularly by the consecutive actions of γ-glutamylcysteine synthetase and glutathione synthetase utilizing adenosine triphosphate. The control point in the synthesis is γ-glutamylcysteine synthetase, which is subject to feedback inhibtion by reduced glutathione.[27,28] Breakdown of glutathione is initiated by γ-glutamyl transpeptidase, which catalyses transfer of the γ-glutamyl group of glutathione to acceptors, e.g., amino acids, dipeptides, and H_2O.[11,28] Cystine is the most active amino acid acceptor, but other neutral amino acids are also acceptors (e.g., methionine and glutamate).[10,11] Cysteinyl-glycine, formed in the transpeptidation reaction, is split by dipeptidases to cysteine and glycine, while the γ-glutamyl amino acids are substrates of γ-glutamyl cyclotransferase, which converts them into 5-oxiproline and the corresponding amino acids.[11,29] Conversion of 5-oxiproline to glutamate is catalyzed by 5-oxiprolinase.[11]

The relative levels of oxidized and reduced glutathione is normally regulated by a series of enzymes, which include the glutathione peroxidase and glutathione reductase (Figure 3.3).[11,27] The latter is dependent on NADPH, which is resupplied by a reduction of NADP+ via the pentose-phosphate pathway.[28] Normally, almost all (>99%) of the intracellular glutathione is in the reduced form.[27] However, GSSG can accumulate under certain circumstances such as rapid GSSG production, reduced glutathione reductase activity, or impaired transport of GSSG out of the cell.[27]

It is notable that γ-glutamyl transpeptidase is mainly extracellularly located, whereas glutathione is found principally within cells. It seems that many cells normally export glutathione, which then interacts with γ-glutamyl transpeptidase and dipeptidases bound to the outside of the cell membrane.[30,31]

Substrates (glutamate, cysteine, and glycine) for the synthesis of glutathione are provided by transport of either amino acids or γ-glutamyl amino acids into the cells.[26,27] It seems that cysteine availability is rate-limiting for glutathione synthesis.[26-28]

Liver is an important source of extracellular glutathione.[31] Plasma glutathione is used by many tissues which have high levels of γ-glutamyl transpeptidase, e.g., kidney, lung, and brain.[30] Glutathione itself is not transported into

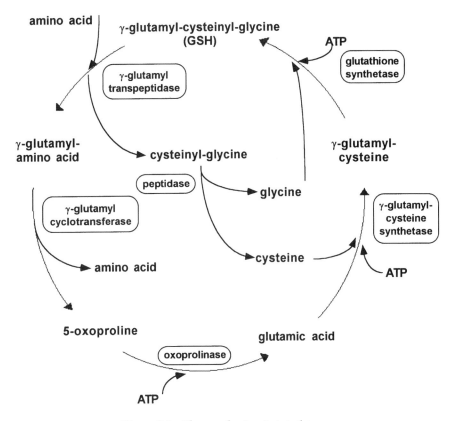

Figure 3.3 The synthesis of glutathione.

most of the cells of these tissues, but is broken down by the membrane-bound γ-glutamyl transpeptidase and dipeptidases, and the breakdown products are transported and utilized for glutathione synthesis. This is an important pathway of glutathione metabolism.[26,28,30] Thus, γ-glutamyl transpeptidase is not only important in the breakdown of glutathione, but also in preventing loss of thiol moieties and in the transport of glutathione precursors into cells.

Homocysteine

Among the plasma thiols, homocystine has recently received considerable attention, especially because hyperhomocysteinemia is a risk factor for early-onset cardiovascular disease[32,33] and is a useful marker of impaired function of cobalamin or folate.[34] Furthermore, ROS formation has been demonstrated during autooxidation of homocysteine.[35,36] Depending on parameters such as pH, concentration, and the presence of metal ions, reduced homocysteine may function either as an antioxidant or as a pro-oxidant.[37,38] In cardiovascular patients with elevated plasma homocysteine, reduced homocysteine has been suggested as a possible atherogenic agent due to its pro-oxidant effect.[38]

Homocysteine is a product of transmethylation and is either remethylated to methionine or converted to cystathionine. The former reaction is in most tissues catalyzed by cobalamin-dependent methionine synthase, which requires 5-methyltetrahydrofolate as co-substrate.[34] Cystathionine is metabolized to cysteine, which is a precursor of glutathione.[31,39] Glutathione in turn is degraded to cysteinylglycine which is further cleaved to cysteine and glycine.[31] Thus, these thiols are metabolically related.

Oxidative stress in disease processes

Oxidative stress has been implicated in the pathogenesis of several noninfectious clinical disorders including heart and brain ischemic diseases, several lung disorders (e.g., asthma, emphysema, and bleomycin toxicity), and seems to be involved in carcinogenesis.[40-43] Oxidative stress may also play a pathogenic role in several autoimmune and inflammatory disorders such as glomerulonephritis, rheumatoid arthritis, drug-induced vasculitis, Crohn's disease, and adult respiratory distress syndrome.[40,41] It has also been suggested that oxidative stress is a major contributor to degenerative diseases of aging such as brain dysfunction and cataract.[14,17]

In addition to HIV infection (see later), increased oxidative stress may also contribute to the pathogenesis of other chronic infections, e.g., chronic hepatitis B and C virus infection and chronic parasitic infections such as schistosomiasis and *Clonorchis sinensis* infection.[17]

The mechanisms by which oxidative stress causes disease include several factors in which induction of glutathione redox disturbances and oxidizing of thiol groups are of major importance and will be discussed below.

Other factors in part related to disturbed glutathione metabolism seem also to be involved in the pathogenesis of various diseases. At least two important transcription factors, nuclear factor (NF)-κB and activator protein (AP)-1, are regulated by the intracellular redox state.[44] DNA binding sites for these factors are located in the promoter region of many genes that are involved in the pathogenesis of various diseases.[44]

A major feature of enhanced oxidative stress is increased DNA strand breakage, and these oxidative DNA lesions may play an important role in the pathogenesis of aging and cancer.[12,17,41]

Oxidative stress is also characterized by a loss of intracellular NADPH, probably related to increased poly (adenosine diphosphate-ribose) polymerase activity, which uses NADPH as substrate.[12,41] This enzyme is activated under conditions of DNA strand breakage.[45] Rise in intracellular Ca^{2+} with secondary activation of Ca^{2+}-dependent enzymes such as proteases and phospholipases leading to worsening of oxidative damage appears also to be a consequence of oxidative stress.[12,18] This rise in intracellular Ca^{2+} may in part be mediated by impaired Ca^{2+}-adenosine triphosphatase and activated mitochondrial pores.[12,46]

Finally, lipid peroxidation caused by oxidative stress gives rise to mutagenic and toxic lipid epoxides, lipid hydroperoxides, lipid alkoxyl, peroxyl radicals, and enals.[17,47]

Formation of nitric oxide, which is a highly reactive free radical, may also contribute to the cytotoxic effects of increased oxidative stress.[48]

Thiol status in patients with HIV infection

In recent years, several reports have suggested that impaired antioxidant defense plays a role in the immunopathogenesis of HIV infection. With regard to glutathione homeostasis, several reports have demonstrated abnormalities *in vivo* during HIV infection, although the results are somewhat conflicting. Decreased levels of reduced glutathione in HIV-infected patients have been found in plasma,[1] in lung epithelial-lining fluid,[1] in PBMC,[2] and in CD4+ and CD8+ lymphocytes.[3,4] On the other hand, in two studies, levels of reduced glutathione in PBMC from HIV-seropositive patients were not different from levels found in healthy controls.[49,50] Furthermore, in one recent study, we demonstrated that increased levels of oxidized glutathione and decreased ratio of reduced to total glutathione rather than decreased levels of reduced glutathione were the major glutathione disturbances in CD4+ lymphocytes from HIV-infected patients (Table 3.1), particularly in patients with advanced clinical and immunological disease.[5]

Table 3.1 Antioxidant Levels in CD4+ Lymphocytes, CD8+ Lymphocytes, Monocytes and Plasma

	CD4+ Lymphocytes	CD8+ Lymphocytes	Monocytes	Plasma
Total glutathione	—	—	↑	—
Oxidized glutathione	↑	—	—	↓
Reduced/total glutathione	↓	↑	—	ND
Total cysteine	ND	ND	ND	—
Reduced/total cysteine	ND	ND	ND	—
Total cysteinylglycine	ND	ND	ND	—
Reduced/total cysteinylglycine	ND	ND	ND	↑
Total homocysteine	ND	ND	ND	—
Reduced/total homocysteine	ND	ND	ND	↑
Glutamate	ND	ND	ND	—

Note: Levels as determined by the authors.[5,62,70] The CD4+ lymphocytes differ from the other cell populations by their enhanced levels of oxidized glutathione and low ratio of reduced/total glutathione. Both are parameters of increased oxidative stress. These alterations were most pronounced in the "naive" subpopulation (CD4+CD45RA+) compared to CD4+CD45RO+ memory subpopulation. In plasma, the elevated ratios of reduced/total homocysteine and cysteinylglycine should be emphasized, possibly contributing to enhanced production of ROS. (—: No significant difference compared to blood donor controls; ↑ or ↓: significant difference compared to blood donor controls; ND: not determined).

It has been claimed that depletion of reduced glutathione in HIV infection is caused by decreased availability of precursor amino acids, particularly of cysteine.[2,49,51] However, in one study, depletion of reduced glutathione in serum was accompanied by normal cysteine levels.[52] Furthermore, except for a slight decrease in oxidized cysteine, recent studies in our group did not demonstrate any abnormalities in plasma cysteine levls in HIV-infected individuals.[5] Thus, although several lines of evidence suggest that there are important glutathione abnormalities in HIV-infected individuals, several controversies exist concerning thiol status during HIV infection.

The discrepancies may at least in part be related to methodological differences. First, it is known that factors such as food intake, [53,54] age,[53,55] gender,[56] smoking,[38,57] family history of coronary heart disease,[39] and circadian fluctuations[58,59] may all influence plasma and possibly cellular levels of various thiol species. These factors have to be controlled for analysis of thiol status in HIV-infected individuals. Second, and most important, due to the high reactivity of thiols, the analysis of reduced, oxidized, and protein-bound forms of these compounds in plasma may be unreliable if proper precautions are not taken.[31,56,60] A period of 2.5 min is sufficient for oxidation of a substantial fraction of glutathione,[60] and cysteine may be oxidized even more rapidly.[61] In several studies by Dröge et al. showing decreased plasma levels of reduced cysteine during HIV infection, the time between blood collection and addition of acid to blood samples was longer than 90 min[2] and this may well lead to erroneous results. In studies from our group[5,62] plasma thiols were immediately derivatized during blood collection ensuring that essentially no oxidation could take place. Third, it has been demonstrated that protein-bound cysteine is the predominant form of this thiol in plasma with only approximately 40% being in the free form.[5,38,60,62] Thus, the results from previous studies only reporting plasma levels of free cysteine species[2,49,63,64] will not reflect the total cysteine status in plasma. Furthermore, by forming mixed disulfides with proteins,[38,56] this free cysteine fraction will further decrease *ex vivo* during storage of whole blood or plasma, both at low (4°C) and high (20°C) temperature if the thiol compounds are not derivatized during blood collection.[60,65]

With regard to measurement of intracellular levels of reduced glutathione in PBMC, a recent study[66] has demonstrated technical flaws when using flow cytometry and monochlorobimane conjugated to glutathione as done in several studies analyzing glutathione levels in lymphocytes during HIV infection.[3,4,67] It was found that a considerable fraction of the glutathione-bimane adducts is released from cells, accumulates extracellularly within minutes, and will not be measured.[66] This extracellular release of the glutathione-bimane adducts may be prevented by adding sulfosalicylic acid to the cells before derivatization with monobromobimane.[31,60] Moreover, it seems that the specificity of the flow cytometry method may be poor compared with that of the chromatographic method used in some other studies.[5,50,56,60,62]

Furthermore, it is conceivable that the degree and rate of the thiol oxidation in plasma *ex vivo* may be altered by disease activity during HIV infection. This will further complicate the interpretation of data from studies comparing plasma cysteine levels or reduced glutathione levels in lymphocyte subsets in HIV-infected patients with levels in healthy controls.

Finally, it should be underscored that the glutathione levels may differ between different cell types, and more importantly, that the response of the glutathione redox cycle to oxidative stress may be differently regulated in different cell types.[9,68] Studies from our group suggest that the regulation of the glutathione metabolism is different in monocytes and CD4+ lymphocytes[5,69] and in CD45RA+ ("naive") and CD45RO+ ("memory") CD4+ lymphocytes.[69,70] Thus, when measuring intracellular glutathione levels in PBMC as has been done in most studies on glutathione disturbances in HIV infection, the findings may merely reflect variable proportions of particular cell types in HIV-infected patients. Barditch-Crovo et al.[71] have recently reported that HIV-infected patients have increased levels of reduced glutathione in PBMC compared with controls when expressed as glutathione levels per number of cells, but decreased levels when expressed as glutathione levels per mg cell protein. We believe that this discrepancy may partly be explained by increased proportions of monocytes in PBMC from HIV-infected patients. Furthermore, our previous report of isolated CD8+ lymphocytes from HIV-infected patients showing normal glutathione redox status[5] seems partly to reflect altered distribution of naive and memory CD8+ lymphocytes in these patients. In fact, we have recently found that while there is an increase in proportion of CD45RO+CD8+ subpopulation comprising normal glutathione redox status, there is a decrease in proportion of CD45RA+CD8+ lymphocytes with raised levels of oxidized glutathione and decreased ratio of reduced to total glutathione in HIV-infected patients.[70]

Increased level of oxidized glutathione — important indicator of increased oxidative stress during HIV infection

It has been suggested that decreased levels of reduced glutathione in PBMC or lymphocyte subpopulations is an important marker of oxidative stress.[72] However, there are also reports of increased levels of this glutathione species during oxidative stress.[73-77] In fact, at least some antioxidant defenses can be induced by increased ROS generation,[78] and an increase in reduced glutathione may represent an adaptive response to oxidative stress mediated by increased activity of enzymes involved in glutathione synthesis, e.g., γ-glutamylcysteine synthetase,[74] increased uptake of precursors (e.g., cysteine), or intact glutathione.[74,77] It seems that increased levels of oxidized glutathione or decreased ratio of reduced to total glutathione are better parameters of increased oxidative stress than decreased levels of reduced glutathione.[27,73,79-82] Interestingly, it has been found that increased intracellular levels of reduced glutathione do not protect cells against oxidative damage if these cells have decreased ratio of reduced to total glutathione.[73] Thus, it appears that the capacity of the glutathione redox cycle, rather than intracellular levels of reduced glutathione, may determine the resistance to oxidative stress, at least in some cell types.[27,73,79]

Most studies analyzing intracellular glutathione status in PBMC or lymphocyte subpopulations in HIV-infected individuals have only measured levels of reduced glutathione. However, we have recently determined the glutathione redox balance in lymphocyte subpopulations and monocytes during HIV infection by measuring intracellular levels of both reduced and total glutathione. We found a marked increase in oxidized glutathione and a considerable decrease in ratio of reduced to total glutathione as the major glutathione redox disturbances in CD4+ lymphocytes from HIV-infected individuals. In resting mammalian cells, only a small fraction of total glutathione exists in the oxidized form.[27,28] However, we found that CD4+ lymphocytes from the majority of patients with symptomatic HIV infection had a ratio of reduced to total glutathione below 0.5. Although a decrease of such magnitude has been found in some intracellular structures such as the endoplasmic reticulum,[83] this has not been reported, to our knowledge, in lymphocyte subpopulations in any human disease. Furthermore, the increase in oxidized glutathione and the decrease in ratio of reduced to total glutathione, but not the moderate decrease in levels of reduced glutathione in CD4+ lymphocytes, were significantly correlated with advanced clinical and immunological disease.[5] These changes, reflecting increased oxidized stress, may well represent important immunopathogenic factors in HIV infection. Interestingly, we have observed similar glutathione disturbances in CD4+ lymphocytes from patients with common variable immunodeficiency (CVI, a primary B-cell deficiency), and this may well be of importance for the pathogenesis of CVI.[69]

Glutathione redox disturbances in CD4+ lymphocytes during HIV infection — reflection of increased "inflammatory stress"?

Several hypotheses have been put forward to explain the disturbed glutathione metabolism during HIV infection. Lymphocytes depend on extracellular concentration of reduced cysteine for glutathione synthesis and provision of cysteine is the rate-limiting step.[31,51] It has been suggested that the decreased plasma levels of cysteine leads to disturbed glutathione homeostasis in HIV infection.[2,51] However, when appropriate methods for measuring circulating thiol levels are used, no abnormalities in plasma cysteine levels seem to be present in any group of HIV-infected patients.[5,62] As an alternative explanation for the deranged thiol status in HIV-infected patients, Dröge et al. have proposed that elevated circulating concentrations of glutamate in HIV infection may inhibit the uptake of oxidized cysteine into monocytes and macrophages which then will make less reduced cysteine available to lymphocytes for synthesis of reduced glutathione.[63,84] However, we and others[5,64] could not confirm these findings [63,84] of increased serum levels of glutamate during HIV infection. In these studies[63,84] there are no reports of glutamine or glutamine + glutamate levels, and one cannot exclude that the demonstration of raised glutamate levels in these studies may represent *ex vivo* interconversion of glutamine to glutamate.[85]

Thus, it appears that increased levels of oxidized glutathione and decreased ratio of reduced to total glutathione are the major intracellular glutathione redox disturbances in CD4+ lymphocytes from HIV-infected individuals. Among the CD4+ lymphocytes, the most pronounced glutathione abnormalities were found in the "naive" (CD45RA+) subpopulation.[70]

Several factors may influence the intracellular levels of oxidized glutathione during oxidative stress, including increased generation, the activities in the glutathione reductase and glutathione transhydrogenase (e.g., thioredoxin), and the ability to export oxidized glutathione from cells.[27,28,83]

Recent studies have focused on the cooperation between the glutathione and the thioredoxin system.[86,87] Indeed, thioredoxin appears to be of importance for maintenance of glutathione in a reduced state and vice versa.[28,88] Furthermore, it seems that some of the effects seen after increasing the intracellular ratio of reduced to total glutathione may at least in part be mediated by raised thioredoxin levels (e.g., inhibition of apoptosis).[86,89] Masutani et al. found that thioredoxin high-producer cells were selectively lost in lymph nodes from AIDS patients.[90] In a recent study, elevated plasma thioredoxin levels were found in HIV-infected patients, especially in those with advanced disease.[91] Thus, the combined redox disturbances of the glutathione and the thioredoxin system seen in HIV-infected patients may represent a vicious circle contributing to the markedly disturbed intracellular redox balance.

Oxidative stress may lead to increased formation of oxidized glutathione, and recent studies have suggested that enhanced ROS generation in lymphocytes may be an important immunopathogenic factor in HIV infection as indicated in Figure 3.4.[92] Furthermore, we have recently demonstrated a significant positive correlation between serum level of TNFα and levels of oxidized glutathione in CD4+ lymphocytes from HIV-infected patients.[5,70] This may suggest that increased inflammatory stress, which in turn may result in increased ROS generation,[93] is responsible for disturbed glutathione redox cycle in CD4+ lymphocytes during HIV infection. Indeed, TNFα stimulation both *in vitro* and *in vivo* has been shown to increase the level of oxidized glutathione.[94,95]

The activity of the glutathione reductase system is of particular importance in the defense against oxidative stress by regeneration of reduced from oxidized glutathione.[27] The markedly decreased ratio of reduced to total glutathione in CD4+ lymphocytes from HIV-infected individuals may indicate marked impairment of this enzyme system during HIV infection. The glutathione reductase system is dependent on NADPH, which is resupplied by a reduction in NADP+ via the pentose-phosphate pathway.[28] Interestingly,

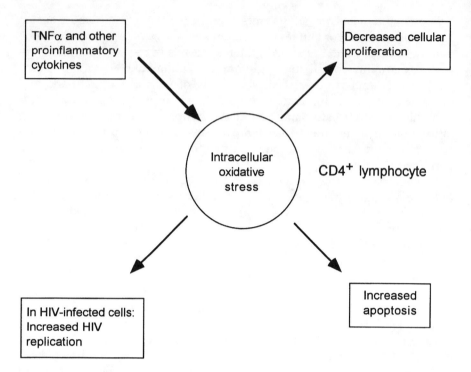

Figure 3.4 Hypothetical scheme regarding the causes and effects of intracellular oxidative stress in CD4+ lymphocytes from HIV patients. Chronic "inflammatory stress" due to overproduction of TNFα and other proinflammatory cytokines causes intracellular oxidative stress. This leads to impaired lymphocyte proliferation and possibly increased apoptosis. In HIV-infected cells, oxidative stress can also result in increased HIV replication due to activation of the transcription factor NF-κB.

low level of NADPH compromising the activity of glutathione reductase has been demonstrated in AIDS-related Kaposi's sarcoma cells.[96]

Last, but not least, TNFα and other pro-inflammatory cytokines, which enhance ROS production, may also inhibit this reductase system by depleting intracellular NADPH levels.[93] Thus, we believe that increased "pro-inflammatory stress", and in particular increased TNFα activity, is of major importance for the glutathione redox disturbances during HIV infection.

Increased TNFα activity and disturbed glutathione redox status — a vicious cycle operating in HIV infection

Several lines of evidence suggest that the correlation between increased TNFα activation and intracellular glutathione redox disturbances in CD4+ lymphocytes from HIV-infected patients[5] may reflect important immuno-pathogenic mechanisms in HIV infection. TNFα stimulation may decrease levels of reduced glutathione by causing enhanced ROS production which in turn leads to consumption of this glutathione species.[94,97,98] TNFα stimulation both *in vivo* and *in vitro* has also been demonstrated to increase oxidized glutathione levels and to impair the activity of the glutathione reductase system.[93-95,99] Moreover, it seems that antioxidants such as *N*-acetylcysteine (NAC) and glutathione impair TNFα production from PBMC.[100,101] Furthermore, glutathione redox disturbances as found in CD4+ lymphocytes from HIV-infected individuals may possibly increase the inflammatory cellular response to TNFα stimulation,[102] and proper glutathione redox status is of major importance in protecting against the toxic effects of TNFα.[6,93]

Thus, at normal glutathione redox status, proliferation and antigenic stimulation will be favored ("antigenic mode"), whereas at lower ratio of reduced to total glutathione, inflammatory-type responses are more likely to occur ("inflammatory mode").[102] Finally, increased TNFα activation may in turn increase the sensitivity of cells to ROS exposure.[94] Thus, TNFα activation with enhanced ROS generation and disturbed glutathione homeostasis may represent a vicious cycle leading to increased levels of oxidative stress with important clinical, immunological, and virological consequences in HIV infection (Figure 3.4).

Immunological consequences of glutathione redox disturbances in HIV infection

Disturbed intracellular glutathione metabolism in lymphocytes may result in immunological dysfunction either as a direct effect of decreased level of reduced glutathione,[103,104] as a direct effect of increased levels of oxidized glutathione,[105,106] or indirectly through intracellular redox disturbances and oxidative stress.[83,107] Furthermore, as enhanced ROS production may induce glutathione redox disturbances, it is difficult to separate the effects of increased ROS generation from disturbed glutathione homeostasis. Thus, while depletion of intracellular reduced glutathione with buthionine sulfoximine (a glutathione synthesis inhibitor) may inhibit lymphocyte proliferation,[103,104] it fails to induce T cell apoptosis.[86] However, ROS generation may lead to glutathione redox disturbances *and* apoptosis in these cells.[86]

Several immunological functions related to HIV infection are dependent on adequate intracellular glutathione redox balance, e.g., lymphocyte activation by mitogens, natural killer cell activation, and T-cell-mediated cytotoxicity.[103,108,109] Furthermore, a shift from Th1 (e.g., IL-2) to a Th2 (e.g., IL-4 and IL-10) cytokine profile has been suggested to be of importance in the immunopathogenesis of HIV infection.[110,111] Interestingly, recent studies have found that thiol supplementation or reducing, in contrast to oxidizing conditions, may suppress Th2 cytokine production.[112,113]

Decreased T cell proliferation or anergy upon antigen stimulation is an important immunological feature of HIV infection.[114] This hypoproliferation may be manifest even long before any decline in the absolute numbers of

CD4+ lymphocytes is observed.[115,116] Disturbed intracellular glutathione homeostasis may be of importance for this defect in T cell proliferation (Figure 3.4), and this will be discussed in somewhat more detail.

Disturbed intracellular redox status may alter functions of several enzymes and cofactors, particularly those with free SH groups in important positions,[28,88] and may also influence other intracellular redox systems.[20,88] Furthermore, optimal concentrations of thiol species are required for rapid and complete refolding of many proteins.[83,107] Thus, important cellular functions may indeed be affected by intracellular glutathione redox disturbances. In fact, a recent study has demonstrated that a decrease in intracellular levels of reduced glutathione by as little as 10 to 30% almost completely abrogated the intracellular calcium flux and the proliferative response when T cells were stimulated through the T cell receptor(TCR)/CD3 complex.[102] This may seem in some contrast with the observed increased or maintained tyrosine phosphorylation after TCR/CD3 stimulation in glutathione depleted cells.[117,118] However, examination of the complex signal transduction pathway triggered by anti-CD3/TCR stimulation indicates that increases in tyrosine phosphorylation of inhibitory sites of p59^{fyn} and p56^{lck}, regulated by CD45 tyrosine phosphatase in concert with p50^{csk}, will suppress the activities of these src kinases and result in decreased phosphorylation of other proteins (e.g., phospholipase C-γ).[119,120] Interestingly, it has been suggested that increased levels of oxidized glutathione may inhibit tyrosine phosphatases and thereby inhibit dephosphorylation of inhibitory sites of src kinases.[106] In fact, decreased CD45 tyrosine phosphatase activity has been found in CD4+ lymphocytes from HIV-infected patients, and this impaired phosphatase activity was partly restored by antioxidant supplementation.[121] Thus, it seems that glutathione redox disturbances with a decreased ratio of reduced to total glutathione may markedly impair stimulation through the TCR/CD3 complex.

IL-2 production is of major importance for an adequate lymphocyte proliferative response, and decreased intracellular levels of reduced glutathione seem to impair IL-2 production in lymphocytes,[122,123] although the results are somewhat conflicting.[124,125] In fact, it has been suggested that H$_2$O$_2$ may stimulate IL-2 production through activation of the transcriptional factor NF-κB in T cell lines.[126] These discrepancies may have several explanations. First, activation of NF-κB through phosphorylation of the inhibitor I-κB, which thereby dissociates from the NK-κB complex, seems to be dependent on increased tyrosine phosphorylation.[127] Although glutathione redox disturbances may enhance phosphorylation of I-κB after some stimuli (e.g., TNFα), this phosphorylation may be impaired after antigenic stimuli.[117,128] Second, although physiological levels of H$_2$O$_2$ may activate NF-κB and induce IL-2 production and proliferation in lymphocytes, unphysiologically high ROS production and increased levels of oxidized glutathione may impair these functions partly by inhibiting DNA binding of NF-κB and NF-AT, another transcriptional factor of importance for IL-2 production.[106,129] Third, it seems that the stimulating effect of H$_2$O$_2$ on NF-κB is restricted to some T cell lines.[130] Fourth, HIV-infected patients are characterized by persistently enhanced oxidative stress *in vivo*.[5,7,131] Although short time (hours) exposure to physiological concentrations of ROS may enhance IL-2 production *in vitro*, chronic exposure to increased oxidative stress seems to impair IL-2 production.[129,132]

It appears that enhanced ROS production and glutathione redox disturbances as found in HIV-infected patients will markedly impair rather than enhance IL-2 production in lymphocytes and will markedly suppress lymphocyte proliferation upon antigen stimulation. Indeed, we have recently demonstrated a significant correlation between intracellular redox disturbances in CD4+ lymphocytes and both impaired lymphocyte proliferation and decreased IL-2 production in HIV-infected patients.[5] Furthermore, recent studies of Cayota et al. have demonstrated that restoration of glutathione redox imbalance by anti-oxidant supplementation was able to revert the impaired proliferative activity of CD4+ lymphocyte from HIV-infected patients on CD3 stimulation.[67]

Glutathione redox disturbances in CD4+ lymphocytes during HIV infection — possible role in apoptosis

Apoptosis has been suggested to play an important immunopathogenic role in HIV infection, both in the depletion of CD4+ and CD8+ lymphocytes in advanced disease.[133-138] Importantly, a recent study demonstrated a significant correlation between disease progression and apoptosis of CD4+ and CD8+ lymphocytes in HIV-infected individuals.[139]

Several lines of evidence suggest that the markedly disturbed intracellular glutathione homeostasis, in particular when combined with increased TNFα activity, may be of major importance for this inappropriate induction of apoptosis (Figure 3.4). TNFα may induce apoptosis in both neoplastic and nonneoplastic cell types.[93,140,141] It seems that the factors determining whether cells will undergo apoptosis after TNFα stimulation at least partly depend on the extent of ROS formation as well as the cell's redox buffering capacity, of which glutathione redox status is of major importance.[93,142] Furthermore, recent studies have suggested that reduction in mitochondrial potential associated with increased ROS production is an early irreversible step of apoptosis in lymphocyte *in vivo*, further supporting a role for redox status in regulation of apoptosis.[82,143] Interestingly, such mitochondrial dysfunction has recently been demonstrated in circulating T lymphocytes from HIV-infected individuals.[92] In addition, independent of TNFα, it seems that intracellular redox disturbances mediated by increased levels of oxidized glutathione may activate redox sensitive transcriptional factors leading to induction of apoptosis.[140] Moreover, the bcl-2 proto-oncogen is rather unique among cellular genes in its ability to block apoptotic death in multiple contexts which include TNF and possibly also fas-ligand mediated apoptosis.[144,145] Hockenbery et al.[146] have suggested that bcl-2 protects against apoptosis by regulating an antioxidant pathway at the sites of ROS production. Interestingly, they also found that overexpression of glutathione peroxidase and supplementation with NAC, but not overexpression of manganese superoxide dismutase, could prevent apoptosis in a similar fashion as bcl-2.[146] Of importance, N-acetylcysteine has also been found to inhibit apoptosis in HIV-infected cells.[147]

The importance of ROS generation in the induction of apoptosis and the role of bcl-2 as an "antioxidant" have recently been questioned. Two laboratories have shown that bcl-2 protects against apoptosis in near-anaerobic conditions.[148,149] Nevertheless, although ROS generation may not represent a final common pathway in induction of apoptosis, it may be of great importance for induction of apoptosis through certain stimuli (e.g., TNF).[93,140,141] Notably, glutathione may be involved in regulation of apoptosis in some other ways than operating as an antioxidant. Glutathione redox status may modify the sulphydryl groups of several proteins including enzymes and thereby alter their functions. The DNA-binding capacity of certain transcriptional factors [e.g., Fos-Jun (AP-1)], with possible function in the induction of apoptosis, may also be influenced by glutathione redox status.

Recently, Herzenberg et al. suggested that Fas antigen stimulation is of major importance for the increased apoptosis of T lymphocytes in HIV-infected patients.[150] Fas- and TNF-induced apoptosis seem to operate at least partly through different intracellular pathways,[141] and the role of glutathione in protection against fas-mediated apoptosis has been questioned.[151] However, in a recent study Chiba et al. found that fas-mediated apoptosis in human T cells, but not perforin-mediated apoptosis, is impaired by increasing intracellular level of reduced glutathione in these cells.[152] Kohno et al. have recently shown that fas-mediated apoptosis is related to GSH in adult T cell leukemia cells,[142] while van den Dobbelsteen et al. found that fas-induced apoptosis in a T cell line was associated with loss of GSH due to enhanced export out of the cells.[153] Further studies are needed to clarify the role of intracellular redox status in fas-mediated apoptosis.

While HIV itself or interaction of CD4+ lymphocytes with gp120 may represent the "priming signal" for subsequent induction of apoptosis,[136] indirect mechanisms, which include activation of the TNF system and intracellular glutathione redox disturbances, appear also to be important in mediating increased apoptosis of T lymphocytes during HIV infection.[154]

Intracellular redox disturbances in combination with persistent immune activation: important role in enhancing HIV replication

Persistent immune activation and, in particular, TNFα activation together with increased oxidative stress seem to be major characteristics of HIV-infected patients. Recent studies indicate that HIV infection, even in the asymptomatic phase, is characterized by an active process in which cells are being infected and dying at a high rate and in large numbers, suggesting that AIDS is primarily a consequence of continuous, high-level replication of HIV.[155-157] However, this view does not exclude an important role for sustained immune activation and intracellular redox disturbances in the immunopathogenesis of HIV infection. There is a growing body of evidence indicating that an activated immune system is needed to maintain a high level of virus replication.[133,158] Both TNFα and ROS are potent stimulators of HIV replication through activation of NF-κB which is essential for the expression of genes controlled by the LTR of HIV.[97,126,159] Interestingly, it has been suggested that increased oxidized glutathione or decreased reduced to total glutathione ratio may directly enhance HIV replication through this mechanism.[160,161]

Furthermore, NAC, glutathione, and glutathione-esters have been demonstrated to inhibit HIV replication *in vitro*, both in acutely and chronically infected cell lines and in lymphocytes and monocyte/macrophages from HIV-seronegative donors.[97,162-168] However, there are to our knowledge no studies demonstrating inhibitory effect of glutathione supplementation on HIV replication in cells from HIV-infected patients, either *in vivo* or *in vitro*. It seems that the antiviral effect of glutathione is mediated by inhibition of NFκB activation.[97,162,166] However, Bergami et al.[163] have reported that cystamine, which may enhance intracellular levels of reduced glutathione,[169] inhibits HIV replication in human lymphocytes and macrophages by interfering with the orderly assembly of HIV virions. Furthermore, oltipraz (4-methyl-5-(2-pyrazinyl)-1,2-dithiole-3-thione), which also may increase intracellular levels of reduced glutathione has been found to be a potent inhibitor of HIV reverse transcriptase.[170,171] By whatever mechanisms, restoring of glutathione redox status in HIV-infected patients may not only have immunomodulating effects such as inhibition of apoptosis and restoring of impaired IL-2 production and lymphocyte proliferation, but may also possibly have direct anti-HIV effects.

Homocysteine in HIV infection

In a recent study, we found that all but one of 21 patients with HIV infection had plasma levels of reduced homocysteine above the range of the control group.[62] However, no difference in the plasma concentration of total homocysteine was found when patients and controls were compared. As a result, the reduced-total homocysteine ratio was considerably increased in the HIV-infected patients. Our data on plasma levels of total homocysteine in HIV patients are in accordance with a previous study showing normal serum levels of total homocysteine in 20 AIDS patients.[52] Elevated levels of reduced homocysteine in plasma have been found in various other conditions such as homocystinuria,[172] cobalamin deficiency,[173] and after administration of homocysteine[174] or methionine.[175] In all these conditions, the elevation of reduced homocysteine has been associated with increased concentrations of total homocysteine in plasma. To our knowledge, the combination of elevated levels of reduced homocysteine and normal total homocysteine concentrations has not previously been observed in any clinical condition.

Depending on parameters such as pH, concentration, and the presence of metal ions, reduced homocysteine may function either as an antioxidant or as a pro-oxidant.[37,38] In patients with elevated plasma concentration of reduced homocysteine and early-onset arteriosclerosis, reduced homocysteine has been suggested as a possible thrombogenic agent due to its pro-oxidant effect.[38]

Our findings of elevated concentration of reduced homocysteine may be relevant for current theories implicating oxidative stress in the immuno-pathogenesis of HIV infection.[5,7,8,72] Elevated levels of reduced homocysteine might contribute to the production of ROS as the sulfhydryl group of homocysteine is believed to act catalytically with cupric or ferric ions to generate hydrogen peroxide and various homocysteinyl radicals.[35,36,61] In one of these studies, homocysteine plus an increasing concentration of copper led to hydrogen peroxide production in a dose-dependent manner.[36] Although data on serum copper levels in HIV patients are discrepant,[176,177] a longitudinal study has shown that patients progressing to AIDS had significantly higher serum copper levels compared to the nonprogressors.[176] In the presence of metal ions, e.g., copper or iron ions, hydrogen peroxide can react to form the highly reactive hydroxyl radical.[61] Recent studies suggest that it is the hydroxyl radical that is responsible for the NF-κB activation causing the stimulation of HIV replication in HIV-infected cells.[178] Thus, one may speculate that elevated circulating levels of reduced homocysteine in HIV patients is one of several contributing factors to an enhanced production of ROS, which in turn could lead to stimulation of HIV replication through NF-κB activation. Alternative to the hypothesis suggested above, elevated levels of reduced homocysteine might be a consequence of other redox disturbances in patients with HIV infection. Also, it is uncertain whether the measured reduced homocysteine in plasma from these patients is trapped in a form reacting with the derivatizing agent or exists as authentic homocysteine in the circulation.

No significant differences in reduced homocysteine levels were noted when asymptomatic and symptomatic HIV patients were compared, and we did not find any relationship between reduced homocysteine levels and other markers of immunodeficiency.[62]

Cobalamin or folate deficiency leads to hyperhomocysteinemia.[39,173] Most patients in our study had cobalamin levels in the lower normal range. While only two of the patients had cobalamin levels in serum below normal, their plasma concentration of total homocysteine was slightly elevated. Our findings of subnormal cobalamin levels in some HIV-infected patients are in accordance with recent studies.[177,179,180] However, the total homocysteine concentrations in the patient and control groups were similar.

Also, the HIV-infected patients in our study had reduced methionine concentration in plasma. This is in accordance with previous reports.[2,64] As methionine is an essential amino acid, malabsorption may lead to methionine deficiency. However, none of the patients in this study had clinical signs or symptoms suggesting malabsorption.

A significant but modest decrease in the total cysteinylglycine plasma concentration was found in the HIV patients compared to controls. As cysteinylglycine is a degradation product of glutathione,[27] the decreased concentration of cysteinylglycine might reflect low glutathione turnover. In fact, plasma glutathione tended to be lower in this group of HIV patients compared to controls.[5] The concentration of reduced cysteinylglycine tended to be slightly elevated in the patient group resulting in an increased reduced-total ratio. As with homocysteine, elevated levels of reduced cysteinylglycine might contribute to ROS generation due to the presence of a free sulfhydryl group.[61]

Correction of thiol redox status — therapeutic approaches in HIV-infected patients

The cornerstone in treatment of HIV-infected patients is antiviral agents such as nucleoside analogs and protease inhibitors.[181-183] However, there is a growing body of evidence suggesting that immunomodulating agents may be of importance in combination with antiviral agents in the treatment of these patients.[114,184] One immunomodulatory strategy is treatment that restores the dysregulated thiol redox balance in patients with HIV infection. In particular, modulation of the intracellular glutathione redox status in CD4+ lymphocytes is promising.

Cysteine prodrugs

N-acetyl-L-cysteine (NAC) is a direct ROS scavenger and is metabolized *in vivo* to cysteine that restores intracellular GSH levels.[185,186] Presently, NAC is used as an antidote for paracetamol (acetaminophen) overdose[187] and in the treatment of various respiratory diseases.[188,189] It can be given orally and is well tolerated.[190] NAC effectively inhibits TNFα-induced activation of the HIV long terminal repeat, leading to reduced HIV replication in infected cells.[162,166] This effect of NAC is due to a specific blocking of the induction of NF-κB.[97,191] Also, NAC has been shown to enhance antibody-dependent cellular cytotoxicity of cells from patients with HIV infection.[192] In a recent *in vitro* study, the impaired proliferative capacity of CD4+ lymphocytes from HIV-infected patients was restored by NAC.[67] In cultured T cells from HIV-seronegative donors, NAC enhanced both the proliferative capacity and IL-2 production.[122] Furthermore, NAC has been shown to inhibit apoptosis of T lymphocytes and monocytoid cells[193,194] and also in HIV-infected monocytoid cells.[147,195] However, this anti-apoptotic effect of NAC may not be mediated by increase in intracellular GSH.[196]

Only a few trials with NAC have been performed in patients with HIV infection. de Quay et al. treated 9 HIV-infected patients with a single oral dose of NAC and found a transient and moderate increase in GSH in mononuclear cells in some patients.[49] However, the glutathione redox balance in CD4+ lymphocytes was not assessed in this study. In a study over 14 weeks, Walker et al. treated HIV patients with 4 different dosage levels of NAC and did not observe serious toxicities.[138] Finally, Witschi et al. treated 6 AIDS patients with oral NAC for 2 weeks and found a significant increase of plasma cysteine, while the GSH level in mononuclear cells and plasma was unaltered[197]

There may be several reasons for the lack of GSH response to NAC treatment. First, the bioavailability of NAC is low by oral treatment.[190] Second, the control point in glutathione synthesis, γ-glutamylcysteine synthetase, is subject to feedback inhibition by GSH, and this may inhibit the effect of supplementation with NAC or other cysteine prodrugs.[27] Third, it has been suggested that the glutathione imbalance in HIV-infected patients is due to inhibition of systemic synthesis of GSH.[181,198] If so, it is not likely that GSH precursors such as NAC would lead to a marked increase in GSH concentration.

Another cysteine prodrug, L-2-oxothiazolidine-4-carboxylic acid (OTC; also called Procysteine) has been shown to increase GSH levels in lymphocytes when given to healthy volunteers.[199] OTC enters the cells independently of the cystine transport pathway and is converted to cysteine by oxoprolinase inside the cell.[188] While NAC has the dual ability to replenish GSH and scavenge oxidants, OTC is a strict glutathione precursor. When NAC and OTC were compared with respect to inhibition of cytokine-induced HIV replication in various cell lines, it was observed that NAC was far more effective than OTC.[167] Also, NAC fully replenished intracellular GSH, while OTC did not.[167] In a phase I/II trial of intravenous OTC for 6 weeks in 24 asymptomatic HIV-infected patients, no change in CD4+ lymphocyte count or HIV viral load was observed, although in the subgroup of patients receiving the highest OTC dose, whole blood glutathione was significantly higher at the end of the study compared to baseline levels.[200]

Another thiol compound, *cystamine*, has been shown to inhibit HIV replication both in lymphocytes and macrophages *in vitro*.[163,201] Cystamine can increase GSH.[169] In addition, cystamine inhibits HIV replication by interference with two steps of the viral life cycle, namely inhibition of proviral DNA formation and assembly of HIV virions, causing the production of defective viral particles.[163] Interestingly, cystamine also inhibited lipopolysaccharide (LPS)-induced TNFα production in macrophages.[201] However, cystamine has not been used in humans while the structurally related form, cysteamine, has a low toxicity in man.[202] In a recent study, cysteamine was found to be a potent inhibitor of HIV replication *in vitro* at similar concentrations to those obtained by oral administration for the treatment of cystinosis, an inherited disorder.[203]

Treatment with glutathione

In one study, intravenous infusion of GSH was given to eight HIV-infected patients, the plasma level of both cysteine and GSH increased, but the intracellular GSH concentration in *mononuclear cells* did not increase.[198] The authors suggest that GSH remained low due to a decreased systemic synthesis of GSH.[198] However, as we have underscored above, glutathione levels may differ between different cell types, and measurements of intracellular glutathione in *mononuclear cells* may thus merely reflect increased or decreased proportions of particular cell types.

Modulation of glutathione peroxidase

The activity of the selenium-dependent glutathione peroxidases is important for the intracellular protection against oxidative damage. Patients with HIV infection have an impaired selenium status,[204-206] and this may well affect the glutathione peroxidase activity. In fact, selenium supplementation has been shown to increase glutathione peroxidase activity in HIV-infected T lymphocytes.[207] Thus, selenium supplementation in patients with HIV infection may be of importance and may also have a synergistic effect in combination with GSH replenishment, e.g., with NAC.

Modulation of glutathione reductase

The elevated intracellular level of oxidized glutathione in CD4+ lymphocytes from HIV-infected patients may well be due to impaired activity of glutathione reductase. FAD is synthesized from riboflavin and is required as cofactor for glutathione reductase. Thus, one might speculate that reduced uptake of riboflavin due to malabsorption could lead to reduced activity of glutathione reductase. However, no data are available from HIV patients regarding this subject.

Also, glutathione reductase is dependent on NADPH, and it is of importance that pro-inflammatory cytokines such as TNFα deplete intracellular NADPH levels[93] and thus may inhibit the reductase. The effects of TNFα are further potentiated by the HIV regulatory protein tat.[208] Furthermore, tat caused a decrease in the intracellular glutathione level in different T cell lines.[208]

Thus, anti-TNFα treatment may well enhance the activity of glutathione reductase in HIV-infected patients. Several clinical trials with thalidomide[209,210] or pentoxifylline[211-213] have been performed, but glutathione status has not been evaluated in these trials. It is thus important that the intracellular glutathione redox balance is evaluated in future trials where anti-TNFα treatment is given.

Other antioxidants with effects on the glutathione redox balance

In vitro studies with alpha-lipoic acid and vitamin E derivatives have shown that they inhibit TNFα induced NF-κB activation in T cell lines, and it has been suggested that these compounds may be possible candidates for clinical trials in HIV-infected patients.[214,215]

Ascorbic acid inhibits HIV replication *in vitro*.[164,216] Furthermore, ascorbic acid has a synergistic effect in combination with NAC with regard to reduction of HIV replication.[164] The antiviral effect of ascorbic acid seems not to be mediated by suppression of NF-κB activation.[217]

Based on these data and the fact that ascorbic acid has a low toxicity,[218] it would be interesting to evaluate ascorbic acid in combination with thiols such as NAC in clinical trials of HIV-infected patients. In a current study in our department, HIV-patients receive a combination of NAC and ascorbic acid while clinical, immunological, and virological parameters are evaluated.

Conclusion

Two lines of evidence suggest that patients with HIV infection may benefit from antioxidant treatment: First, the impaired glutathione status in their CD4+ lymphocytes, and second, *in vitro* data indicating that oxidative stress leads to impairment of important lymphocyte functions and causes increased HIV replication in infected cells. Whether treatment with antioxidants such as *N*-acetylcysteine will prove to be useful in the treatment of patients with HIV infection awaits the results of future clinical trials.

References

1. Buhl, R., Jaffe, H.A., Holroyd, K.J., Wells, F.B., Mastrangeli, A., Saltini, C., Cantin, A.M., and Crystal, R.G., Systemic glutathione deficiency in symptom-free HIV-seropositive individuals, *Lancet*, 2, 1294, 1989.
2. Eck, H.P., Gmünder, H., Hartmann, M., Petzoldt, D., Daniel, V., and Dröge, W., Low concentrations of acid-soluble thiol (cysteine) in the blood plasma of HIV-1-infected patients, *Biol. Chem. Hoppe-Seyler*, 370, 101, 1989.
3. Staal, F.J.T., Roederer, M., Israelski, D.M., Bubp, J., Mole, L.A., Mcshane, D., Deresinski, S.C., Ross, W., Sussman, H., Raju, P.A., Anderson, M.T., Moore, W., Ela, S.W., and Herzenberg, L.A., Intracellular glutathione levels in T-Cell subsets decrease in HIV-infected individuals, *AIDS Res. Hum. Retroviruses*, 8, 305, 1992.
4. Roederer, M., Staal, F.J.T., Osada, H., and Herzenberg, L.A., CD4 and CD8 T Cells with high intracellular glutathione levels are selectively lost as the HIV infection progresses, *Int. Immunol.*, 3, 933, 1991.
5. Aukrust, P., Svardal, A.M., Müller, F., Lunden, B., Ueland, P.M., and Frøland, S.S., Increased levels of oxidized glutathione in CD4+ lymphocytes associated with disturbed intracellular redox balance in human immunodeficiency virus type 1 infection, *Blood*, 86, 258, 1995.

6. Roederer, M., Ela, S.W., Staal, F.J.T., and Herzenberg, L.A., N-Acetylcysteine — A new approach to anti-HIV therapy, *AIDS Res. Hum Retroviruses*, 8, 209, 1992.

7. Müller, F., Reactive oxygen intermediates and human immunodeficiency virus (HIV) infection, *Free Radical Biol. Med.*, 13, 651, 1992.

8. Dröge, W., Cysteine and glutathione deficiency in AIDS patients — a rationale for the treatment with N-acetyl-cysteine, *Pharmacology*, 46, 61, 1993.

9. Halliwell, B. and Cross, C.E., Reactive oxygen species, antioxidants, and acquired immunodeficiency syndrome. Sense or speculation, *Arch. Intern. Med.*, 151, 29, 1991.

10. Halliwell, B. and Gutteridge, J.M.C., Role of free radicals and catalytic metal ions in human disease: an overview, *Methods Enzymol.*, 186, 1, 1990.

11. de Bono, D.P., Free radicals and antioxydants in vascular biology: the roles of reaction kinetics, environment and substrate turnover, *Q.J. Med.*, 87, 445, 1994.

12. Bast, A., Haenen, G.R.M.M., and Doelman, C.J.A., Oxidants and antioxidants: state of art, *Am. J. Med.*, 91, 4S, 1991.

13. Halliwell, B., Drug antioxidant effects, *Drug*, 42, 569, 1991.

14. Yu, B.P., Cellular defenses against damage from reactive oxygen species, *Physiol. Rev.*, 74, 139, 1994.

15. Rosen, G.M., Pou, S.P., Ramos, C.L., Cohen, M.S., and Britigan, B.E., Free radicals and phagocytic cells, *FASEB J.*, 9, 200, 1995.

16. Halliwell, B., Reactive oxygen species in living systems — source, biochemistry, and role in human disease, *Am. J. Med.*, 91(suppl. 3C), 14S, 1991.

17. Ames, B.N., Shigenaga, M.K., and Hagen, T.M., Oxidants, antioxidants, and the degenerative diseases of aging, *Proc. Natl. Acad. Sci. U.S.A.*, 90, 7915, 1993.

18. Frei, B., Reactive oxygen species and antioxidant vitamins: mechanism of action, *Am. J. Med.*, 97, 5S, 1994.

19. Sinclair, A.J., Barnett, A.H., and Lunec, J., Free radicals and antioxidant systems in health and disease, *Br. J. Hosp. Med.*, 43, 334, 1990.

20. Meister, A., Glutathione ascorbic acid antioxidant system in animals, *J. Biol. Chem.*, 269, 9397, 1994.

21. Meister, A., On the antioxidant effects of ascorbic acid and glutathione, *Biochem. Pharm.*, 44, 1905, 1992.

22. Jain, A., Mārtensson, J., Mehta, T., Krauss, A.N., Auld, P.A.M., and Meister, A., Ascorbic acid prevents oxidative stress in glutathione-deficient mice: effects on lung type II cell lamellar bodies, lung surfactant, and skeletal muscle, *Proc. Natl. Acad. Sci. U.S.A.*, 89, 5093, 1992.

23. Packer, L., New horizons in vitamin E research — the vitamin E cycle, biochemistry, and clinical applications. In *Lipid Soluble Antioxidants: Biochemistry and Clinical Applications*, Ong, A.S.H. and Packer, L., Eds., Birkhäuser Verlag, Basel, 1-16, 1992.

24. Packer, L., Witt, E.H., and Tritschler, H.J., Alpha-lipoic acid as a biological antioxidant, *Free Radical. Biol. Med.*, 19, 227, 1995.

25. Han, D., Tritschler, H.J., and Packer, L., Alpha-lipoic acid increases intracellular glutathione in a human T-lymphocyte Jurkat cell line, *Biochem. Biophys. Res. Commun.*, 207, 258, 1995.

26. Meister, A., Glutathione deficiency produced by inhibition of its synthesis, and its reversal; applications in research and therapy. *Pharmac. Ther.*, 51, 155, 1991.

27. Deneke, S.M. and Fanburg, B.L., Regulation of cellular glutathione, *Am. J. Physiol.*, 257, L163, 1989.
28. Meister, A., Glutathione metabolism and its selective modification, *J. Biol. Chem.*, 263, 17206, 1988.
29. Thompson, G.A. and Meister, A., Utilization of L-cystine by the gamma-glutamyl transpeptidase gamma-glutamyl cyclotransferase pathway, *Proc. Natl. Acad. Sci. U.S.A.*, 72, 1985, 1975.
30. Meister, A., Glutathione, ascorbate, and cellular protection, *Cancer Res.*, 54(suppl.), 1969S, 1994.
31. Meister, A. and Anderson, M.E., Glutathione, *Annu. Rev. Biochem.*, 52, 711, 1983.
32. Kang, S.-S., Wong, P.W.K., and Malinow, M.R., Hyperhomocyst(e)inemia as a risk factor for occlusive vascular disease, *Annu. Rev. Nutr.*, 12, 279, 1992.
33. Boushey, C.J., Beresford, S.A., Omenn, G.S., and Motulsky, A.G., A quantitative assessment of plasma homocysteine as a risk factor for vascular disease. Probable benefits of increasing folic acid intakes, *JAMA*, 274, 1049, 1995.
34. Ueland, P.M., Refsum, H., Stabler, S.P., Malinow, M.R., Andersson, A., and Allen, R.H., Total homocysteine in plasma or serum. Methods and clinical applications, *Clin. Chem.*, 39, 1764, 1993.
35. Wall, R.T., Harlan, J.M., Harker, L.A., and Striker, G.E., Homocysteine-induced endothelial cell injury *in vitro*: a model for the study of vascular injury, *Thrombosis Res.*, 18, 113, 1980.
36. Starkebaum, G. and Harlan, J.M., Endothelial cell injury due to copper-catalyzed hydrogen peroxide generation from homocysteine, *J. Clin. Invest.*, 77, 1370, 1986.
37. Preibisch, G., Küffner, C., and Elstner, E.F., Biochemical model reactions on the prooxidative activity of homocysteine, *Z. Naturforsch*, 48c, 58, 1993.
38. Mansoor, M.A., Bergmark, C., Svardal, A.M., Lønning, P.E., and Ueland, P.M., Redox status and protein binding of plasma homocysteine and other aminothiols in patients with early-onset peripheral vascular disease, *Arterioscler. Thromb. Vasc. Biol.*, 15, 232, 1995.
39. Ueland, P.M. and Refsum, H., Plasma homocysteine, a risk factor for vascular disease: plasma levels in health, disease, and therapy, *J. Lab. Clin. Med.*, 114, 473, 1989.
40. Lunec, J. Free radicals: their involvement in disease processes, *Ann. Clin. Biochem.*, 27, 173, 1990.
41. Halliwell, B., Gutteridge, J.M.C., and Ross, C.E., Free radicals, antioxidants, and human disease: where are we now? *J. Lab. Clin. Med.*, 119, 598, 1992.
42. Floyd, R.A., Role of oxygen free radicals in carcinogenesis and brain ischemia, *FASEB J.*, 4, 2587, 1990.
43. Cross, C.E., van der Vliet, A., ONeill, C.A., and Eiserich, J.P., Reactive oxygen species and the lung, *Lancet*, 344, 930, 1994.
44. Sen, C.K. and Packer, L., Antioxidant and redox regulation of gene transcriptionn, *FASEB J.*, 10, 709, 1996.
45. Schraufstatter, I.U., Hyslop, P.A., Hinshaw, D.B., Spragg, R.G., Sklar, R.A., and Cochrane, C.G., Hydrogen peroxide-induced injury of cells and its prevention by inhibitors of poly (ADB-ribose) polymerase, *Proc. Natl. Acad. Sci. U.S.A.*, 83, 4908, 1986.
46. Crompton, M., Costi, A., and Hayat, L., Evidence for the presence of reversible Ca^{2+} dependent pore activitated by oxidative stress in heart mitochondria, *Biochem. J.*, 245, 915, 1987.

47. Sandstrom, P.A., Tebbey, P.W., van Cleave, S., and Buttke, T. M., Lipid hydroperoxides induce apoptosis in T cells displaying a HIV associated glutathione peroxidase deficiency, *J. Biol. Chem.*, 269, 798, 1994.

48. Walker, M.W., Kinter, M.T., Roberts, R.J., and Spitz, D.R., Nitric oxide-induced cytotoxicity: involvement of cellular resistance to oxidative stress and the role of glutathione in protection, *Pediatr. Res.*, 37, 41, 1995.

49. de Quay, B., Malinverni, R., and Lauterburg, B.H., Glutathione depletion in HIV-infected patients — role of cysteine deficiency and effect of oral N-acetylcysteine, *AIDS*, 6, 815, 1992.

50. Pirmohamed, M., Williams, D., Tingle, M.D., Barry, M., Khoo, S.H., OMahony, C., Wilkins, E.G.L., Breckenridge, A.M., and Park, B.K., Intracellular glutathione in the peripheral blood cells of HIV-infected patients: failure to show a deficiency, *AIDS*, 10, 501, 1996.

51. Dröge, W., Eck, H.P., and Mihm, S., HIV-induced cysteine deficiency and T-cell dysfunction — a rationale for treatment with N-acetylcysteine, *Immunol. Today*, 13, 211, 1992.

52. Jacobsen, D.W., Green, R., Herbert, V., Longworth, D.L, and Rehm, S., Decreased serum glutathione with normal cysteine and homocysteine levels in patients with AIDS, *Clin. Res.*, 38, 556A, 1990.

53. Ubbink, J.B., Vermaak, W.J.H., van der Merwe, A., and Becker, P.J., The effect of blood sample aging and food consumption on plasma total homocysteine levels, *Clin. Chim. Acta*, 207, 119, 1992.

54. Hum, S., Koski, K.G., and Hoffer, L.J., Varied protein intake alters glutathione metabolism in rats, *J. Nutr.*, 122, 2010, 1992.

55. Lang, C.A., Naryshkin, S., Schneider, D.L., Mills, B.J., and Lindeman, R.D., Low blood glutathione levels in healthy aging adults, *J. Lab. Clin. Med.*, 120, 720, 1992.

56. Mansoor, M.A., Svardal, A.M., and Ueland, P.M., Determination of the *in vivo* redox status of cysteine, cysteinylglycine, homocysteine, and glutathione in human plasma, *Anal. Biochem.*, 200, 218, 1992.

57. Duthie, G.G., Arthur, J.R., and James, W.P., Effects of smoking and vitamin E on blood antioxidant status, *Am. J. Clin. Nutr.*, 53, 1061S, 1991.

58. Smaland, R., Svardal, A.M., Lote, K., Ueland, P.M., and Lærum, O.D., Glutathione content in human bone marrow and circadian stage relation to DNA synthesis, *J. Natl. Cancer Inst.*, 83, 1092, 1991.

59. Farooqui, M.Y.H. and Ahmed, A.E., Circadian periodicity of tissue glutathione and its relationship with lipid peroxidation in rats, *Life Sci.*, 34, 2413, 1984.

60. Svardal, A.M., Mansoor, M.A., and Ueland, P.M., Determination of reduced oxidized, and protein-bound glutathione in human plasma with precolumn derivatization with monobromobimane and liquid chromatography, *Anal. Biochem.*, 184, 338, 1990.

61. Munday, R., Toxicity of thiols and disulphides: involvement of free-radical species, *Free Radical Biol. Med.*, 7, 659, 1989.

62. Müller, F, Svardal, A.M., Aukrust, P., Berge, R.K., Ueland, P.M., and Frøland, S.S., Elevated plasma concentration of reduced homocysteine in patients with human immunodeficiency virus infection, *Am. J. Clin. Nutr.*, 63, 242, 1996.

63. Eck, H.P., Mertens, T., Rosokat, H., Fatkenheuer, G., Pohl, C., Schrappe, M., Daniel, V., Naher, H., Petzoldt, D., Drings, P., et al., T4+ cell numbers are correlated with plasma glutamate and cystine levels: association of hyperglutamataemia with immunodeficiency in diseases with different aetiologies, *Int. Immunol.*, 4, 7, 1992.

64. Hortin, G., Landt, M., and Powderly, W.G., Changes in plasma amino acid concentrations in response to HIV-1, *Clin. Chem.*, 40, 785, 1994.
65. Fiskerstrand, T., Refsum, H., Kvalheim, G., and Ueland, P.M., Homocysteine and other thiols in plasma and urine: automated determination and sample stability, *Clin. Chem.*, 39, 263, 1993.
66. van der Ven, A.J.A.M., Mier, P., Peters, W.H.M., Dolstra, H., van Erp, P.E.J., Koopmans, P.P., and van der Meer, J.W., Monochlorobimane does not selectively label glutathione in peripheral blood mononuclear cells, *Anal. Biochem.*, 217, 41, 1994.
67. Cayota, A., Vuillier, F., Gonzalez, G., and Dighiero, G., *In vitro* antioxidant treatment recovers proliferative responses of anergic CD4+ lymphocytes from human immunodeficiency virus-infected individuals, *Blood*, 87, 4746, 1996.
68. Kavanagh, T.J., Grossmann, A., Jaecks, E.P., Jinneman, J.C., Eaton, D.L, Martin, G.M., and Rabinovitch, P.S., Proliferative capacity of human peripheral blood lymphocytes sorted on basis of glutathione content, *J. Cell. Physiol.*, 145, 472, 1990.
69. Aukrust, P., Svardal, A.M., Müller, F., Lunden, B., Berge, R.K., and Frøland, S.S., Decreased levels of total and reduced glutathione in CD4(+) lymphocytes in common variable immunodeficiency are associated with activation of the tumor necrosis factor system: possible immunopathogenic role of oxidative stress, *Blood*, 86, 1383, 1995.
70. Aukrust, P., Svardal, A.M., Müller, F., Lunden, B., Nordøy, I., and Frøland, S.S., Markedly disturbed glutathione redox status in CD45RA+CD4+ lymphocytes in human immunodeficiency virus type 1 infection is associated with selective depletion of this lymphocyte subset, *Blood*, 88, 2626, 1996.
71. Barditch-Crovo, P., Svobodova, V., and Lietman, P., Apparent deficiency of glutathionine in the PBMCs of people with AIDS depends on method of expression, *J. Acq. Immun. Defic. Synd. Hum. R.*, 8, 313, 1995.
72. Staal, F.J.T., Ela, S.W., Roederer, M., Anderson, M.T., and Herzenberg, L.A., Glutathione deficiency and human immunodeficiency virus infection, *Lancet*, 339, 909, 1992.
73. Jenkinson, S.G., Lawrence, R.A., Zamora, C.A., and Deneke, S.M., Reduction of intracellular glutathione in alveolar type II pneumocytes following BCNU exposure, *Am. J. Physiol.*, 266, L125, 1994.
74. Miura, K. Ishii, T., Sugita, Y., and Bannai, S., Cystine uptake and glutathione level in endothelial cells exposed to oxidative stress, *Am. J. Physiol.*, 262, C50, 1992.
75. Cantin, A.M., North, S.L., Hubbard, R.C., and Crystal, R.G., Normal alveolar epithelial lining fluid contains high levels of glutathione, *J. Appl. Physiol.*, 63, 152, 1987.
76. Shi, M.M., Iwamoto, T., and Forman, H.J., Gamma-glutamylcysteine synthetase and GSH increase in quinone-induced oxidative stress in BPAEC, *Am. J. Physiol.*, 267, L414, 1994.
77. Benard, O. and Balasubramanian, K.A., Effect of oxidant exposure on thiol status in the intestinal mucosa, *Biochem. Pharmacol.*, 45, 2011, 1993.
78. Harris, E.D., Regulation of antioxidant enzymes, *FASEB J.*, 6, 2675, 1992.
79. Suttorp, N., Kästle, S., and Neuhof, H., Glutathione redox cycle is an important defense system of endothelial cells against chronic hyperoxia, *Lung*, 169, 203, 1991.

80. Irita, K., Okabe, H., Koga, A., Kurosawa, K., Tagawa, K., Yamakawa, M., Yoshitake, J.-I., and Takahashi, S., Increased sinusidal efflux of reduced and oxidized glutathione in rats with endotoxin/D-galactosamine hepatitis, *Circ. Shock*, 42, 115, 1994.
81. Hughes, H.H., Jaeschke, H., and Mitchell, J.R., Measurement of oxidative stress *in vivo*, *Methods Enzymol.*, 186, 681, 1990.
82. Garcia de la Asuncion, J., Millan, A., Pla, R., Bruseghini, L., Esteras, A., Pallardo, F.V., Sastre, J., and Vina, J., Mitochondrial glutathione oxidation correlates with age-associated oxidative damage to mitochondrial DNA, *FASEB J.*, 10, 333, 1996.
83. Hwang, C., Sinskey, A. J., and Lodish, H.F., Oxidized redox state of glutathione in the endoplasmic reticulum, *Science*, 257, 1496, 1992.
84. Dröge, W., Eck, H.P., Näher, H., Pekar, U., and Daniel, V., Abnormal amino acid concentrations in the blood of patients with acquired immunodeficiency syndrome (AIDS) may contribute to the immunological defect, *Biol. Chem. Hoppe-Seyler*, 369, 143, 1988.
85. Parvy, P., Bardet, J., Rabier, D., Gasquet, M., and Kamoon, P., Intra- and interlaboratory quality control for assay of amino acids in biological fluids: 14 years of French experience, *Clin. Chem.*, 39, 1831, 1993.
86. Sato, J., Iwata, S., Nakamura, K., Hori, T., Mori, K., and Yodo, J., Thiol-mediated redox regulation of apoptosis, *J. Immunol.*, 154, 3194, 1995.
87. Iwata, S., Hori, T., Sato, N., Uedataniguchi, Y., Yamabe, T., Nakamura, H., Masutani, H., and Yodoi, J., Thiol-mediated redox regulation of lymphocyte proliferation — possible involvement of adult T cell leukemia-derived factor and glutathione in transferrin receptor expression, *J. Immunol.*, 152, 5633, 1994.
88. Holmgren, A., Thioredoxin and glutaredoxin systems, *J. Biol. Chem.*, 264, 13963, 1989.
89. Newman, G.W., Balcewicz-Salbinska, M.K., Guarnaccia, J.R., Remold, H.G., and Silberstein, D.S., Opposing regulatory effects of thioredoxin and eosinophil cytotoxicity-enhancing factor on the development of human immunodeficiency virus 1, *J. Exp. Med.*, 180, 359, 1994.
90. Masutani, H., Naito, M., Takahashi, K., Hattori, T., Koito, A., Takatsuki, K., Go, T., Nakamura, H., Fujii, S., Yoshida, Y., Okuma, M., and Yodor, J., Dysregulation of adult T-cell leukemia-derived factor (ADF)/thioredoxin in HIV infection: loss of ADF high producer cells in lymphoid tissues of AIDS patients, *AIDS Res. Hum. Retrovirus.*, 8, 1707, 1992.
91. Nakamura, H., DeRosa, S., Roederer, M., Anderson, M.T., Dubs, J.G., Yodoi, J., Holmgren, A., and Herzenberg, L.A., Elevation of plasma thioredoxin levels in HIV-infected individuals, *Int. Immunol.*, 8, 603, 1996.
92. Macho, A., Castedo, M., Marchetti, P., Aguilar, J.J., Decaudin, D., Zamzami, N., Girard, P.M., Uriel, J., and Kroemer, G., Mitochondrial dysfunctions in circulating T lymphocytes from human immunodeficiency virus-1 carriers, *Blood*, 86, 2481, 1995.
93. Buttke, T.M. and Sandstrom, P.A., Oxidative stress as a mediator of apoptosis, *Immunol. Today*, 15, 7, 1994.
94. Ishii, Y., Partridge, C.A., del Vecchio, P.J., and Malik, A. B., Tumor necrosis factor-α-mediated decrease in glutathione increases the sensitivity of pulmonary vascular endothelial cells to H_2O_2, *J. Clin. Invest.*, 89, 794, 1992.

95. Chang, S.W., Ohara, N., Kuo, G., and Voelkel, N.F., Tumor necrosis factor-induced lung injury is not mediated by platelet-activating factor, *Am J. Physiol.*, 257, L232, 1989.
96. Mallery, S.R., Bailer, R.T., Hohl, C.M., Ngbautista, C.L., Ness, G.M., Livingston, B.E., Hout, B.L., Stephens, R.E., and Brierley, G.P., Cultured AIDS-related Kaposi's sarcoma (AIDS-KS) cells demonstrate impaired bioenergetic adaptation to oxidant challenge: implication for oxidant stress in AIDS-KS pathogenesis, *J. Cell Biochem.*, 59, 317, 1995.
97. Staal, F.J.T., Roederer, M., Herzenberg, L.A., and Herzenberg, L., Intracellular thiols regulate activation of nuclear factor kappa B and transcription of human immunodeficiency virus, *Proc. Natl. Acad. Sci. U.S.A.*, 87, 9943, 1990.
98. Bilzer, M. and Lauterberg, B.H., Glutathione metabolism in activated human neutrophils: stimulation of glutathione synthesis and consumption of glutathione by reactive oxygen species, *Eur. J. Clin. Invest.*, 21, 316, 1991.
99. Adamson, G.M. and Billings, R.E., Tumor necrosis factor induced oxidative stress in isolated mouse hepatocytes, *Arch. Biochem. Biophys.*, 294, 223, 1992.
100. Eugul, E.M., deLustro, B., Rouhafza, S., Ilnicka, M., Lee, S.W., Wilhelm, R., and Allison, A.C., Some antioxidants inhibit, in a co-ordinate fashion, the production of tumor necrosis factor-α, IL-1β and IL-6 by human peripheral blood mononuclear cells, *Int. Immunol.*, 6, 409, 1994.
101. Peristeris, P., Clark, B.D., Gatti, S., Faggioni, R., Mantovani, A., Mengozzi, M., Orencole, S.F., Sironi, M., and Ghezzi, P., N-acetylcysteine and glutathione as inhibitors of tumor necrosis factor production, *Cell. Immunol.*, 240, 390, 1992.
102. Staal, F.J.T., Anderson, M.T., Staal, G.E.J., Herzenberg, L.A., and Gitler, C., Redox regulation of signal transduction — tyrosine phosphorylation and calcium influx, *Proc. Natl. Acad. Sci. U.S.A.*, 91, 3619, 1994.
103. Hamilos, D.L. and Wedner, H.J., The role of glutathione in lymphocyte activation. I. Comparison of inhibitory effects of buthionine sulfoximine and 2-cyclohexene-1-one by nuclear size formation, *J. Immunol.*, 135, 2740, 1985.
104. Suthanthiran, M., Anderson, M.D., Sharma, V.K., and Meister, A., Glutathione regulates activation-dependent DNA synthesis in highly purified normal human T lymphocytes stimulated via CD2 and CD3 antigen, *Proc. Natl. Acad. Sci. U.S.A.*, 87, 3343, 1990.
105. Hilly, M., Piétri-Rouxel, F., Coquil, J.-F., Guy, M., and Mauger, J.-P., Thiol reagents increase the affinity of the inositol 1,4,6-triphosphate receptor, *J. Biol. Chem.*, 268, 16488, 1993.
106. Dröge, W., Schulze-Osthoff, K., Mihm, S., Galter, D., Schenk, H., Eck, H.P., Roth, S., and Gmünder, H., Functions of glutathione and glutathione disulfide in immunology and immunopathology, *FASEB J.*, 8, 1131, 1994.
107. Ziegler, D.M., Role of reversible oxidation-reduction of enzyme thiol-disulphides in metabolic regulation, *Annu. Rev. Biochem.*, 54, 305, 1985.
108. Yamauchi, A. and Bloom, E.T., Requirement of thiol compounds as reducing agents for IL-2 mediated induction of LAK activity and proliferation of human NK cells, *J. Immunol.*, 151, 5535, 1993.
109. Dröge, W., Pottmeyer-Greber, C., Schmidt, H., and Nick, S., Glutathione augments the activation of cytotoxic T lymphocytes *in vivo*, *Immunobiology*, 171, 151, 1986.
110. Clerici, M., Via, C.S., Lucey, D.R., Roilides, E., Pizzo, P.A., and Shearer, G.M., Functional dichotomy of CD4+ T-helper lymphocytes in asymptomatic human immunodeficiency virus infection, *Eur. J. Immunol.*, 21, 665, 1991.

111. Clerici, M. and Shearer, G.M., The Th1-Th2 hypothesis of HIV infection: new insights, *Immunol. Today,* 15, 575, 1994.
112. Apostolopoulos, V., Pietersz, G.A., Loveland, B.E., Sandrin, M.S., and McKenzie, I.F., Oxidative/reductive conjugation of mannan to antigen selects for T1 or T2 immune responses, *Proc. Natl. Acad. Sci. U.S.A.,* 92, 10128, 1995.
113. Jeannin, P., Delneste, Y., Lecoanethenchoz, S., Gauchat, J.F., Life, P., Holmes, D., and Bonnefoy, J.Y., Thiols decrease human interleukin (IL) 4 production and IL-4-induced immunoglobulin synthesis, *J. Exp. Med.,* 182, 1785, 1995.
114. Pantaleo, G. and Fauci, A.S., New concepts in the pathogenesis of HIV infection, *Annu. Rev. Immunol.,* 13, 487, 1995.
115. Clerici, M., Stocks, N.I., Zajac, R.A., Boswell, R.N., Lucey, D.R., Via, C.S., and Shearer, G.M., Detection of three distinct patterns of T helper cell dysfunction in asymptomatic, human immunodeficiency virus-seropositive patients. Independence of CD4+ cell numbers and clinical staging, *J. Clin. Invest.,* 84, 1892, 1989.
116. Lane, H.C., Depper, J.M., Greene, W.C., Whalen, G., Waldmann, T.A., and Fauci, A.S., Qualitative analysis of immune function in patients with the acquired immunodeficiency syndrome: evidence for a selective defect in soluble antigen recognition, *N. Engl. J. Med.,* 313, 79, 1985.
117. Koretzky, G.A., Picus, J., Thomas, M.L., and Weiss, A., Tyrosin phosphatase CD45 is essential for coupling T-cell antigen receptor to the phosphatidyl inositol pathway, *Nature,* 346, 66, 1990.
118. June, C.H., Fletcher, M.C., Ledbetter, J.A., Schieven, G.I., Siegel, J.N., Phillips, A.F., and Samelson, L.E., Inhibition of tyrosine phosphorylation prevents T-cell receptor-mediated signal transduction, *Proc. Natl. Acad. Sci. U.S.A.,* 87, 7722, 1990.
119. Anderson, S.J., Levin, S.D., and Perlmutter, R.M., Involvement of the protein tyrosin kinase p56[lck] in T cell signalling and thymocyte development, *Adv. Immunol.* 56, 151, 1994.
120. Weiss, A. and Littman, D.R., Signal transduction by lymphocyte antigen receptors, *Cell,* 76, 263, 1994.
121. Cayota, A., Vuillier, F., Gonzalez, G., and Dighiero, G., CD4(+) lymphocytes from HIV-infected patients display impaired CD45-associated tyrosine phosphatase activity which is enhanced by anti-oxidants, *Blood,* 87, 4746, 1996.
122. Eylar, E., Riveraquinones, C., Molina, C., Baez, I., Molina, F., and Mercado, C.M., N-acetylcysteine enhances T-cell functions and T-cell growth in culture, *Int. Immunol.,* 5, 97, 1993.
123. Wu, D., Meydani, S.N., Sastre, J., Hayek, M., and Meydani, M., *In vitro* glutathione supplementation enhances IL-2 production and mitogenic response of peripheral blood mononuclear cells from young and old subjects, *J. Nutr.,* 124, 655, 1994.
124. Gmünder, H., Roth, S., Eck, H.P., Gallas, H., Mihm, S., and Dröge, W., Interleukin-2 mRNA expression, lymphokine production and DNA synthesis in glutathione depleted T cells, *Cell. Immunol.,* 130, 520, 1990.
125. Roth, S., and Dröge, W., Regulation of interleukin-2 production, interleukin-2 mRNA expression and intracellular glutathione levels in *ex vivo* derived T lymphocytes by lactate, *Eur. J. Immunol.,* 21, 1933, 1991.
126. Schreck, R., Rieber, P., and Baeuerle, P.A., Reactive oxygen intermediates as apparently widely used messengers in the activation of the NF-κB transcription factor and HIV-1, *EMBO J.,* 10, 2247, 1991.

127. Naumann, M. and Scheidereit, C., Activation of NF-κB *in vivo* is regulated by multiple phosphorylations, *EMBO J.*, 13, 4597, 1994.
128. Muroi, M., Muroi, Y., and Suzuki, T., The binding of immobilized IgG2a to Fcgamma2a receptor activates NF-κB via reactive oxygen intermediates and tumor necrosis factor-α, *J. Biol. Chem.*, 48, 30561, 1994.
129. Flescher, E., Ledbetter, J.A., Schieven, G.L., Velaroch, N., Fossum, D., Dang, H., Ogawa, N., and Talal, N., Longitudinal exposure of human T lymphocytes to weak oxidative stress suppresses transmembrane and nuclear signal transduction, *J. Immunol.*, 153, 4880, 1994.
130. Anderson, M.T., Staal, F.J.T., Gitler, C., Herzenberg, L.A., and Herzenberg, L., Separation of oxidant-initiated and redox-regulated steps in the NF-κB signal transduction pathway, *Proc. Natl. Acad. Sci. U.S.A.*, 91, 11527, 1994.
131. Pace, G. W. and Leaf, C.D., The role of oxidative stress in HIV disease, *Free Radical Biol. Med.*, 19, 523, 1995.
132. Dypbukt, J.M., Ankarcrona, M., Burkitt, M., Sjöholm, A., Ström, K., Orrenius, S., and Nicotera, P., Different prooxidant levels stimulate growth, trigger apoptosis or produce necrosis of insulin-secreting RINm5F cells, *J. Biol. Chem.*, 269, 30553, 1994.
133. Fauci, A.S., Multifactorial nature of human immunodeficiency virus disease — implications for therapy, *Science*, 262, 1011, 1993.
134. Ameisen, J.D., Estaquier, J., and Idziorek, T., From AIDS to parasite infection: pathogen-mediated subversion of programmed cell death as a mechanism for immune dysregulation, *Immunol. Rev.*, 142, 9, 1994.
135. Estaquier, J., Idziorek, T., Debels, F., Barresinoussi, F., Hurtel, B., Aubertin, A.M., Venet, A., Mehtali, M., Muchmore, E., Michel, P., Mouton, Y., Girard, M., and Ameisen, J.C., Programmed cell death and AIDS: significance of T-cell apoptosis in pathogenic and nonpathogenic primate lentiviral infections, *Proc. Natl. Acad. Sci. U.S.A.*, 91, 9431, 1994.
136. Pantaleo, G. and Fauci, A.S., Apoptosis in HIV infection, *Nature Med.* 1, 118, 1995.
137. Roederer, M., Dubs, J.G., Anderson, M.T., Raju, P.A., and Herzenberg, L.A., CD8 naive T cell counts decrease progressively in HIV-infected adults, *J. Clin. Invest.*, 95, 2061, 1995.
138. Walker, R.E., Lane, H.C., Boenning, C.M., and Fauci, A.S., The safety, pharmacokinetics, and antiviral activity of N-acetylcysteine in HIV-infected individuals, *J. Cell. Biochem.*, 16, 89, 1992.
139. Gougeon, M.L., Lecoeur, H., Dulioust, A., Enouf, M.G., Crouvoisier, M., Goujard, C., Debord, T., and Montagnier, L., Programmed cell death in peripheral lymphocytes from HIV-infected persons — increased susceptibility to apoptosis of CD4 and CD8 T cells correlates with lymphocyte activation and with disease progression, *J. Immunol.*, 156, 3509, 1996.
140. Sarafian, T.A. and Bredesen, D.E., Invited commentary: is apoptosis mediated by reactive oxygen species? *Free Radical Res.*, 21, 1, 1994.
141. Wong, G.H.W. and Goeddel, D.V., Fas antigen and P55 TNF receptor signal apoptosis through distinct pathways, *J. Immunol.*, 152, 1751, 1994.
142. Kohno, T., Yamada, Y., Hata, T., Mori, H., Yamamura, M., Tomonaga, M., Urata, Y., Goto, S., and Kondo, T., Relation of oxidative stress and glutathione synthesis to CD95(Fas/APO-1) -mediated apoptosis of adult T cell leukemia cells, *J. Immunol.*, 156, 4722, 1996.

143. Henkart, P.A. and Grinstein, S., Apoptosis: mitochondria resurrected? *J. Exp. Med.*, 183, 1293, 1996.
144. Korsmeyer, S.J., Bcl-2 initiates a new category of oncogenes: regulators of cell death, *Blood*, 80, 879, 1992.
145. Itoh, N., Tsujimoto, Y., and Nagata, S., Effects of bcl-2 on Fas antigen-mediated cell death, *J. Immunol.*, 151, 621, 1993.
146. Hockenbery, D.M., Oltvai, Z.N., Yin, X.M., Milliman, C.L., and Korsmeyer, S.J., Bcl-2 functions in an antioxidant pathway to prevent apoptosis, *Cell*, 75, 241, 1993.
147. Malorni, W., Rivabene, R., Santini, M.T., and Donelli, G., N-acetylcysteine inhibits apoptosis and decreases viral particles in HIV-chronicaly infected U937 cells, *FEBS Lett.*, 327, 75, 1993.
148. Jacobson, M.D. and Raff, M.C., Programmed cell death and Bcl-2 protection in very low oxygen, *Nature*, 374, 814, 1995.
149. Shimizu, S., Eguchi, Y., Kosaka, H., Kamiike, W., Matsuda, H., and Tsujimoto, Y., Prevention of hypoxia-induced cell death by Bcl-2 and Bcl-xL, *Nature*, 374, 811, 1995.
150. Katsikis, P.D., Wunderlich, E.S., Smith, C.A., and Herzenberg, L.A., Fas antigen stimulation induces marked apoptosis of T lymphocytes in human immunodeficiency virus-infected individuals, *J. Exp. Med.*, 181, 2029, 1995.
151. Hug, H., Enari, M., and Nagata, S., No requirement of reactive oxygen intermediates in Fas-mediated apoptosis, *FEBS Lett.*, 351, 311, 1994.
152. Chiba, T., Takahashi, S., Sato, N., Ishii, S., and Kikuchi, K., Fas-mediated apoptosis is modulated by intracellular glutathione in human T cells, *Eur. J. Immunol.*, 26, 1164, 1996.
153. van den Dobblesteen, D.J., Nobel, C.S.I., Schlegel, J., Cotgreave, I.A., Orrenius, S., and Slater, A.F.G., Rapid and specific efflux of reduced glutathione during apoptosis induced by anti-fas/APO-1 antibody, *J. Biol. Chem.*, 271, 15420, 1996.
154. Finkel, T.H., Tudorwilliams, G., Banda, N.K., Cotton, M.F., Curiel, T., Monks, C., Baba, T.W., Ruprecht, R.M., and Kupfer, A., Apoptosis occurs predominantly in bystander cells and not in productively infected cells of HIV- and SIV-infected lymph nodes, *Nature Med.*, 1, 129, 1995.
155. Wei, X., Ghosh, S.K., Taylor, M.E., Johnson, V.A., Emini, E.A., Deutsch, P., Lifson, J.D., Bonhoeffer, S., Nowak, M.A., Hahn, B.H., Saag, M.S., and Shaw, G.M., Viral dynamics in human immunodeficiency virus type 1 infection, *Nature*, 373, 117, 1995.
156. Ho, D.D., Neumann, A.U., Perelson, A.S., Chen, W., Leonard, J.M., and Markowitz, M., Rapid turnover of plasma virions and CD4 lymphocytes in HIV-1 infection, *Nature*, 373, 123, 1995.
157. Coffin, J.M., HIV population dynamics *in vivo*: implications for genetic variation, pathogenesis and therapy, *Science*, 267, 483, 1994.
158. Levy, J.A., Pathogenesis of human immunodeficiency virus infection, *Microbiol. Rev.*, 57, 183, 1993.
159. Matsuyama, T., Kobayashi, N., and Yamamoto, N., Cytokines and HIV infection — is AIDS a tumor necrosis factor disease, *AIDS*, 5, 1405, 1991.
160. Israel, N., Gougerotpocidalo, M.A., Aillet, F., and Virelizier, J.L., Redox status of cells influences constitutive or induced NF-κB translocation and HIV long terminal repeat activity in human T-cell and monocytic cell lines, *J. Immunol.*, 149, 3386, 1992.

161. Simon, G., Moog, C., and Obert, G., Valproic acid reduces the intracellular level of glutathione and stimulates human immunodeficiency virus, *Chem.-Biol. Interact.*, 91, 111, 1994.

162. Kalebic, T., Kinter, A., Poli, G., Anderson, M.E., Meister, A., and Fauci, A.S., Suppression of human immunodeficiency virus expression in chronically infected monocytic cells by glutathione, glutathione ester, and N-acetylcysteine, *Proc. Natl. Acad. Sci. U.S.A.*, 88, 986, 1991.

163. Bergamini, A., Capozzi, M., Ghibelli, L., Dini, L., Salanitro, A., Milanese, G., Wagner, T., Beninati, S., Pesce, C.D., Amici, C., and Rocchi, G., Cystamine potently suppresses *in vitro* HIV replication in acutely and chronically infected human cells, *J. Clin. Invest.*, 93, 2251, 1994.

164. Harakeh, S. and Jariwalla, R.J., Comparative study of the anti-HIV activities of ascorbate and thiol-containing reducing agents in chronically HIV-infected cells, *Am. J. Clin. Nutr.*, 54, S1231, 1991.

165. Ho. W.-Z. and Douglas, S.D., Glutathione and normal-acetylcysteine suppression of human immunodeficiency virus replication in human monocyte/macrophages *in vitro*, *AIDS Res. Hum. Retrovirus.*, 8, 1249, 1992.

166. Roederer, M., Staal, F.J.T., Raju, P.A., Ela, S.W., Herzenberg, L.A., and Herzenberg, L., Cytokine-stimulated human immunodeficiency virus replication is inhibited by N-acetyl-L-cysteine, *Proc Natl. Acad. Sci. U.S.A.*, 87, 4884, 1990.

167. Raju, P.A., Herzenberg, L.A., and Roederer, M., Glutathione precursor and antioxidant activities of N-acetylcysteine and oxothiazolidine carboxylate compared in *in vitro* studies of HIV replication, *AIDS Res. Hum. Retrovirus.*, 10, 961, 1994.

168. Lioy, J., Ho, W.-Z., Cutilli, J.R., Polin, R.A., and Douglas, S.D., Thiol suppression of human immunodeficiency virus type-1 replication in primary cord blood monocyte-derived macrophages *in vitro*, *J. Clin. Invest.*, 91, 495, 1993.

169. Djurhuus, R., Svardal, A.M., Mansoor, M.A., and Ueland, P.M., Modulation of glutathione content and the effect of methionine auxotrophy and cellular distribution of homocysteine and cysteine in mouse cell lines, *Carcinogenesis*, 12, 241, 1991.

170. Prochaska, H.J., Yeh, Y., Baron, P., and Polsky, B., Oltipraz, an inhibitor of human immunodeficiency virus type 1 replication, *Proc. Natl. Acad. Sci. U.S.A.*, 90, 3953, 1993.

171. Prochaska, H.J., Chavan, S.J., Baron, P., and Polsky, B., Oltipraz, a novel inhibitor of human immunodeficiency virus type 1 (HIV-1) replication, *J. Cell Biochem.*, 117, 1995.

172. Mansoor, M.A., Ueland, P.M., Aarsland, A., and Svardal, A.M., Redox status and protein binding of plasma homocysteine and other aminothiols in patients with homocystinuria, *Metabolism*, 42, 1481, 1993.

173. Mansoor, M.A., Ueland, P.M., and Svardal, A.M., Redox status and protein binding of plasma homocysteine and other aminothiols in patients with hyperhomocysteinemia due to cobalamin deficiency, *Am. J. Clin. Nutr.*, 59, 631, 1994.

174. Mansoor, M.A., Guttormsen, A.B., Fiskerstrand, T., Refsum, H., Ueland, P.M., and Svardal, A.M., Redox status and protein binding of plasma aminothiols during the transient hyperhomocysteinemia that follows homocysteine adminstration, *Clin. Chem.*, 39, 980, 1993.

175. Mansoor, M.A., Svardal, A.M., Schneede, J., and Ueland, P.M., Dynamic relation between reduced, oxidized, and protein-bound homocysteine and other thiol components in plasma during methionine loading in healthy men, *Clin. Chem.*, 38, 1316, 1992.
176. Graham, N.M., Sorensen, D., Odaka, N., Brookmeyer, R., Chan, D., Willett, W.C., Morris, J.S., and Saah, A.J., Relationship of serum copper and zinc levels to HIV-1 seropositivity and progression to AIDS, *J. Acq. Immun. Defic. Synd. Hum. R.*, 4, 976, 1991.
177. Beach, R.S., Mantero-Atienza, E., Shor-Posner, G., Javier, J.J., Szapocznik, J., Morgan, R., Sauberlich, H.E., Cornwell, P.E., Eisdorfer, C., and Baum, M.K., Specific nutrient abnormalities in asymptomatic HIV-1 infection, *AIDS*, 6, 701, 1992.
178. Schreck, R.., Meier, B., Mannel, D.N., Dröge, W., and Baeuerle, P.A., Dithiocarbamates as potent inhibitors of nuclear factor kappaB activation in intact cells, *J. Exp. Med.*, 175, 1181, 1992.
179. Rule, S.A.J., Hooker, M., Costello, C., Luck, W., and Hoffbrand, A.V., Serum vitamin B-12 and transcobalamin levels in early HIV disease, *Am. J. Hematol.*, 47, 167, 1994.
180. Beach, R.S., Morgan, R., Wilkie, F., Mantero-Atienza, E., Blaney, N., Shor-Posner, G., Lu, Y., Eisdorfer, C., and Baum, M.K., Plasma vitamin B12 level as a potential cofactor in studies of human immunodeficiency viurs type 1-related cognitive changes, *Arch. Neurol.*, 49, 501, 1992.
181. Helbling, B., Von Overbeck, J., and Lauterburg, B.H., Decreased synthesis of glutathione in patients with AIDS, *Eur. J. Clin. Invest.*, 24, A38, 1994.
182. Markowitz, M., Saag, M., Powderly, W.G., Hurley, A.M., Hsu, A., Valdes, J.M., Henry, D., Sattler, F., Lamarca, A., Leonard, J.M., and Ho, D.D., A preliminary study of ritonavir, an inhibitor of HIV-1 protease, to treat HIV-1 infection, *N. Engl. J. Med.*, 333, 1534, 1995.
183. Collier, A.C., Coombs, R.W., Schoenfeld, D.A., Bassett, R.L., Timpone, J., Baruch, A., Jones, M., Facey, K., Whitacre, C., McAuliffe, V.J., Friedman, H.M., Merigan, T.C., Reichman, R.C., Hooper, C., and Corey, L., Treatment of human immunodeficiency virus infection with saquinavir, zidovudine, and zalcitabine, *N. Engl. J. Med.*, 334, 1011, 1996.
184. Dalgleish, A.G., The immune response to HIV: potential for immunotherapy? *Immunol. Today*, 16, 356, 1995.
185. Aruoma, O.I., Halliwell, B., Hoey, B.D., and Butler, J., The antioxidant action of N-acetylcysteine: its reaction with hydrogen peroxide, hydroxyl radical, superoxide, and hypochlorous acid, *Free Radical. Biol. Med.*, 6, 593, 1989.
186. Burgunder, J.M., Varriale, A., and Lauterburg, B.H., Effect of N-acetylcysteine on plasma cysteine and glutathione following paracetamol administration, *Eur. J. Clin. Pharmacol.*, 36, 127, 1989.
187. Smilkstein, M.J., Knapp, G.L., Kulig, K.W., and Rumack, B.H., Efficacy of oral N-acetylcysteine in the treatment of acetaminophen overdose, *N. Engl. J. Med.*, 319, 1557, 1988.
188. Meister, A., Anderson, M.E., and Hwang, O., Intracellular cysteine and glutathione delivery systems, *J. Am. Coll. Nutr.*, 5, 137, 1986.
189. Meyer, A., Buhl, R., Kampf, S., and Magnussen, H., Intravenous N-acetylcysteine and lung glutathione of patients with pulmonary fibrosis and normals, *Am. J. Respir. Crit. Care Med.*, 152, 1055, 1995.

190. Holdiness, M.R., Clinical pharmacokinetics of N-acetylcysteine, *Clin. Pharma-cokinet.*, 20, 123, 1991.
191. Mihm, S., Ennen, J., Pessara, U., Kurth, R., and Dröge, W., Inhibition of HIV-1 replication and NF-κB activity by cysteine and cysteine derivatives, *AIDS*, 5, 497, 1991.
192. Roberts, R.L., Aroda, V.R., and Ank, B.J., N-acetylcysteine enhances antibody-dependent cellular cytotoxicity in neutrophils and mononuclear cells from healthy adults and human immunodeficiency virus-infected patients, *J. Infect. Dis.*, 172, 1492, 1995.
193. Sandstrom, P.A., Mannie, M.D., and Buttke, T.M., Inhibition of activation-induced death in T cell hybridomas by thiol antioxidants — oxidative stress as a mediator of apoptosis, *J. Leukocyte Biol.*, 55, 221, 1994.
194. Cossarizza, A., Franceschi, C., Monti, D., Salvioli, S., Bellesia, E., Rivabene, R., Biondo, L., Rainaldi, G., Tinari, A., and Malorni, W., Protective effect of N-acetylcysteine in tumor necrosis factor-alpha-induced apoptosis in U937 cells: the role of mitochondra, *Exp. Cell Res.*, 220, 232, 1995.
195. Malorni, W., Rivabene, R., Santini, M.T., Rainaldi, G., and Donelli, G., N-acetylcysteine prevents TNF-induced mitochondrial damage, apoptosis and viral particle production in HIV-infected U937 cells, *Redox. Rep.*, 1, 57, 1994.
196. Jones, D.P., Maellaro, E., Jiang, S.N., Slater, A.F.G., and Orrenius, S., Effects of N-acetyl-L-cysteine on T-cell apoptosis are not mediated by increased cellular glutathione, *Immunol. Lett.*, 45, 205, 1995.
197. Witschi, A., Junker, E., Schranz, C., Speck, R.F., and Lauterburg, B.H., Supple-mentation of N-acetylcysteine fails to increase glutathione in lymphocytes and plasma of patients with AIDS, *AIDS Res. Hum. Retrovirus.*, 11, 141, 1995.
198. Helbling, B., VonOverbeck, J., and Lauterburg, B.H., Decreased release of glutathione into the systemic circulation of patients with HIV infection, *Eur. J. Clin. Invest.*, 26, 38, 1996.
199. Porta, P., Aebi, S., Summer, K., and Lauterburg, B.H., L-2-oxothiazolidine-4-carboxylic acid, a cysteine prodrug: pharmacokinetics and effects on thiols in plasma and lymphocytes in human, *J. Pharmacol. Exp. Ther.*, 257, 331, 1991.
200. Kalayjian, R.C., Skowron, G., Emgushov. R.T., Chance, M, Spell, S.A., Borum, P.R., Webb, L.S., Mayer, K.H., Jackson, J.B., Yenlieberman, B., Story, K.O., Rowe, W.B., Thompson, K., Goldberg, D., Trimbo, S., and Lederman, M.M., A phase I/II trial of intravenous L-2-oxothiazolidine-4-carboxylic acid (pro-cysteine) in asymptomatic HIV-infected subjects, *J. Acq. Immun. Defic. Synd. Hum. R.*, 7, 369, 1994.
201. Ho. W.-Z., Zhu, X.-H., Song, L., Lee, H.-R., Cutilli, J.R., and Douglas, S.D., Cystamine inhibits HIV type 1 replication in cells of monocyte/macrophage and T cell lineages, *AIDS Res. Hum. Retrovirus.*, 11, 451, 1995.
202. Markello, T.C., Bernardini, M.E., and Gahl, W.A., Improved renal function in children with cystinosis treated with cysteamine, *N. Engl. J. Med.*, 328, 1157, 1993.
203. Bergamini, A., Ventura, L., Mancino, G., Capozzi, M., Placido, R., Salanitro, A., Cappannoli, L., Faggioli, E., Stoler, A., and Rocchi, G., *In vitro* inhibition of the replication of human immunodeficiency virus type 1 by β-mercapto-ethylamine (cysteamine), *J. Infect. Dis.*, 174, 214, 1996.
204. Fuchs, J., Schofer, H., Ochsendorf, F., Janka, S., Milbradt, R., Buhl, R., Unkel-bach, U., Freisleben, H.J., Oster, O., Siems, W., Grune, T., and Esterbauer, H., Antioxidants and peroxidation products in the blood of HIV-1 infected pa-tients with HIV associated skin diseases, *Eur. J. Dermatol.*, 4, 148, 1994.

205. Sappey, C., Leclercq, P., Coudray, C., Faure, P., Micoud, M., and Favier, A., Vitamin, trace element and peroxide status in HIV seropositive patients: asymptomatic patients present a severe beta-carotene deficiency, *Clin. Chim. Acta*, 230, 35, 1994.

206. Allavena, C., Dousset, B., May, T., Dubois, F., Canton, P., and Belleville, F., Relationship of trace element, immunological markers, and HIV-1 infection progression, *Biol. Tr. Elem. Res.*, 47, 133, 1995.

207. Sappey, C., Legrandpoels, S., Bestbelpomme, M., Favier, A., Rentier, B., and Piette, J., Stimulation of glutathione peroxidase activity decreases HIV type 1 activation after oxidative stress, *AIDS Res. Hum. Retrovirus.*, 10, 1451, 1994.

208. Westendorp, M.O., Shatrov, V.A., Schulze-Osthoff, K., Frank, R., Kraft, M., Los, M., Krammer, P.H., Dröge, W., and Lehmann, V., HIV-1 tat potentiates TNF-induced NF-κB activation and cytotoxicity by altering the cellular redox state, *EMBO J.*, 14, 546, 1995.

209. Tramontana, J.M., Utaipat, U., Molloy, A., Akarasewi, P., Burroughs, M., Makonkawkeyoon, S., Johnson, B., Klausner, J.D., Rom, W., and Kaplan, G., Thalidomide treatment reduces tumor necrosis factor alpha production and enhances weight gain in patients with pulmonary tuberculosis, *Mol. Med.*, 1, 384, 1995.

210. Klausner, J.D., Makonkawkeyoon, S., Akarasewi, P., Nakata, K., Kasinrerk, W., Corral, L., Dewar, R.L., Lane, H.C., Freedman, V.H., and Kaplan, G., The effect of thalidomide on the pathogenesis of human immunodeficiency virus type 1 and M-tuberculosis infection, *J. Acq. Immun. Defic. Synd. Hum. R.* 11, 247, 1996.

211. Kruse, A., Rieneck, K., Kappel, M., Orholm, M., Bruunsgaard, H., Ullum, H., Skinhoj, P., and Pedersen, B.K., Pentoxifylline therapy in HIV seropositive subjects with elevated TNF, *Immunopharmacology*, 31, 85, 1995.

212. Dezube, B.J., Pardee, A.B., Chapman, B., Beckett, L.A., Korvick, J.A., Novick, W.J., Chiurco, J., Kasdan, P., Ahlers, C.M., Ecto, L.T., and Crumpacker, C.S., Pentoxifylline decreases tumor necrosis factor expression and serum triglycerides in people with AIDS, *J. Acq. Immun. Defic. Synd. Hum. R.*, 6, 787, 1993.

213. Dezube, B.J., Lederman, M.M., Spritzler, J.G., Chapman, B., Korvick, J.A., Flexner, C., Dando, S., Mattiacci, M.R., Ahlers, C.M., Zhang, L., Novick, W.J., Kasdan, P., Fahey, J.L., Pardee, A.B., and Crumpacker, C.S., High-dose pentoxifylline in patients with AIDS: inhibition of tumor necrosis factor production, *J. Infect. Dis.*, 171, 1628, 1995.

214. Suzuki, Y.J. and Packer, L., Inhibition of NF-κB activation by vitamin E derivatives, *Biochem. Biophys. Res. Commun.*, 193, 277, 1993.

215. Suzuki, Y.J., Aggarwal, B.B., and Packer, L., Alpha-lipoic acid is a potent inhibitor of NF-κB activation in human T cells, *Biochem. Biophys. Res. Commun.*, 189, 1709, 1992.

216. Harakeh, S., Jariwalla, R.J., and Pauling, L., Suppression of human immunodeficiency virus replication by ascorbate in chronically and acutely infected cells, *Proc. Natl. Acad. Sci U.S.A.*, 87, 7245, 1990.

217. Harakeh, S. and Jariwalla, R.J., Ascorbate effect on cytokine stimulation of HIV production, *Nutrition*, 11, 684, 1995.

218. Sauberlich, H.E., Pharmacology of vitamin C, *Annu. Rev. Nutr.*, 14, 371, 1994.

chapter four

Nutritional aspects of neuropsychological function in HIV/AIDS

Marianna K. Baum and Gail Shor-Posner

Nutritional status and central nervous system function

Multiple parameters of nutritional status i.e., both overall protein/energy status, as well as specific micronutrient status, have been demonstrated to play an important role in nervous system function. Prolonged inadequate nutrition can lead to neurologic diseases that affect the central, peripheral, or both nervous systems.[17] Nutrient deficiencies of thiamin, pyridoxine, niacin, pantothenic acid, biotin, cobalamin, and folate are frequently associated with psychoneurological symptoms ranging from peripheral neuropathies to spinal cord degeneration and global cognitive impairment.[17]

Neurologic manifestations of pellagra, the classical disease of niacin deficiency, for example, include peripheral neuropathy, diminished taste and smell, proprioceptive alterations, and encephalopathy. Depression is common, and as the deficiency continues, cells of the motor cortex, peripheral nerves, and white matter of the dorsal columns may degenerate.[20] Beriberi, a vitamin-deficiency disease caused by inadequate thiamin intake, is also characterized by degenerative changes in the nervous system, ranging from peripheral neuropathy to encephalopathy (known as Wernicke's encephalopathy) and psychosis.[17]

In a number of clinical settings, cobalamin (vitamin B_{12}) deficiency, in the absence of HIV-1 infection, has been associated with a wide range of neurological, psychiatric and cognitive alterations.[13,18,27,35,47] Malabsorption of cobalamin from the gastrointestinal tract can result in subacute degeneration of the spinal cord, optic nerves, cerebral white matter, and peripheral nerves.[35,60] In addition to the neurological complications, psychological symptoms may range from apathy, irritability, and depression, to confusion, and frank dementia.[27,32]

Central nervous system changes and the occurrence of abnormal electroencephalograms are also evident with pyridoxine (vitamin B_6) deficiency.[15,49,50] Moreover, a number of neuropsychiatric complications including peripheral neuropathies, attention deficit disorder, seizures, and mental retardation, as well as depressive illness, have been related to low pyridoxine levels.[6,14,17,54]

Cognitive dysfunction in HIV/AIDS

Neurological complications of HIV infection cause substantial morbidity and are frequently associated with high mortality.[43] The damage to the central nervous system in HIV-1 infection is manifested by many neurological symptoms similar to those associated with nutritional deficiencies, including diffuse and regional encephalopathies, myelopathy, meningitis, intraaxial cranial neuropathies, and retinopathy.[34a,40,42]

Evidence of HIV-1 infection in the brain can be found throughout the course of the disease and often leads to the devastating loss of cognitive function.[10] Along with depression and poor social support, central nervous system deficits can significantly affect the ability to maintain adequate nutrition.[55] Dementia or motor impairment may render an HIV-infected patient incapable of preparing and eating meals. Additionally, psychological factors such as anxiety and depression can contribute to anorexia,[46] which left untreated may result in a decline in body weight, fat, and cell mass.[33]

Moderate cognitive impairment has been estimated to occur in approximately 75% of HIV-infected individuals during the late symptomatic stage, and 50% of individuals during the early symptomatic stage.[22] Although there has been considerable debate regarding the prevalence of cognitive alterations during the asymptomatic stages of HIV-1 infection, due, in part, to the methodological differences between studies, definitions of cognitive impairment, and subject populations, approximately 35% of asymptomatic HIV-1 infected individuals have been reported to exhibit moderate cognitive deficits.[57] Thus, the majority of HIV-1 infected adults may experience some degree of cognitive impairment during the course of their illness. The loss of cognitive capacity in HIV-1 infected persons is of major clinical and public health concern as it has been associated with decreased functional capacity[26] along with an increased risk of mortality.[37,59]

Cognitive performance, cobalamin status, and HIV-1 infection

The precise underlying mechanisms that account for HIV-1 associated cognitive impairment are presently unknown. The functional integrity of neurons or astrocytes may be affected by the production of either cell- or virus-coded toxins as well as immune activation.[30,42] Cobalamin (vitamin B_{12}) levels, which may also influence neurological function are frequently low among HIV/AIDS infected patients,[1,4,9,12,25,28,34,41,45] suggesting that some of the neuropsychological symptoms noted in HIV-1 infection may be linked to inadequate nutritional status.

Our investigations of nutritional status in relationship to neuropsychological function indicate that inadequate vitamin B_{12} status is associated with cognitive deficits in HIV-1 infected adults. Specifically, HIV-1 infected individuals with low vitamin B_{12} levels (<240 pg/ml) demonstrate significantly poorer performance on memory tasks and decreased visuospatial problem solving abilities.[5] Furthermore, our longitudinal studies indicate that normalization of vitamin B_{12} status is associated with significant improvement while becoming cobalamin deficient (<200 pg/ml), in contrast, is related to a significant decline in the speed of accessing information from semantic memory.[52] The differences in information processing speed between the groups that varied in their cobalamin status were not associated with a clinically significant degeneration in overall cognitive performance and did not appear to be explained by clinical or immunological status. Additionally, use of zidovudine, self-reported alcohol use, measures of psychological distress, age, education of the participants, and individual differences in two-choice reaction time did not appear to influence the results, supporting an important role for nutrition in this domain of neuropsychological function.

Cobalamin therapy — therapeutic responses

Nutritional supplementation studies to enhance neuropsychological function in HIV-1 infected individuals are limited. Cobalamin treatment has been reported to resolve symptoms of HIV-associated dementia complex in a patient with low serum vitamin B_{12} levels[29] and has been associated with a therapeutic response in HIV-1 infected subjects referred for neurological evaluation.[34] In other clinical settings, a dramatic neurologic improvement has also been demonstrated following parenteral cobalamin treatment in patients with neuropsychiatric disorders.[35] In elderly patients who presented with the diagnosis of dementia and had low serum vitamin B_{12} levels improvement in cognitive functions as well as in activities of daily living was shown after parenteral cobalamin injections.[23] Cobalamin administration does not seem useful, however, in preventing or reducing zidovudine-associated neutropenia[39] or zidovudine-induced myelotoxicity in the overall treated population.[19]

Psychological function, pyridoxine status, and HIV-1 infection

In addition to its important role in cognitive function, nutritional status has also been shown to have a significant influence on psychological functioning in HIV-1 infected individuals. Our longitudinal studies in HIV-1 infected homosexual men have demonstrated improved mood (decline in psychological distress) with normalization of vitamin B_6 status in inadequate subjects, and with increased tryptophan intake in vitamin B_6 adequate individuals.[53] Significant effects for the nutritional variables remained even when controlling for life stressors (events with a negative impact), social support and coping style, which have previously been associated with levels of psychological distress in HIV-1 infected individuals.[7,8]

These results suggest that vitamin B_6 status may be an important cofactor in mediating psychological distress over time in HIV-1 infected individuals. Inadequate vitamin B_6 status is prevalent in HIV-1 infected men and women who abuse drugs[51] and HIV-1 infected homosexual men, even during the early stages of disease.[3,4] These findings are of particular concern in light of the important function of vitamin B_6 in the control of metabolic processes of the nervous system.[24,38] Deficiency of pyridoxine has been associated with a variety of neuropsychiatric complications, specifically peripheral neuropathies, attention deficit disorder, seizures, and mental retardation as well as depressive illness, cognitive dysfunction, and psychological distress.[6,14,17,47,53,54]

Vitamin B_6 status and neurotransmitter function

One possible mechanism by which vitamin B_6 deficiency could be affecting brain function is through its effect on the metabolism of neurotransmitters, particularly the synthesis of serotonin.[16] The synthesis of serotonin, specifically, depends on dietary intake of L-tryptophan followed by hydroxylation and vitamin B_6 dependent decarboxylation. Dietary pyridoxine deficiency has been demonstrated to affect the principal serotonergic pathways of tryptophan degradation and be associated with an increase in the excretion of quinolinic acid, an endogenous neurotoxin.[11,48] Because of decreased anabolism to serotonin increased tryptophan is available, in this context, for catabolism to quinolinic acid. Administration of vitamin B_6, on the other hand, appears to reverse changes in tryptophan metabolites and increase levels of serotonin in ADD patients[6] and children with Down's syndrome.[44]

Marked disturbances in serotonin/tryptophan pathways have been reported in patients with AIDS,[31,56] in association with neuropsychological deficits.[30] Although the cause of altered serotonergic levels in HIV-1 infected individuals remains unknown, inadequate vitamin B_6 status would be expected to result in low levels of serotonin synthesis and may thus contribute to a degenerative change in mental function. In light of evidence that changes in tryptophan metabolites may be reversed and levels of serotonin increased with vitamin B_6 therapy, the need for clinical-intervention studies to determine whether nutritional supplementation enhances psychological functioning in HIV-1 disease becomes particularly important.

Plasma nutrient levels and dietary intake

Our early studies[4] revealed that plasma levels are associated, at least in part, with dietary intake for several nutrients, suggesting that normalization may be achieved through dietary supplementation.[2] The presence of abnormal nutrient values, despite high levels of supplementation, indicates that additional factors may be involved including nutrient-malabsorption, altered nutrient excretion, or metabolic factors that could potentially influence vitamin metabolism. The possible negative effects of oversupplementation must be carefully considered in determining the appropriate dietary recommendations for individuals with adequate or inadequate absorption.

Significant Sources of Nutrients Important in Brain Function

Nutrient	Sources
Thiamin (vitamin B_1)	Occurs in all nutritious foods in moderate amounts; pork, ham, bacon, liver, whole grains, legumes, nuts
Niacin	Milk, eggs, meat, poultry, fish, whole-grain and enriched breads and cereals, nuts, and all protein-containing foods
Pyridoxine (vitamin B_6)	Green and leafy vegetables, meats, fish, poultry, shellfish, legumes, fruits, whole grains
Cobalamin (vitamin B_{12})	Animal products (meat, fish, poultry, shellfish, milk, cheese, eggs)
Folate	Leafy green vegetables, legumes, seeds, liver

From Whitney, E.N., Hamilton, E.M.N., and Rolfes, S.R., *Understanding Nutrition*, 5th ed., West Publishing, St. Paul, MN, 1990.

Summary

Longitudinal studies conducted in HIV-1 infected individuals suggest that nutritional deficiency is an important contributory factor of HIV-1 associated cognitive impairment and psychological distress. Clinical trials are needed to confirm that restoration of adequate plasma vitamin B_{12} and B_6 levels can improve cognitive function and mood state in HIV-1 disease. Dysphoric mood and cognitive impairment may play a role in quality of life as well as treatment compliance, underscoring the critical need for further studies.

References

1. Baum, M.K., Shor-Posner, G., Lu, Y., Rosner, B., Sauberlich, H.E., Fletcher, M.A., Szapocznik, J., Eisdorfer, C., Buring, J.E., and Hennekens, C.H., Micronutrients and HIV-1 disease progression, *AIDS*, 9, 1051, 1995.
2. Baum, M.K., Cassetti, L., Bonvehi, P., Shor-Posner, G., Lu, Y., and Sauberlich, H., Inadequate dietary intake and altered nutrition status in early HIV-1 infection, *Nutrition*, 10, 16, 1994.

3. Baum, M.K., Mantero-Atienza, E., Shor-Posner, G., Fletcher, M.A., Morgan, R., Eisdorfer, C., Sauberlich, H., Cornwell, P.E., and Beach, R.S., Association of vitamin B_6 status with parameters of immune function in early HIV-1 infection, *J. Acquir. Immune Def. Syndr.*, 4, 1122, 1991.
4. Beach, R.S., Mantero-Atienza, E., Shor-Posner, G., Javier, J.J., Szapocznik, J., Morgan, R., Sauberlich, H.E., Cornwell, P.E., Eisdorfer, C., and Baum, M.K., Specific nutrient abnormalities in asymptomatic HIV-1 infection, *AIDS*, 6, 701, 1992a.
5. Beach, R.S., Morgan, R., Wilkie, F., Mantero-Atienza, E., Blaney, N., Shor-Posner, G., Lu, Y., Eisdorfer, C., and Baum, M.K., Plasma vitamin B_{12} level as a potential cofactor in studies of human immunodeficiency virus type 1-related cognitive changes, *Arch. Neurol.*, 49, 501, 1992b.
6. Bhagavan, H.N., Coleman, M., and Coursin, D.B., The effect of pyridoxine hydrochloride on blood serotonin and pyridoxal phosphate contents in hyperactive children, *Pediatrics*, 55, 437, 1975.
7. Blaney, N.T., Goodkin, K., Feaster, D., Morgan. R., Millon, C., Szapocznik, J., and Eisdorfer, C., A longitudinal stress moderator model of distress in early HIV-1 infection: the role of social support and coping, *Psychology and Health*, 12, 633, 1997.
8. Blaney, N.T., Goodkin, K., Morgan, R., Feaster, D., Millon, C., Szapocznik, J., and Eisdorfer, C., A stress moderator model of distress in early HIV-1 infection: concurrent analysis of life events, hardiness and social support, *J. Psychosom. Res.*, 35, 297, 1991.
9. Boudes, P., Zittoun, J., and Sobel, A., Folate, vitamin B_{12}, and HIV infection, *Lancet*, 335, 1401, 1990.
10. Brew, B.J., HIV-1 related neurological disease, *AIDS*, 6 (suppl. 1), S10, 1993.
11. Brown, R.R., Yess, N., Price, J.M., Linswiler, H., Swan, P., and Hankes, L.V., Vitamin B_6 depletion in man: urinary excretion of quinolinic acid and niacin metabolites, *J. Nutr.*, 87, 419, 1965.
12. Burkes, R.L., Cohen, H., Krailo, M., Snow, R.M., and Carmel, R., Low serum cobalamin levels occur frequently in the acquired immune deficiency syndrome and related disorders, *Eur. J. Haematol.*, 38, 141, 1987.
13. Carmel, R., Karnaze, D.S., and Weiner, J.M., Neurologic abnormalities in cobalamin deficiency are associated with higher cobalamin 'analogue' values than are hematologic abnormalities, *J. Lab. Clin. Med.*, 111, 57, 1988.
14. Carney, M.W.P., Williams, D.G., and Sheffield, B.F., Thiamine and pyridoxine lack in newly-admitted psychiatric patients, *Brit. J. Psychiat.*, 135, 249, 1979.
15. Coursin, D.B., Vitamin B_6 metabolism in infants and children, *Vit. Hormones*, 22, 755, 1964.
16. Dakshinamurti, K. and Paulose, C.S., Consequences of decreased brain serotonin in the pyridoxine-deficient young rat, *Prog. Neuropsychopharmacol. Biol. Psych.*, 7, 743, 1983.
17. Dreyfus, P.M., Diet and nutrition in neurologic disorders, in Shils, M.E. and Young, V.R., Eds., *Modern Nutrition in Health and Disease*, Lea & Febiger, Philadelphia, 1458, 1988.
18. Elsborg, L., Hansen, T., and Rafaelsen, O.J., Vitamin B_{12} concentrations in psychiatric patients, *Acta Psychiatr. Scand.*, 59, 145, 1979.
19. Falguera, M., Perez-Mur, J., Puig, T., and Cao, G., Study of the role of vitamin B_{12} and folinic acid supplementation in preventing hematologic toxicity of zidovudine, *Eur. J. Haematol.*, 55, 97, 1995.

20. Feldman, E.B., *Essentials of Clinical Nutrition*, F.A. Davis, Philadelphia, 333, 1988.
21. Foresti, V. and Confalonieri, F., Wernicke's encephalopathy in AIDS, *Lancet*, i, 1499, 1987.
22. Grant, I. and Martin, A., Eds., *Neuropsychology of HIV Infection*, Oxford Univ. Press, New York, 1994.
23. Gross, J.S., Weintraub, N.T., Neufeld, R.R., and Libow, L.S., Pernicious anemia in the demented patients without anemia or macrocytosis, *J. Am. Geriatr. Soc.*, 34, 612, 1986.
24. Guilarte, T.R. and Wagner, H.N. Jr., Increased concentrations of 3-hydroxykynurenine in vitamin B_6 deficient neonatal rat brain, *J. Neurochem.*, 49, 1918, 1987.
25. Harriman, G.R., Smith, P.D., Horne, M.K., and Fox, C.H., Vitamin B_{12} malabsorption in patients with acquired immunodeficiency syndrome, *Arch. Intern. Med.*, 149, 2039, 1989.
26. Heaton, R.K., Velin, R.A., McCutchan, J.A., Gulevich, S.J., Atkinson, H., Wallance, M.R., Godfrey, H.P.D., Kirson, D.A., Grant, I., and the H.N.R.C., Neuropsychological impairment in human immunodeficiency virus-infection: implications for employment, *Psychosomat. Med.*, 56, 8, 1994.
27. Hector, M. and Burton, J.R., What are the psychiatric manifestations of vitamin B_{12} deficiency?, *J. Am. Geriatr. Soc.*, 36, 1105, 1988.
28. Herbert, V., Fong, W., Gulle, V., and Stopler, T., Low holotranscobalamin II is the earliest serum marker for subnormal vitamin B_{12} (cobalamin) absorption in patients with AIDS, *Am. J. Hematology*, 34, 132, 1990.
29. Herzlich, B.C. and Schiano, T.D., Reversal of apparent AIDS dementia complex following treatment with vitamin B_{12}, *J. Intern. Med.*, 233, 495, 1993.
30. Heyes, M.P., Brew, B.J., Martin, A., Price, R.W., Salazar, A.M., Sidtis, J.J., Yergey, A., Mouradian, M., Sadler, A.E., Deilp, J., Rubinow, D., and Markey, S.P. Quinolinic acid in cerebrospinal fluid and serum in HIV-1 infection: relationship to clinical and neurological status, *Ann. Neurol.*, 29, 202, 1991.
31. Heyes, M.P., Rubinow, D., Lane, C., and Markey, S.P., Cerebrospinal fluid quinolinic acid concentrations are increased in acquired immune deficiency syndrome, *Ann. Neurol.*, 26, 275, 1989.
32. Karnaze, D.S. and Carmel, R., Low serum cobalamin levels in primary degenerative dementia. Do some patients harbor a typical cobalamin deficiency state? *Arch. Intern. Med.*, 147, 429, 1987.
33. Kern, K.A. and Norton, J.A., Cancer cachexia, *JPEN*, 12, 286, 1988.
34. Kieburtz, K.D., Giang, D.W., Schiffer, R.B., and Vakil, N., Abnormal vitamin B_{12} metabolism in human immunodeficiency virus infection. Association with neurological dysfunction, *Arch. Neurol.*, 48, 312, 1991.
34a. Levy, R.H. and Bredesen, D.E., Central nervous system dysfunction in acquired immunodeficiency syndrome, *AIDS*, 1, 41, 1988.
35. Lindenbaum, J., Healton, E.B., Savage, D.G., Brust, J.C.M., Garrett, T.J., Podell, E.R., Marcell, P.D., Stabler, S.P., and Allen, R.H., Neuropsychiatric disorders caused by cobalamin deficiency in the absence of anemia or macrocytosis, *N. Engl. J. Med.*, 318, 1720, 1988.
36. Martin, A., Basal ganglia and HIV infection. in Grant, I. and Martin, A., Eds., *Neuropsychology of HIV Infection*, Oxford Univ. Press, New York, 1994.

37. Mayeux, R., Stern, Y., Tang, M., Todak, G., Masarder, K., Sano, M., Richards, M., Stein, Z., Ehrhardt, A.A., and Gorman, J.M., Mortality risks in gay men with human immunodeficiency virus infection and cognitive impairment, *Neurology*, 43, 176, 1991.

38. McCormick, D.B., Vitamin B_6 in Shils, M.E. and Young, V.R., Eds., *Modern Nutrition in Health and Disease*, Lea & Febiger, Philadelphia, 1988.

39. McCutchan, J., Allen, J., Ballard, Z., Freeman, B., Bartok, A., and Richman, D., Cobalamin (vitamin B_{12}) supplementation does not prevent the hematologic toxicity of azidothymidine (AZT), *Proc. 5th Int. Conf. AIDS*, Montreal, June 4–9, 1989.

40. Navia, B.A., Jordan, B.D., and Price, R.W., The AIDS dementia complex: I. Clinical features, *Ann. Neurol.*, 19, 517, 1986.

41. Paltiel, O., Falutz, J., Veilleux, M., Rosenblatt, D.S., and Gordon, K., Clinical correlates of subnormal vitamin B_{12} level in paients infected with the human immunodeficiency virus, *Am. J. Hematol.*, 49, 318, 1995.

42. Price, R.W., Sidtis, J., Rosenblum, M., Scheck, A.C., and Cleary, P., The brain in AIDS: central nervous system HIV-1 infection and AIDS dementia complex, *Science*, 239, 586, 1988.

43. Price, R.W., Neurological complications of HIV infection, *Lancet*, 348, 445, 1996.

44. Pueschel, S.M., Reed, R.B., Cronk, C.E., and Goldstein, B.I., 5-Hydroxytryptophan and pyridoxine, *Am. J. Dis. Child.*, 134, 838, 1980.

45. Remacha, A.F., Riera, A., Cadafalch, J., and Gimferrer, E., Vitamin B-12 abnormalities in HIV-infected patients, *Eur. J. Haematol.*, 47, 60, 1991.

46. Ressler, S.S., Nutrition care of AIDS patients, *J. Am. Diet. Assoc.*, 88, 828, 1988.

47. Riggs, K.M., Spiro,A., III, Tucker, K., and Rush, R., Relations of vitamin B-12, vitamin B-6, folate and homocysteine to cognitive performance in the Normative Aging Study, *Am. J. Clin. Nutr.*, 63, 306, 1996..

48. Rose, D.P. and Toseland, P.A., Urinary excretion of quinolinic acid and other tryptophan metabolites after deoxypridoxine or oral contraceptive administration, *Metabolism*, 22, 165, 1973.

49. Sauberlich, H.E., Human requirements for vitamin B_6, *Vitam. Horm.*, 22, 807, 1964.

50. Sauberlich, H.E., Vitamin B_6 status assessment: past and present. in Leklen, J.E. and Reynolds, R.D., Eds., *Methods in Vitamin B_6 Nutrition*, Plenum Pub., New York, 1981.

51. Shor-Posner, G. and Baum, M.K., Nutritional alterations in HIV-1 seropositive and seronegative drug users, *Nutrition*, 12, 555, 1996.

52. Shor-Posner, G., Morgan, R., Wilkie, F., Eisdorfer, C., and Baum, M.K., Plasma cobalamin levels affect information processing speed in a longitudinal study of HIV-1 disease, *Arch. Neurol.*, 52, 195, 1995.

53. Shor-Posner, G., Feaster, D., Blaney, N.T., Rocca, H., Mantero-Atienza, E., Szapocznik, J., Eisdorfer, C., Goodkin, K., and Baum, M.K., Impact of vitamin B_6 status on psychological distress in a longitudinal study of HIV-1 infection, *Int. J. Psychiatry Med.*, 24, 209, 1994.

54. Vir, S.C. and Love, A.H.G., Vitamin B_6 status of the hospitalized aged, *Amer. J. Clin. Nutr.*, 31, 1383, 1978.

55. Weaver, K.E., Psychosocial aspects pertaining to nutrition, in Kotler, D.P., Ed., *Gastrointestinal and Nutritional Manifestations of the Acquired Immunodeficiency Syndrome*, Raven Press, New York, 1991.

56. Werner, E.R., Fuchs, D., Hausen, A. et al., Tryptophan degradation in patients infected by human immunodeficiency virus, *Biol. Chem. Hoppe Seyler,* 369, 337, 1988.
57. White, D.A., Heaton, R.K., Monsch. A.U., Neuropsychological studies of asymptomatic human immunodeficiency virus type 1 infected individuals, *JINS*, 1, 304, 1995.
58. Whitney, E.N., Hamilton, E.M.N., and Rolfes, S.R., *Understanding Nutrition*, 5th ed., West Publishing, St. Paul, MN, 1990.
59. Wilkie, F.L., Goodkin, K., Eisdorfer, C., Feaster, D., Morgan, R., Fletcher, M.A., Blaney, N., Baum, M., and Szapocznik, J., Mild cognitive impairment and risk of mortality, Presentation: *Neurosciences of HIV-1 Infection. Basic and Clinical Frontiers*, Vancouver, British Columbia, 1994.
60. Zegers, de Beyl, D., Delecluse, F., Verbanck, P., Borenstein, S., Capel, P., and Brunko, E., Somatosensory conduction in vitamin B_{12} deficiency, *Electroencephalog. Clin. Neurophysiol.*, 69, 313, 1988.

chapter five

Lauric oils as antimicrobial agents: theory of effect, scientific rationale, and dietary application as adjunct nutritional support for HIV-infected individuals

Mary G. Enig

Introduction

More than a decade and a half after the beginning of the AIDS epidemic there is still general agreement in the medical community that there "remains an urgent need for interventions" that include, in addition to an effective vaccine, safe and inexpensive drug therapies to treat individuals already infected with HIV-1.[1] Such therapies should include effective adjunct nutritional support regimens.

Since the current research[2] suggests that individuals infected with the HIV-1 virus progress more rapidly to AIDS when they have higher levels of the virus RNA, it is clear that alternative treatment modalities that help to lower the virus load would be useful. Although some of the recent studies (reported in 1996), using multiple drug cocktails, have been shown to lower viral load and look promising, the expense of such treatment is considerable (more that $15,000 per person per year).[3] There are also concerns that there may be increased risk that such treatment might lead to drug-resistant viral strains.[4] Thus, the potential benefit of regularly including in diets inexpensive and safe components that can help to lower the viral load, such as the lauric oils, represents a desirable nutritional support regimen for HIV-infected individuals worth investigating.

Medium-chain saturated fatty acids are well known for their virucidal effects against viruses with lipid membranes as well as against numerous other pathogenic microorganisms.[5] These antimicrobial fatty acids and their derivatives are essentially nontoxic to man; they are produced *in vivo* by humans when they ingest those foods that contain adequate levels of the appropriate medium-chain saturated fatty acids such as lauric acid.

In this chapter, a diet regimen that utilizes adequate sources of those anti-viral, anti-bacterial, and anti-protozoal monoglycerides and their fatty acid precursors that are found principally in lauric oils is proposed and described. The lauric oils such as coconut oil or palm kernel oil, both of which are GRAS, can provide a unique source of both antimicrobial lipids and needed calories. The scientific rationale for their use is reviewed and documented.

Nutritional needs during HIV infection

Information about the nutritional needs, and development of systems of nutritional support for individuals infected with the human immunodeficiency virus known as HIV-1 (or HIV+ for short), or those suffering from the frank autoimmune deficiency syndrome (AIDS), has been gradually increasing over the past several years. In part, recognition of the importance of this specialized nutrition information has come about because of the realization that nutrition plays a critical role in maintaining an efficiently functioning immune system.

The individual with HIV+/AIDS, whose immune system is already compromised by being HIV+ or who has progressed to a frank AIDS, is further disadvantaged by a diet that is inadequate in calories or a diet that has inappropriate balance of macro and micro nutrients. The individual with AIDS will become readily malnourished as well as progressively more immune-compromised under circumstances with frequent bouts of infection such as those precipitated by opportunistic microorganisms, e.g., cytomegalovirus, candida, and cryptosporidium.

A comprehensive review in 1990 by Raiten[6] was directed at providing "…a scientific report on all aspects of nutrition and HIV-related disease for the use of health care providers." The review was prepared by the Life Sciences Research Office of the Federation of American Societies for Experimental Biology for the Center for Food Safety and Applied Nutrition of the Food and Drug Administration. Although the review included discussions of both conventional and unconventional diet therapies, information on antimicrobial lipids was not included.

Nutritional interventions during HIV infection

Aron[7] has reviewed the use of nutritional interventions in early HIV disease, latent stage HIV, and late stage HIV/AIDS. During early HIV infection there is an increase in resting energy expenditure (REE), a decrease in lean body mass, and altered triglyceride status. Recommendations during this early stage include increased energy intake with emphasis on avoidance of low or no-calorie foods and beverages. Also recommended is supplementation with certain vitamins and trace elements, as well as experimental fish oil supplementation.

During latent stage HIV infection there are further increases in REE as well as futile lipid cycling with difficulty maintaining body weight. Recommendations during this stage include the addition of enteral feeding supplementation using intact formulas (e.g., Ensure, Nutren, Replete, etc.) or special formulas (e.g., Impact, Peptamen) and various digestive aids.

Further metabolic disturbances during late stage HIV disease — AIDS — include the problems of major lipid futile cycling with increased *de novo* lipogenesis, increased whole body fat oxidation, increased endogenous cholesterogenesis, increased free fatty acid production, greatly increased REE, decreased nitrogen balance, and increased hepatic gluconeogenesis. Further complications stem from multiple infections caused by opportunistic microorganisms (e.g., cytomegalovirus, candida, *cryptosporidia*). Nutritional intervention in this late stage disease has been focused on aggressive parenteral nutrition; an upper daily limit for lipids given parenterally has been set at $0.11 \text{ g/kg} \cdot \text{h}$.

Aron[7] also notes that "the use of nutrient components for their pharmacologic properties rather than for their nutrient effects warrants investigation," and suggests the attractiveness of studying a "superlipid" composed of fish oil, medium chain triglyceride and phospholipid in AIDS patients who require TPN.

Current published dietary recommendations for individuals with HIV/AIDS

Current published dietary regimens for individuals infected with HIV invariably address the concept of "eating right" as a means of improving immune status, since, as noted by Dwyer,[8] "...conventional or standard treatments are relatively ineffective in halting the underlying immunodeficiency." Different clinicians understand the meaning of "eating right" differently. For example, Dwyer et al.[8] consider the Dietary Guidelines for Americans an appropriate basic diet; Wickwire,[9] on the other hand, points to the inappropriateness of such a diet for individuals with AIDS.

These two approaches are in diametric opposition with respect to the dietary fat. Dwyer et al.[8] encourage a lower fat regimen, in part because of the anecdotal information about problems with fat digestion in AIDS patients, and in part because of the current anti-fat rhetoric from government agencies and certain consumer groups. Wickwire[9] recognizes the need for a higher fat regimen to provide additional caloric density to the diet.

Low fat dietary regimens are not appropriate for individuals
with HIV+/AIDS

With the exception of a few special diet booklets written for HIV+/AIDS patients, which recognize the need for "fats in moderation," writers of current foods and nutrition texts who use government- and industry-promoted recommendations either ignore the issue of fats or are rather uniform in their advocacy of the selection of low-fat foods. However, these writers usually recommend high-calorie diets. High-calorie diets cannot be made palatable without using adequate levels of fat.

Automatic acceptance by health and nutrition professionals of U.S. government recommendations for lowering dietary fat consumption to 30% of energy (calories), which are applied to all fats regardless of type, should be ignored by the individual who is HIV+ or has progressed to AIDS as long as the fat in the diet is high lauric fat. Fats that should be avoided are those oils that are partially hydrogenated and oils that are high in omega-6 fatty acids without adequate levels of omega-3 fatty acids. It is important to maintain an appropriate omega-6/omega-3 balance, i.e., no less than 4:1 and no greater than 10:1.[10]

Rationale for adding antiviral lipids to diets

None of the clinicians from the mainstream nutrition/dietetics community seems to have recognized the added potential to be gained by use of antimicrobial lipids in the nutritional support treatment of HIV-infected individuals or patients who have progressed to AIDS. These antimicrobial fatty acids and their derivatives are essentially nontoxic to man; they are produced *in vivo* by humans when they ingest those commonly available foods that contain adequate levels of medium-chain fatty acids such as lauric acid. According to published research, lauric acid is one of the best "inactivating" fatty acids, and its monoglyceride is an even more effective antimicrobial than the fatty acid alone.[11-15]

Antimicrobial activity of monolaurin, the monoglyceride of lauric acid

Recognition of the antimicrobial activity of the monoglyceride of lauric acid (monolaurin) has been reported since 1966. The seminal work can be credited to Jon Kabara at Michigan State University.[11] Some of the early work by Kabara that showed virucidal effects of monolaurin on enveloped RNA and DNA viruses was done with selected prototypes or recognized representative strains of enveloped human viruses; the envelope of these viruses is a lipid membrane. This early research was directed at the virucidal effects of monolaurin because there were concerns about viral contamination in foods, and monolaurin was seen as having potential related benefits to food preservation.[16]

Table 1   Viruses and Bacteria Inactivated
by Monolaurin

Viruses
Human immunodeficiency virus HIV-1 or HIV+
Measles virus
Herpes simplex virus-1 (HSV-1)
Vesicular stomatitis virus (VSV)
Visna virus
Cytomegalovirus (CMV)
Influenza virus
Pneumonovirus
Syncytial virus
Rubeola virus
Bacteria
Listeria monocytogenes
Staphylococcus aureus
Streptococcus agalactiae
Groups A,B,F & G streptococci
Gram-positive organisms
Gram-negative organisms if pretreated with chelator

From Refs. 5, 11, 13, 17–25.

Kabara and others have reported that certain fatty acids (e.g., medium-chain saturates) and their derivatives (e.g., monoglycerides) can have adverse effects on a variety of microorganisms. Those microorganisms that are inactivated by monolaurin include bacteria, yeast, fungi, and enveloped viruses (Table 1).[5,11,13,17-25]

The medium-chain saturated fatty acids and their derivatives act by disrupting the lipid membranes of the organisms.[19,20] In particular, enveloped viruses are inactivated in both human and bovine milk by added fatty acids (FAs) and monoglycerides (MGs)[21] as well as by endogenous FAs and MGs(11).[11,22-24] All three monoesters of lauric acid are shown to be active antimicrobials, i.e., α-, α'-, and β-MG. Additionally, it is reported that the antimicrobial effects of the FAs and MGs are additive and total concentration is critical for inactivating viruses.[25]

Some of the viruses inactivated by the lauric acid monoglycerides, in addition to HIV, are the measles virus, herpes simplex virus-1 (HSV-1), vesicular stomatitis virus (VSV), visna virus, and cytomegalovirus (CMV). Many of the pathogenic organisms reported to be inactivated by these antimicrobial lipids are those known to be responsible for opportunistic infections in HIV-positive individuals. For example, concurrent infection with cytomegalovirus is recognized as a serious complication for HIV+ individuals.[26] Thus, it would appear to be important to investigate the practical aspects and the potential benefit of an adjunct nutritional support regimen for HIV-infected individuals, which will utilize those dietary fats that are sources of known antiviral, antimicrobial, and antiprotozoal monoglycerides and fatty acids.

The properties that determine the anti-infective action of these lipids are related to their structure, e.g., monoglycerides, free fatty acids. The monoglycerides are active; diglycerides and triglycerides are inactive. Of the saturated fatty acids, lauric acid has greater antiviral activity than either caprylic acid (C-8), capric acid (C-10) or myristic acid (C-14) for these viruses.

The action attributed to monolaurin is that of solubilizing the lipids and phospholipids in the envelope of the virus causing the disintegration of the virus envelope. In effect, it is reported that the fatty acids and monoglycerides produce their killing/inactivating effect by lysing the (lipid bilayer) plasma membrane. However, there is evidence from recent studies that one antimicrobial effect is related to its interference with signal transduction.[27]

Lauric acid in the diet: historical and current status

What is the current use of lauric-rich diets as antiviral modalities for adjunct nutrition support in HIV?

Except for the use of commercially available enteral feeding supplements (e.g., Ensure-type liquids) that utilize medium-chain triglyceride (MCT) oils, and one enteral product (Impact®, Sandoz Nutrition) that contains palm kernel oil as part of its structured lipid, novel or unusual dietary treatments related to fats in the diet appear not to have been systematically investigated for HIV adjunct treatment, although there is a substantial research supporting their potential. At least one of the commercial lipid formulas (High MCT Supplement®, Corpak, Inc.) is based on coconut oil. This product is listed as an incomplete medical food in tables of enteral formulas and does not appear to have been utilized in treatment of AIDS patients.

The American Foundation for AIDS Research (AMFAR) did a preliminary review of the antiviral lipid monolaurin in 1987 but did not pursue this adjunct treatment modality (AMFAR office, personal communication 1994). Also in 1987, an alternative medical journal published an extensive discussion of the properties and clinical use of monolaurin.[28] However, as noted above, the review by Raiten[6] did not indicate use of or knowledge of monolaurin.

Most dietary recommendations published for HIV+/AIDS patients are directed at prevention of weight loss. All the diets currently being formally recommended by the professional dietetic groups, government agencies, or organizations involved in support for individuals with AIDS are structured from foods that are missing lauric acid. Thus any benefit that might accrue to an individual who is HIV+ or has AIDS, from the substantial utilization of lauric acid-rich foods, is missing.

The potential benefits that can be derived from feeding antimicrobial lipids need to be investigated in humans on a systematic basis, the lauric oils need to be made more readily available in the general food supply, and the rationale for use of these lipids needs to be explained to the food and nutrition professionals as well as the medical and lay community.

Loss of lauric acid from the American diet

Increasingly, over the past 40 years, the American diet has undergone major changes. Many of these changes involve changes of fats and oils. There has been an increasing supply of the partially hydrogenated *trans*-containing vegetable oils and a decreasing amount of the lauric acid-containing fats and oils. As a result of these shifts in fats usage, there has been an increased consumption of *trans* fatty acids and linoleic acid and a decrease in the consumption of lauric acid. There has also been a decrease in some of the other antimicrobial fatty acids. This type of change in the diet has an important effect on the fatty acids the body has available for its metabolic activities.

The lipid coated (envelop) viruses are dependent on host lipids for their lipid constituents. Given this fact, it becomes important to evaluate the variability of the fatty acids in an individual patient's diet, since such variability is reflected in the changes in the lipid membrane of the virus envelope, leads to the variability of glycoprotein expression, and plays a role in the aspects of mutation that interfere with successful vaccine development.

Lauric acid intake in selected Asian countries

Based on the per capita intake of coconut oil in 1985 as reported by Kaunitz,[29] the per capita daily intake of lauric acid can be approximated. For those major producing countries such as the Philippines, Indonesia, and Sri Lanka, and consuming countries such as Singapore, the daily intakes of lauric acid were approximately 7.3 grams (Philippines), 4.9 grams (Sri Lanka), 4.7 grams (Indonesia), and 2.8 grams (Singapore). In India, intake of lauric acid from coconut oil in the coconut growing areas (e.g., Kerala) range from about 12 to 20 grams per day,[30] whereas the average for the rest of the country is less than half a gram. An average high of approximately 68 grams of lauric acid is calculated from the coconut oil intake previously reported by Prior et al.[31] in 1981 for the Tokelau Islands. Other coconut producing countries may also have intakes of lauric acid in the same range.

Lauric acid intake in the U.S.

In the U.S. today, there is very little lauric acid in most of the foods. During the early part of the 20th century and up until the late 1950s many people consumed heavy cream and high-fat milk. These foods could have provided approximately 3 grams of lauric acid per day to many individuals. In addition, desiccated coconut was a popular food in homemade cakes, pies, and cookies, as well as in commercial baked goods, and 1 to 2 tablespoons of desiccated coconut would have supplied 1 to 2 grams of lauric acid. Those foods made with the coconut oil based shortenings would have provided additional amounts. Until two years ago, some of the commercially sold popcorn, at least in movie theaters, had coconut oil as the oil. This means that for those people who did consume this type of popcorn, the possible lauric acid intake was 6 grams or more in a 3-cup order.

Some infant formulas (but not all) have been good sources of lauric acid for infants. However, in the past 3 to 4 years there has been reformulation with a loss of a portion of coconut oil in these formulas and a subsequent lowering of the lauric acid levels. Only one U.S. manufactured enteral formula contains lauric acid (e.g., Impact®) and this is normally used in hospitals for enteral tube feeding. It is reported to be very effective in reversing severe weight loss in AIDS patients, but it is discontinued when the patients leave the hospital because it is not sufficiently palatable for continued oral use (D.P. Kotler, private communication, 1995) The more widely promoted enteral formulas (e.g., Ensure®, Nutren®) are not made with lauric oils, and, in fact, many are made with partially hydrogenated oils.

There are currently some candies sold in the U.S. that are made with palm kernel oil and a few specialty candies made with coconut oil and desiccated coconut. These can supply small amounts of lauric acid. Cookies such as macaroons, if made with desiccated coconut, are good sources of lauric acid, supplying as much as 6 grams of lauric acid per macaroon (Red Mill Farms's Jennies® is apparently the only brand in the U.S. that supplies this amount). However, these cookies make up a small portion of the cookie market. Most cookies in the United States are no longer made with coconut oil shortenings; however, there was a time when the fat in many U.S. cookies (e.g., Pepperidge Farm) was about 25% lauric acid.

Originally, one of the largest manufacturers of cream soups used coconut oil in the soup formulations. Many popular cracker manufacturers also used coconut oil as a spray coating. These products supplied a small amount of lauric acid on a daily basis for some people.

Sources of lauric acid

There are only a few basic foods that contain lauric acid in more than trace amounts. These foods include the following (listed in descending order from the largest to the smallest amount in a practical serving): extracted lauric oils (coconut, palm kernel), whole coconut, creamed coconut (bar), coconut cream (fresh or canned), coconut milk (fresh or canned), heavy cream, table cream, half and half, whole milk (see Table 2). Creamed coconut in a 200-gram bar is readily available in the refrigerator case in markets that sell Indian (Asian) foods. Derivative foods such as macaroons or granola, both of which are made with desiccated coconut, can provide substantial amounts of lauric acid as can enteral drinks if they are high-fat and made with lauric oils. These are the only food sources that are readily available in the U.S., and granola manufactured by major cereal manufacturers is no longer made with coconut oil nor does most of it have added coconut flakes (Table 3). Appropriate margarine spreads are not currently made of lauric-rich oils, but could be formulated as shown in Table 4. Such blended formulations would provide adequate essential fatty acids (i.e., omega-3 and omega-6) at the same time they supply appropriate amounts of lauric acid.

Table 2   Lauric Acid Content of Selected Foods

Food	Grams/Cup
Coconut cream, raw	37.0
Coconut cream, canned	23.3
Fresh grated coconut, packed	19.4
Fresh coconut, grated, loose	11.9
Granola cereal (with coconut oil and coconut)	6.05
Coconut cream pudding	1.29
Whole milk	0.23

From *U.S. Department of Agriculture Handbook* Nos. 8-1 (1976), 8-8 (1982), 8-12 (1984), and 8-19 (1991).

Table 3   Granola and Whole Milk as Potential Sources of Lauric Acid

Prior to 1990	6.28 grams of lauric acid
After 1990	0.23 grams of lauric acid

Table 4   Examples of Lauric Acid Content of Proposed Lauric-Rich Margarine Spreads

Spread	Grams/TBS
Coconut/flax "et al."[a] blend; 90/10	5–6
Palm kernel/soy blend; 90/10	6–7

[a] Flax "et al." = mixture of flax/sunflower/sesame/pumpkin/borage oils (commercially available from Omega Nutrition).

Diets to maximize the dietary intake of lauric acid

In the U.S. in 1995, it was usually necessary to add fats such as coconut oil or creamed coconut to foods in order to have a source of lauric acid in the diet. Other than macaroons made with desiccated coconut, desiccated coconut itself, and candies made with coconut oil or palm kernel oil, there are very few food items readily available in supermarkets that are made with coconut oil. An occasional snack chip may be found that is still made with coconut oil. Such was not the case 20, 30, or 40 years or more ago when many commercial food items included coconut oil in their formulations.

Probable levels of lauric acid required for antimicrobial effect

Based on the amount of lauric acid found in human milk, which is known to be effective in its role as an antimicrobial component for the infant, the percent of calories that would be appropriate can be determined. For example, human milk provides at least 3.5% of calories as lauric acid for the human infant. Mature human milk has been noted to have up to 12% of the total fat as lauric acid (approximately 6.6% of calories.[32] The upper end of this range represents approximately twice the amount of calories as lauric acid (i.e., 7% of calories) as does the minimum.

When developing lauric-rich diets for adults, one can use this range as the starting point for calculating the amount of lauric fat to be consumed. Based on the upper end of the range, we see that this would entail providing an adult consuming 3,000 kilocalories a day with 52 grams of coconut oil (approximately 24 grams of lauric acid). This could be accomplished by use, for example, of two 250-ml cans of a calorically dense enteral formula (e.g., Carnation Nutren 2.0) *if* that product was made with full coconut oil. As it is, that product is made with MCT oil and corn oil and provides no lauric acid.

Lauric acid-rich diets can be developed readily for infants and children. For infants, a formula made with coconut oil that supplies at least 7% of the calories as lauric acid would be needed. When infants progress to solid food, these foods can be enriched with added coconut oil. Cereals and strained baby foods make ideal bases for 2 to 5 gram additions of coconut oil (0.5 to 1.0 teaspoons). This would add approximately 1 to 2 grams of lauric acid. Children can utilize the same protocol as outlined for adults with alterations in the portions of food depending on the caloric needs of the child.

General ways to incorporate coconut oil or creamed coconut into the diet

Foods that are very palatable with added coconut oil, and thus have the potential to become regular lauric acid sources in home preparation, include the following: all cooked cereals, all baked goods, blender drinks (fruit based), steamed puddings, creamed soups, rice and beans, stews (meat, poultry, fish, or vegetable), main dishes such as chili and lasagna, spaghetti and noodles, potatoes (e.g., scalloped, mashed), and rich sauces with equal amounts of flour and fat.

Creamed coconut can be melted into most of the mixed dishes; it will supply only two-thirds the amount of lauric acid as coconut oil. When coconut oil-based margarine spreads are available, these spreads can be used on bread as any spread or in any of the applications listed above. Depending on the amount of coconut oil contained in the spread formulation, the amount of lauric acid will vary, but will be less than the amount in whole coconut oil.

A probable margarine spread, which would be 80% fat with a certain portion of that fat coming from nonlauric oil, could provide about 3.7 grams of lauric acid in a tablespoon, whereas the whole coconut oil, which is 100% fat, will provide 6.7 grams of lauric acid. This means that larger amounts of the spread would need to be used to reach the same lauric acid goal. For fortifying cereals, creamed soups, or other cooked dishes, 3-tablespoon portions of coconut-based margarine need to be used in place of the 2-tablespoon portions of coconut oil.

Enriching main dishes with lauric acid

Any food served as a main dish that is enhanced by an added sauce can be enriched with coconut oil. A rich sauce can be made with 2 tablespoons coconut oil (or 3 tablespoons of coconut oil margarine), 2 tablespoons flour, and 1 cup of milk (or broth) plus flavoring such as salt and pepper or curry, etc. Coconut oil can be used for sauteing fish, poultry, meat, or any vegetables.

Coconut oil or a coconut oil margarine spread can be used in preparation of any recipe that calls for butter, margarine, or shortening. Rice dishes, bean dishes, spaghetti dishes, noodle dishes, and mashed or scalloped potato dishes are all appropriate foods for enrichment with coconut oil or creamed coconut. Lasagna is a good dish to use for incorporating additional lauric oils. The amount of lauric acid that will be consumed will depend on the amount put into the dish and the number of servings available from each dish.

Enriching cereals with lauric acid

Enriching cooked cereals with lauric acid sources can be readily accomplished by adding coconut oil, creamed coconut, or a margarine spread made with coconut oil and high in lauric acid to the finished cereal. Cereals that adapt well to added coconut oil include Cream of Rye, oatmeal, farina, Malt O Meal, Maypo, Roman Meal, Cream of Rice, Wheatena, Ralston, Cream of Wheat, and various multigrain cereals. These cereals are best when they have been cooked in milk.

For those individuals with milk intolerance, water, coconut milk, rice milk, or soy milk can be substituted. Soy milk is not without its own intolerance though, and it is recommended only as a last suggestion. Good quality whole milk should be well tolerated; in fact it is better tolerated by individuals with milk intolerance than is skim milk.

A cooked cereal with 2 tablespoons of coconut oil added will provide about 12.4 grams of lauric acid.

Blender drinks as sources of lauric acid

The fruit/fruit juice exchange can be used to increase the lauric acid content of the diet by making blender drinks with added coconut cream, coconut milk, or coconut oil.

A blender drink will provide 10 to 11 grams of lauric acid when it is made with ½ cup of canned coconut milk.

Nut butters as sources of lauric acid

The meat exchange (together with the fat exchange) can be considered to include nut butters. These nut butters can be made with any nut of choice (peanut, cashew, and almond are popular) combined with creamed coconut or with regular coconut oil.

Two tablespoons of nut butter blends made with creamed coconut in a 1:1 ratio (or made with 2 parts of coconut oil to 3 parts of other ground nuts) will provide approximately 4 grams of lauric acid.

Desserts and baked goods as lauric acid sources

All recipes for biscuits, bread and rolls, muffins, or pizza dough can be adapted to use either coconut oil or a coconut oil margarine spread as the shortening in place of any other oil or fat. Commercial macaroons served as a dessert or snack provide 6.5 grams of lauric acid for each macaroon if the macaroon is made from desiccated coconut and is labeled as containing 14 grams of fat.

Individuals whose digestion is not functioning in top form should use coconut oil and coconut milk and cream, or creamed coconut as their preferred source of lauric acid since they may not properly digest and extract adequate lauric acid from the dried coconut unless it is very finely ground.

Model diet incorporating sources of lauric acid

Alteration of 1800 kilocalorie basic diet to add lauric acid

An 1,800 kilocalorie (kcal) diet would be short 200 to 600 kcal for an adequate diet for most people. As noted by Aron[7] a more appropriate caloric level is likely to be 3,000 kcal. Adding coconut oil and/or products containing coconut (e.g., desiccated coconut, coconut cream, coconut milk) as given in Table 5 will increase the caloric density by approximately 600 kcal and will add appropriate amounts of lauric acid to the diet.

In the example in Table 5 of an adapted menu, coconut oil or coconut oil spread has been added to cooked cereal, blender drinks, rice, and other vegetables and a macaroon has been included. This menu would provide 30 to 36 grams of lauric acid.

This meal plan outlined in Table 5 is based on the exchange system as shown in Table 6. The original meal plan contained approximately 1,800 kcal. The caloric intake has been increased by approximately 600 kcal to approximately 2,400 kcal by increasing the number of fat exchanges three times. As a result, 30.3 grams of lauric acid has been incorporated into the day's diet (36 grams with a macaroon instead of muffin for an evening snack), whereas the original diet contained less than 0.1 grams of lauric acid. The enrichment has been accomplished by adding coconut oil to cereal, adding creamed coconut or coconut milk to blender fruit drinks, and by adding coconut oil to rice and vegetables.

With the enriched food plan, the fat equals 41% of energy, which is typical of moderate-fat, natural-foods diets recommended by medical and nutrition texts 50 to 60 years ago.[33,34] Of the 75 grams of saturated fat contained in this food plan, approximately 40 grams come from the complete medium chain saturates, i.e., caprylic, capric, and lauric acids.

Table 5 A 2400-Kilocalorie Meal Plan Adapted
from an 1800-Kilocalorie Meal Exchange Plan

Sample Menu

Breakfast
1(2) Fruit exchange(s)   ½ cup orange (apple) juice
3 Bread exchanges   1 cup cooked cereal (oatmeal, Wheatena, etc.);
                          1 slice of bread (toasted if desired) or roll
2–4 Fat exchanges   1–2 tbsp coconut oil added to cereal;
                          1 tsp butter or coconut oil spread for bread or roll
1 Milk exchange   1 cup whole milk

Lunch
2 Meat exchanges   1 roast beef sandwich made w/2 oz roast beef, thin sliced
  (lean–medium fat)
2 Bread exchanges   2 slices whole wheat or sourdough bread
1 Vegetable exchange   ½ tomato, sliced
2–3 Fat exchanges   1 tsp mayonnaise;
                          Blender drink made w/1 tbsp creamed coconut
                          or ¼ cup of coconut milk/cream or 1 tbsp of coconut oil
2 Fruit exchanges   ½ banana;
                          1 cup strawberries;
1 Milk exchange   ½ cup whole milk

Dinner
3 Meat exchanges   3 oz roasted chicken
  (lean–medium fat)
3 Bread exchanges   1 cup rice;
                          1 dinner roll
2 Vegetable exchanges   ½ cup carrot slices;
                          ½ cup peas
2–3 Fat exchanges   2 tsp coconut oil for vegetables/rice;
                          1 tsp butter or coconut oil spread for roll

Afternoon or Evening Snack
1 Bread exchange   1 whole grain muffin or 1 macaroon cookie
2 Fruit exchanges   Blender drink made w/
                          ½ banana;
                          1 cup strawberries;
½ Milk exchange   ½ cup whole milk;
1–2 Fat exchanges   1 tbsp coconut oil

Government-Endorsed Dietary Recommendations

Most of the current government-endorsed dietary recommendations (1995)
in the U.S. are based on the federal government dietary guidelines mandated
in 1977. These guidelines reflect some biases against the consumption of
adequate amounts of natural fats.

Table 6 Exchange Protocol

Basic starch/bread exchanges average approximately 80 kcal each. These starch/bread exchanges include most breads and rolls, many crackers, cereals, rice, macaroni and other pasta, and starchy vegetables such as potatoes, corn, lima beans, peas, pumpkin, parsnips, winter squash, dried peas, beans, and lentils.

Some starch/bread foods are made with added fat (crackers, etc.) and count as a combination of starch/bread serving and fat serving; such a serving would total approximately 125 kcal and would include such foods as biscuits, muffins, pancakes, and crackers with added fat.

Meat exchanges can be measured on a per ounce basis. For example, an average one ounce serving of lean meat is approximately 55 kcal; you would count 75 kcal for one ounce of medium-fat meat; and 100 kcal for one ounce of high-fat meat. One ounce of medium fat meat is the equivalent of one lean meat exchange plus one fat exchange. In addition to traditional beef, pork, lamb, veal, and game, fish and other seafood, all types of poultry, eggs, cheese, and certain legume dishes (e.g., peanut butter) are considered meat exchanges.

Vegetable exchanges average approximately 25 kcal per ½ cup serving. (Starchy vegetables average approximately 80 kcal per serving and are really counted in the bread category.) Protective vitamins, minerals, and beneficial phenolic compounds vary among the different vegetables.

Fruit exchanges provide approximately 60 kcal per serving. Protective vitamins, minerals, and beneficial phenolic compounds vary among the different fruits.

Skim milk (or very low-fat milk) **exchanges** provide approximately 90 to 100 kcal; low-fat (2%) milk and whole (3–3.5%) milk exchanges provide approximately 120 and 150 kcal respectively. Skim and low fat milk as usually consumed are not sufficiently high in fat to provide the beneficial antimicrobial or immune stimulating lipid factors. One cup of 2% milk has one fat exchange; one cup of whole milk has 1½ fat exchanges

Fat exchanges average 45 kcal for 5 grams which is approximately 1 teaspoon. Caloric value is the same for most fats whether natural or manufactured except that butter, coconut oil, and palm kernel oil have slightly fewer calories because of their short- and medium-chain fatty acids.

Typical daily diet plans based on the present U.S. government recommendations aim at the inclusion of: 8 to 9 starch/bread exchanges, 5 to 6 meat exchanges (lean to medium fat), 3 to 5 vegetable exchanges, 4 to 5 fruit exchanges, 2 skim milk exchanges, and 6 fat exchanges in an 1,800 kcal diet; or 15 starch/bread exchanges, 8 meat exchanges (lean to medium fat), 6 vegetable exchanges, 6 fruit exchanges, 3 skim milk exchanges, and 12 fat exchanges in a 3,000 kcal diet.

Summary

Well into the second decade of the AIDS epidemic, clinicians and researchers acknowledge that nutritional support of individuals who are HIV+ remains an important priority and that this nutritional support should include alternative therapies. The nutritional support may take various forms, e.g., added supplements of vitamins and minerals, and phytochemicals. In this chapter the added benefit of antimicrobial fatty acids from food has been reviewed, and dietary regimens that include antimicrobial fatty acids has been proposed.

There is potential for use of a more effective nutritional support regimen for HIV-infected individuals utilizing sources of antiviral, antimicrobial, and antiprotozoal monoglycerides and fatty acids that are found principally in lauric oils. These antimicrobial fatty acids and their derivatives are essentially nontoxic to man; they are produced *in vivo* by humans when they ingest those foods that contain adequate levels of medium-chain fatty acids such as lauric acid.

In addition to the HIV virus, other enveloped viruses inactivated by the antimicrobial lipids are the measles virus, herpes simplex virus-1, vesicular stomatitis virus, visna virus, and cytomegalovirus. Many of these pathogenic organisms are those known to be responsible for opportunistic infections in HIV+ individuals.

According to several decades of research, lauric acid is one of the best "inactivating" fatty acids, and its monoglyceride is even more effective than the fatty acid alone. Enteral feeding supplements that utilize medium-chain triglyceride (MCT) oils are commercially available. However, comparable commercial sources that provide lauric acid have not been available. Thus, the potential benefits from consuming antimicrobial lipids have not been widespread.

The use of lauric oils such as coconut oil or palm kernel oil, both of which are GRAS, is proposed as a unique source of both antimicrobial lipids and calories. These lauric oils can be readily incorporated into regular diets to provide a steady source of lauric acid.

Note added in proof

The usefulness of coconut oil as a source of lauric acid and its derivative monolaurin for lowering the viral load in individuals who are HIV+ has recently been "documented" in several individuals who had records of their viral load status prior to starting a dietary regimen that included coconut or coconut oil. The reported drop in viral load was greater than 2 log, e.g., from >400,000 to 2400 copies/mL or to undetectable levels, which would be in the significant range according to the current convention (i.e., less than 0.5 log change is not considered significant).

The individuals who reported beneficial lowering of their viral loads from coconut oil were consuming approximately 20 to 25 g of lauric acid from approximately 40 to 50 g (3–3.5 tbsp) of coconut oil. This likely represents about 14% of the kcal as coconut oil, and 7% of kcal as lauric acid.

References

1. Blattner, W.A., HIV epidemiology: past, present, and future, *FASEB J.* 5, 2340, 1991.
2. O'Brien, T.R., Blattner, W.A., Waters, D., et al. Serum HIV-1 levels and time to development of AIDS in the multicenter hemophilia cohort study, *J. Am. Med. Assoc.*, 276, 105, 1996.
3. Wilson, E.K., AIDS conference highlights hope of drug cocktails, chemokine research, *Chem. Eng. News*, 74, 42, 1996.
4. Schoofs, M., Drug resistance: the next AIDS crisis, *Village Voice*, 41, 15, 1996.
5. Isaacs, C.E., Kim, K.S, and Thormar, H., Inactivation of enveloped viruses in human bodiily fluids by purified lipids, *Ann. N.Y. Acad. Sci.*, 724, 457, 1994.
6. Raiten, D.J., Nutrition and HIV infection: a review and evaluation of the extant knowledge of the relationship between nutrition and HIV infection. Prepared for the Food and Drug Administration under Contract No. 223-88-2124 by the Life Sciences Research Office, Special Publications Office, Federation of American Societies for Experimental Biology, Bethesda, MD. (Reprinted in *Nutrition in Clinical Practice* Suppl., Vol. 6, No. 3, June 1991.)
7. Aron, J.M., Optimization of Nutritional Support in HIV Disease, Chap. 14 in *Nutrition and AIDS*, Watson, R.R., Ed., CRC Press, Boca Raton, FL, 215, 1994.
8. Dwyer, J.T., Bye, R.L., Holt, P.L., and Lauze, S.R., Unproven nutrition therapies for AIDS: what is the evidence? *Nutr. Today*, 23(2), 25, 1988.
9. Wickwire, P.A., Nutrition and HIV: your choices make a difference, Tennessee Department of Health and Environment, Tennessee Office of the East Central AIDS Education and Training Center (ECAETC), 1991.
10. Ferrier, L.K., Caston, L.J., Leeson, S., Squires, J., Weaver, B.J., and Holub, B.J., α-Linolenic acid- and docosahexaenoic acid-enriched eggs from hens fed flaxseed: influence on blood lipids and platelet phospholipid fatty acids in humans, *Am. J. Clin. Nutr.* 62, 81, 1995.
11. Kabara, J.J., Fatty acids and derivatives as antimicrobial agents — a review, in *The Pharmacological Effect of Lipids*, Kabara, J.J., Ed., American Oil Chemists' Society, Champaign IL, 1, 1978.
12. Sands, J.A., Auperin, D.D., Landin, P.D., Reinhardt, A., and Cadden, S.P., Antiviral effects of fatty acids and derivatives: lipid-containing bacteriophages as a model system, in *The Pharmacological Effect of Lipids*, Kabara, J.J., Ed., American Oil Chemists' Society, Champaign IL, 75, 1978.
13. Kabara, J.J., Antimicrobial agents derived from fatty acids, *J. Am. Oil Chem. Soc.*, 61, 397, 1984.
14. Kabara, J.J., Inhibition of *staphylococcus aureus*, in *The Pharmacological Effect of Lipids II*, Kabara, J.J., Ed., American Oil Chemists' Society, Champaign IL, 71, 1985.
15. Fletcher, R.D., Albers, A.C., Albertson, J.N., and Kabara, J.J., Effects of monoglycerides on *mycoplasma pneumoniae* growth, in *The Pharmacological Effect of Lipids II*, Kabara, J.J., Ed., American Oil Chemists' Society, Champaign IL, 59, 1985.
16. Hierholzer, J.C. and Kabara, J.J., *In vitro* effects of monolaurin compounds on enveloped RNA and DNA viruses, *J. Food Safety*, 4, 1, 1982.
17. Boddie, R.L. and Nickerson, S.C., Evaluation of postmilking teat germicides containing Lauricidin, saturated fatty acids, and lactic acid, *J. Dairy Sci.*, 75, 1725, 1992.

18. Wang, L.L. and Johnson, E.A., Inhibition of Listeria monocytogenes by fatty acids and monoglycerides, *Appl. Environ. Microbiol.*, 58, 624, 1992.
19. Isaacs, C.E. and Thormar, H., The role of milk-derived antimicrobial lipids as antiviral and antibacterial agents, in *Immunology of Milk and the Neonate*, Mestecky, J., et al., Eds., Plenum Press, New York, 1991.
20. Isaacs, C.E., Litov, R.E., Marie, P., and Thormar, H., Addition of lipases to infant formulas produces antiviral and antibacterial activity, *J. Nutr. Biochem.*, 3, 304, 1992.
21. Isaacs, C.E. and Schneidman, K., Enveloped viruses in human and bovine milk are inactivated by added fatty acids(FAs) and monoglycerides(MGs), *FASEB J.* Abstr. 5325, p. A1288, 1991.
22. Isaacs, C.E. and Thormar, H., Membrane-disruptive effect of human milk: inactivation of enveloped viruses, *J. Infect. Dis.* 154, 966, 1986.
23. Thormar, H., Isaacs, E.C., Brown, H.R., Barshatzky, M.R., and Pessolano, T., Inactivation of enveloped viruses and killing of cells by fatty acids and monoglycerides, *Antimicrob. Agents Chemother.*, 31, 27, 1987.
24. Isaacs, C.E., Kashyap, S., Heird, W.C., Thormar, H., Antiviral and antibacterial lipids in human milk and infant formula feeds, *Arch. Dis. Child.*, 65, 861, 1990.
25. Isaacs, E.C. and Thormar, H., Human milk lipids inactivated enveloped viruses, in *Breastfeeding, Nutrition, Infection and Infant Growth in Developed and Emerging Countries*, Atkinson, S.A., Hanson, L.A., and Chandra, R.K., Eds., Arts Biomedical Publishers and Distributors, St. John's NF, Canada, 1990.
26. Macallan, D.C., Noble, C., Baldwin, C., Foskett, M., McManus, T., and Griffin, G.E. Prospective analysis of patterns of weight change in stage IV human immunodeficiency virus infection, *Am. J. Clin. Nutr.*, 58, 417, 1993.
27. Projan, S.J., Brown-Skrobot, S., Schlievert, P.M., Vandenesch, F., and Novick, R.P., Glycerol monolaurate inhibits the production of beta-lactamase, toxic shock toxin-1, and other staphylococcal exoproteins by interfering with signal transduction, *J. Bacteriol.*, 176, 4204, 1994.
28. Anti-viral effects of monolaurin, *JAQA*, 2, 4, 1987.
29. Kaunitz, H., Dayrit, C.S. Coconut oil consumption and coronary heart disease. *Philipp. J. Intern. Med.*, 30, 165, 1992.
30. Eraly, M.G., IV., Coconut oil and heart attack, in *Proc. Symp. Coconut and Coconut Oil Human Nutr.*, Mar. 1994, Coconut Development Board, Kochi, India, 1995, pp. 63-64.
31. Prior, I.A., Davidson, F., Salmond, C.E., and Czochanska, Z., Cholesterol, coconuts, and diet on Polynesian atolls, a natural experiment: the Pukapuka and Tokelau Island studies, *Am. J. Clin. Nutr.*, 34, 1552, 1981.
32. Chen, Z.-Y., Pelletier, G., Hollywood, R., and Ratnayake, W.M.N., *Trans* fatty acids isomers in Canadian human milk, *Lipids*, 30, 15, 1995.
33. *De Re Medicina*, Eli Lilly, Indianapolis, IN, 1941.
34. Proudfit, F.T., *Nutrition and Diet Therapy, 8th Ed.*, Macmillan, New York. 1942.

chapter six

Experimental studies with antioxidants

Raxit J. Jariwalla

Abstract: A reduced intracellular state is vital to homeostatic control of cellular growth and function. Recent studies have shown that HIV infection is characterized by a state of oxidative stress associated with deficiencies in blood serum of exogenous (dietary) and endogenous antioxidants as well as overproduction of reactive free radicals. Such abnormalities may foster increased virus production and contribute to impairment of immune-cell proliferation and function. Experimental studies have demonstrated that supplementary concentrations of dietary, endogenous, and synthetic antioxidants can suppress virus replication and influence immune-cell function and survival. Antioxidants manifesting such effects are promising candidates for developing new complementary therapies for treatment of HIV/AIDS.

Introduction

It is now well recognized that oxidative imbalance is a central abnormality underlying HIV infection and AIDS (for recent reviews see References 1, 2). The prooxidant state associated with HIV/AIDS results not only from overproduction of oxygen free radicals but also from progressive depletion of the body's antioxidant reserves. Free radical overproduction results from hyperactivation of immune cells involved in host-defense and inflammatory reactions. The hyperactivity of such cells has been detected early in HIV infection and has been associated with increased generation of both oxygen

radicals[3] and pro-inflammatory products which include prostaglandins, leukotrienes, and cytokines.[1,2] In addition to these primary markers of the oxidative state, abnormalities in secondary and tertiary markers are also common in HIV infection. Secondary markers arise from oxidative reactions
mediated by the primary free radicals that involve generation of lipid/pro-
tein peroxides and clastogenic factors capable of damaging DNA. Among
the peroxidative products, malondialdehyde, 4-hydroxyalkenals and protein
carbonyls are frequently found to be elevated in early HIV infection. Their
prevalence reflects an overactivity of the oxidant-generating immune cells
which in turn leads to depletion of the body's vital antioxidant stores.

Antioxidant abnormalities associated with HIV/AIDS include deficiencies in the serum or intracellular level of endogenous and exogenous
(dietary) antioxidant stores, both of which are prevalent early in asymptomatic infection. Endogenous antioxidants commonly affected are amino acid
peptide thiols which include cysteine, methionine, glutathione, and intracellular enzymes such as glutathione peroxidase, catalase, and superoxide
dismutase. Among the dietary antioxidants, deficiencies are commonly
found in vitamins A, B-complex, C, E, and carotenoids, trace elements such
as selenium, copper, and zinc, and fat soluble compounds including coenzyme Q_{10} and fatty acids. These abnormalities, together with overproduction
of free radicals and increase in resting energy expenditure,[4] converge to
exacerbate the prooxidant state in HIV infection.

The increased oxidative stress associated with HIV infection has provided the experimental basis for studies with antioxidants. Recent reviews
have described the oxidative imbalance and micronutrient abnormalities
associated with HIV infection.[1,2] This review will focus on experimental
studies of endogenous, exogenous, and synthetic antioxidants that may have
potential clinical applications in HIV infection. The potential of plant-derived
antioxidants was described by Greenspan and Aruoma.[1]

Endogenous antioxidants

Glutathione

Glutathione (GSH) is a peptide thiol composed of three amino acids —
cysteine, glutamate, and glycine. It is a major antioxidant defense mechanism
in aerobic living cells where it functions to protect cellular structures from
oxidative damage by neutralizing toxic peroxides in the reaction catalyzed
by the selenium-containing enzyme glutathione peroxidase. As a reducing
agent, it also functions to maintain ascorbate (and other antioxidants such
as alpha-tocopherol) in their reduced state.[5] During the reduction process,
GSH is itself oxidized to GSSG from which it is readily reduced back to GSH
through the activity of the enzyme, GSH reductase. GSH is also utilized in
detoxification of cytoxic byproducts via conjugation of electrophilic compounds in a reaction catalyzed by GSH transferase. Aside from this role in
protecting against oxidative stress, GSH is an important immuno-modulator,

shown essential to maintaining normal cell-mediated immune responses. Adequate levels of GSH have been found to be necessary for T-cell activation, cellular and antibody-dependent cytotoxicity, and phagocytic activity.[6]

HIV-infected individuals and AIDS patients manifest severe GSH deficiency. Asymptomatic persons were reported to have significantly depressed levels of extracellular GSH.[7] Total glutathione concentration in plasma was lowered in HIV-seropositive persons to about one-third of that in HIV-negative controls.[7] GSH level in lung epithelial lining fluid was about 60% of that in controls.[7] In addition to a systemic GSH deficiency, HIV-infected persons were also reported to manifest low intracellular GSH levels in their T-cell subsets that declined progressively with the advancement of disease.[8] In persons with AIDS-related complex, GSH levels were reported to be 66% of normal in helper (CD4) lymphocytes and 69% of normal in suppressor (CD8) lymphocytes. In AIDS patients, GSH levels were 63% of normal in CD4 cells and 62% of normal in CD8 cells. Intracellular GSH deficiency was attributed to selective loss of high GSH-containing cells.[8] Since cytotoxic T lymphocytes are at the forefront of an immune attack during viral infection, the incremental loss of intracellular GSH may contribute to a progressively weakened immune response in AIDS. Furthermore, sytemic GSH depletion may weaken the body's antioxidant defense leading to cellular damage and organ failure. In this context, GSH depletion in the lungs has been linked to the pathological effects characteristic of pneumonia caused by *Pneumocystis*.[7]

The cause of GSH deficiency in HIV infection is not known. GSH synthesis in cells is catalyzed by the enzymes, gamma-glutamyl-cysteine synthetase and glutathione synthetase. Plasma glutathione has a high turnover and is the main source of transport for cellular glutathione, whose primary site of synthesis is the liver.[9] Animal studies have shown that intracellular GSH levels are dependent on protein intake — especially intake of sulfur-containing amino acids, specifically, cysteine.[10] The latter is a rate limiting substrate in GSH synthesis as its level is about 10 times lower than that of other substrates such as glutamate. It has been reported that HIV-infected persons have decreased plasma cysteine levels.[11] Since cysteine can influence rate of GSH synthesis, its depletion may contribute, at least in part, to the GSH deficiency seen in HIV infection.

The GSH/GSSG couple is a major redox buffer within cells, with ratios ranging from 30:1 to 100:1 in different cell types. Besides counteracting oxidants and maintaining reduced pools of vitamins C and E, the GSH/GSSG couple is involved in redox reactions associated with protein folding and conversion of ribonucleotides to deoxyribonucleotides for DNA synthesis. Additionally, it plays a direct role in transduction of cellular signals through thiol/disulfide exchange reactions with receptor proteins and transcription regulatory factors within cells.

Among the transcription factors affected by GSH are nuclear factor-κB (NF-κB) and activation protein-1 (AP-1), both of which play important roles in induction of HIV gene expression and inflammatory factors. In lymphocytes exposed to mitogens, the response to proliferation was highest in cells having a high intracellular GSH content.[12] On the other hand, depletion of intracellular GSH by various biochemical inhibitors was shown to be accompanied by NF-κB activation with attendant induction of NF-κB-responsive genes including inflammatory cytokines (TNF-α, IL-1), receptor chains for Il-2, and latent HIV provirus.[13]

Several studies have examined the influence of GSH restoration on HIV-infected cells at different stages of virus expression. In latently infected monocytic or T-lymphocytic cell lines, expressing little or no virus, stimulation with TNF-α or phorbol ester (PMA) was associated with GSH depletion, NF-κB activation, and enhancement of HIV gene expression.[14] Exposure of such cell lines to reduced GSH and GSH monoester resulted in inhibition of NF-κB activation and suppression of HIV activity.[15] Similar effects were observed on increase in the intracellular levels of GSH peroxidase induced by supplementation of PMA or cytokine-stimulated T-lymphocytic cells with selenium selenite.[16] In contrast, treatment with GSH of unstimulated chronically-infected T cells did not affect virus production.[17]

Changes in intracellular GSH levels have also been linked to alterations in cell growth and death. Inhibition of GSH synthesis in human lymphoid cells by exposure to L-buthionine-(SR)-sulfoximine was shown to increase their sensitivity to cell killing by gamma radiation.[18] GSH depletion induced by BSO was recently linked to increased rate of neuronal cell death.[19] This effect was blocked by the oncogene Bcl-2 whose expression resulted in the doubling of the intracellular GSH concentration.[19] Bcl-2 also protected a T-cell human hybridoma cell line from oxidative stress (lipid peroxidation) and programmed cell death (apoptosis) induced by glucocorticoids.[20]

In view of the pathological effects of GSH deficiency, several investigators have focused on GSH restoration as a therapeutic strategy to control the progression of HIV infection and AIDS. However, GSH per se has limitations and its direct use has not proven to be efficacious.[2] First, oral GSH is unstable and therefore not optimally active in the body. Second, although GSH can be administered as an aerosol, it is not readily taken up by cells as it has to be in an acetylated form for transport. Accordingly, some researchers have synthesized and utilized esterified derivatives of GSH. Among these, GSH monoester is bioavailable; however, only limited amounts of this compound can be tolerated before it produces toxicity.[21] Hence, therapeutic efforts aimed at restoring intracellular GSH have shifted to exploring other means such as testing precursors of GSH or other nonthiol-based antioxidants (see below).

Cysteine

Aside from its role as a component and precursor of GSH, cysteine is an antioxidant in its own right. In addition, extracellular cysteine has been shown to influence macromolecular (protein and DNA) and cellular viability in stimulated lymphocytes. The latter readily take up cysteine released by macrophages, which have been postulated to influence lymphocyte activation through this mechanism.[22] It has been reported that HIV-infected and

AIDS patients have a plasma cysteine deficiency. The levels of cysteine in blood plasma of patients with lymphadenopathy or AIDS were 66% lower than that in heathy controls. Plasma cysteine levels in infected asymptomatic persons were approximately one-half of that in controls.[11]

The cause of cysteine deficiency in AIDS is not known. Cysteine is a nonessential amino acid, normally synthesized in the liver from the conversion of methionine through the action of the enzyme cystathionine synthase, which requires pyridoxine (vitamin B_6) as a cofactor. Under conditions of pyridoxine deficiency, cysteine may be required as an essential amino acid. Pyridoxine deficiency was reported in about one-half of persons with asymptomatic HIV infection.[23] HIV-infected persons with CD4 deficiencies also have 5 to 6 times higher levels of serum glutamate than uninfected controls.[22] Extracellular glutamate has been shown to compete with the transport of cystine into macrophages resulting in a reduced capacity of these cells to release cysteine and its supply to lymphocytes.[22] These abnormalities may contribute to the cysteine and GSH deficiencies prevalent in AIDS.

Because cysteine is a precursor of GSH, it has been considered as a possible approach to restoring intracellular GSH. *In vitro*, the addition of cysteine to the growth medium of HIV-infected lymphocytic cells was shown to suppress constitutive virus production.[24] However, like oral GSH, cysteine supplementation *in vivo* has its limitations.[2,25] Orally administered cysteine readily oxidizes to cystine and other oxidation products. Whereas cystine can be readily absorbed through the gut, its uptake can be competitively inhibited by dibasic amino acids in the diet. Unlike cystine, other oxidation products of cysteine have been shown to be cytotoxic.[26]

Cysteine derivatives

Because of limitations of cysteine supplemetation, derivatives of cysteine and cysteine prodrugs have been experimentally explored as possible alternatives agents in HIV/AIDS therapy. A widely studied derivative is N-acetylcysteine (NAC) which has been used as an antidote against acetoaminophen overdose and in the treatment of respiratory distress syndrome. It has been shown to function as an antioxidant via its ability to increase intracellular GSH levels[27] as well as through direct scavenging of oxidants.[6] NAC was shown to enhance colony formation in T cells derived from patients with ARC and AIDS. *In vitro*, NAC supplementation to culture medium also blocked NF-κB activation and HIV expression in cytokine-stimulated lymphocytic and monocytic cell lines.[15,28] In unstimulated HIV-infected cells, constitutively producing virus, NAC exerted only a two-fold inhibition of extracellular reverse transcriptase activity but caused over ten-fold suppression in p24 antigen levels.[17]

The efficacy of NAC has also been investigated *in vivo*. Unlike *in vitro* studies, results from clinical investigations have been conflicting. In AIDS patients administered intravenous NAC,[29] the p24 antigen level was significantly lowered over a 15-day infusion period consistent with data from *in vitro* studies. However, in the same clinical investigation, other surrogate markers such as CD4 cell number and β-2-microglobulin level were not affected. In a small study of asymptomatic HIV-infected patients, oral NAC was shown to confer clinical stabilization over a 44-week observation period. Most unexpectedly, mononuclear cells of treated patients showed depletion of GSH and increase in lipid peroxides, suggestive of enhanced free radical production.[30] In another report from the same group, enhanced HIV replication by NAC was also observed in macrophages.[31] In a recent report by a different group, adminstration of NAC to HIV-infected persons did not affect the GSH concentration in plasma or lymphocytes.[32]

Unlike the ambiguous data of NAC effects on surrogate markers, its action on the apoptosis phenotype seems to be consistently uniform. NAC treatment was shown to reduce the rate of apoptosis induced by TNF-α in U937 monocytic cells.[33] A similar effect of NAC was also seen in lymphocytes of HIV-infected persons in a study conducted at the Pasteur Institute.[34] Administration of NAC at 1800 mg/d for >6 months resulted in reduced rate of lymphocyte apoptosis in the treated group compared to that observed in the seronegative controls. This effect of NAC seems to hold promise and needs to be further investigated.

Another alternative to cysteine supplementation is the cysteine prodrug procysteine (l-2-oxothialzolidine-4-carboxylic acid or OTC). Like NAC, it was shown to inhibit TNF-stimulated HIV expression in U1 monocytic cells.[35] Furthermore, in combination with AZT, procysteine administration resulted in significant lowering of AZT toxicity along with potentiation of the antiviral activity in peripheral blood mononuclear cells.[36] In a phase 1 trial of orally administered procysteine in early HIV infection, the cysteine prodrug was found to improve percentage of CD4+ cells and CD4/CD8 ratio in a dose-dependent manner.[37] Viral load seemed to be unaffected as no changes in this parameter were reported. In a separate study of intravenous procysteine, the prodrug was found to produce noticeable side effects.[38] Further work is required on the tolerance and safety of oral procysteine in long-term studies.

Antioxidant enzymes

HIV-infected and AIDS patients also exhibit weakened antioxidant enzyme defenses. Enzymes involved in detoxification of reactive oxidants are located primarily within intracellular compartments. The three main detoxifying enzymes, namely, superoxide dismutase (SOD, cytoplasmic and mitochondrial), catalase, and glutathione peroxidase protect cells from oxidative damage by preventing the initiation and branching of chain reactions of free radicals. In contrast to this function, repair enzymes such as GSH and met.hemoglobin reductases form a second line of defense aimed at reduction and restoration of oxidized substances.

HIV infection has been linked to deficiencies in glutathione peroxidase, which detoxifies peroxides,[39] and mitochondrial MnSOD, a scavenger of superoxide radicals.[40] In lymphocytic T-cell lines cultured *in vitro*, the activities of enzymes catalase, MnSOD, and GSH peroxidase were reported to drop following virus infection.[1] The depression of antioxidant enzymes may be caused in part by expression of HIV-specific genes. In HeLa cells, transfection with a cloned gene encoding the HIV tat protein was shown to result in the downregulation of MnSOD expression to 25% of the level in uninfected cells.[41] In the same model, intracellular sulphur amino acids were depressed by 75% with concomitant increase in the level of protein carbonyls by nearly 100%. The influence of HIV tat on the activity of antioxidant enzymes in peripheral blood mononuclear cells (PBMC) is not known and needs to be investigated to evaluate the significance of the tat gene effect in relation to GSH and antioxidant enzyme deficiency in HIV infection.

Depression in GSH peroxidase has been associated with increased rate of cellular apoptosis. GSH peroxidase catalyzes the neutralization of toxic peroxides including lipid hydroperoxyacids formed from oxidation of cellular membranes. In the HIV-producing human T-cell line 8E5, which manifests GSH peroxidase deficiency, incubation with hydroperoxy fatty acids was found to induce apoptosis.[42] Such an effect was not seen in parental uninfected cells which remained viable after similar treatment.[42] The influence of toxic lipid hydroperoxides in infected PBMC is not known.

Antioxidant enzyme restoration has been considered for use as a therapeutic target in HIV infection. Most of the experimental approaches have been indirect, using treatments that enhance the antioxidant defense enzymes. Selenium supplementation, which stimulates GSH peroxidase activity, was demonstrated to lower NF-κB activation and HIV expression in latently infected lymphocytic and monocytic cell lines induced by TNF-α, PMA, and H_2O_2.[16] The GSH precursor NAC was shown to block activation-induced apoptosis (mediated by oxidative stress) in T-cell hybridomas.[43] Clinical investigations are needed to correlate changes in induced antioxidant enzyme levels with surrogate markers to assess the relevance of this experimental approach for HIV therapy.

Exogenous dietary antioxidants

A hallmark of HIV infection is the prevalence of micronutrient abnormalities which are detected early in infection. Among the nutrients whose levels are altered in HIV infection include vitamins A, B-complex, C, E, and beta-carotene, and trace elements selenium, copper, and zinc. Such nutrient abnormalities appear to arise from multiple causes including malabsorption, metabolic alteration, and nutritional deprivation associated with the risk factors of AIDS. It has been suggested by several authors that micronutrient abnormalities may contribute to the progression of HIV infection and AIDS (for a recent review see Reference 2). Specific micronutrient abnormalities in HIV infection have been detailed by Bogden et al.,[44] Baum et al.[45] and Graham et al.[46] Vitamin alterations in HIV infection have been reviewed by Coodley.[47] The relevance of micronutrient imbalance to pathogenesis and therapy were previously discussed.[2] This section will focus on experimental studies that have been carried out with dietary antioxidants that have potential clinical application for HIV/AIDS.

Water soluble vitamins

Vitamin C (ascorbic acid or ascorbate) is the major aqueous antioxidant in body fluids and tissues. It is also a powerful antiviral agent with immune-stimulating properties (reviewed in Reference 48). In redox reactions ascorbic acid is oxidized to dehydroascorbate from which it is recycled or degraded depending on the status of other antioxidants. At ordinary concentrations at which it is obtained through the diet, vitamin C is regenerated from dehydroascorbate through the action of glutathione. However, under conditions of GSH deficiency such as that prevalent in HIV infection, oxidized ascorbate can get degraded leading to ascorbate deficiency. Vitamin C deficiency was reported in HIV-infected persons without prior history of vitamin supplementation.[44]

Ascorbate contributes up to 24% of the total antioxidant capacity for trapping peroxy radicals in human blood plasma.[49] In a plasma *in vitro* system, ascorbate was demonstrated to function as an outstanding antioxidant, displaying more effectiveness than protein thiols, bilirubin, urate, or tocopherol in protecting against peroxidation of fatty acids.[50] One of the products of this process is malondialdehyde (MDA), which has been used widely as a measure of lipid peroxidative changes associated with the oxidative state.[51] Elevated plasma levels of MDA have been reported in HIV infection consistent with enhanced lipid peroxidation due to increased production of oxygen metabolites.[52]

In animal models of drug-induced glutathione deficiency, high-dose ascorbate was shown to serve as an essential antioxidant, exerting a sparing effect on GSH accompanied by cellular protection from organ damage with a dose-dependent increase in the mortality rate.[6] In humans, administration of low vitamin C diets, associated with oxidant damage, was shown to produce a significant reduction in total glutathione and the ratio of reduced to oxidized glutathione in plasma, and these values were restored upon ascorbate repletion.[53] In another study, supplementaion with vitamin C was demonstrated to elevate red blood cell glutathione in healthy adults.[54] The effects of supplemental vitamin C on endogenous glutathione and lipid peroxides in populations exhibiting thiol deficiency have not been studied and need to be determined.

In laboratory studies utilizing cultures of HIV-infected cells, ascorbate has been shown to suppress HIV replication and activity without affecting the viability of host cells (reviewed in Reference 48). In chronically infected T cells, constitutively producing virus, incubation with nontoxic concentrations of ascorbic acid caused a dose- and time-dependent suppression in the levels of viral reverse transcriptase and p24 antigen released into the culture supernatant.[55] In acutely infected T cells, ascorbate blocked *de novo* infection as assessed by the formation of giant cell syncytia.[55] More recently, ascorbate was shown to block HIV-directed gene expression in a reporter cell line[56] and activation of HIV provirus in latently infected T cells.[57,58] In the latter studies, ascorbate was demonstrated to confer dose-dependent suppression of virus induction following cell stimulation by a mitogen (PMA) and an inflammatory cytokine (TNF-α). Unlike antioxidant thiols such as NAC and PDTC, which suppress HIV activation via the inhibition of NF-κB activity, ascorbate did not affect the functional levels of this transcription factor, indicating a different mechanism of action.[59] Separate studies in chronically infected cells showed that ascorbate produced an inhibitory effect on HIV by acting at a post-transcriptional step directed at the inactivation of virus-specific protein (enzyme) activity.[60] Ascorbate concentrations conferring virus suppression *in vitro* are attainable in blood plasma as determined from pharmacokinetic studies in healthy uninfected volunteers (discussed in Reference 61). The ascorbate dosage required to attain comparable levels in blood plasma of HIV-infected persons (who manifest a high bowel tolerance) need to be determined. The above experimental observations of anti-HIV effects have provided a compelling rationale for testing large doses of ascorbic acid in HIV-infected persons. A clinical trial, sponsored by the NIH, has been planned to address some of these questions.

Other water-soluble antioxidants important in HIV infection include B-complex vitamins pyridoxine and riboflavin. Pyridoxine functions as an apoenzyme for cystathionine synthetase, which requires adequate levels of this B vitamin for conversion of methionine to cysteine. Riboflavin is an essential component of GSH reductase involved in regeneration of reduced GSH. The levels of both vitamins are depressed in HIV infection. Their status and relationship to immune function has been reviewed and discussed in Baum et al.[45]

Fat soluble vitamins

The members of this group include vitamin E and carotenoids of which the most widely studied is β-carotene. Deficiencies in both vitamin E and carotenes have been reported in HIV infection (reviewed in Reference 2). Such deficiencies may arise from malabsorption caused by elevated levels of inflammatory cytokines such as TNF found along the gastrointestinal tract in HIV-infected persons.[62] TNF has been shown to inhibit lipoprotein lipase, a key enzyme controlling the levels of fat-soluble vitamins and nutrients absorbed through the GI tract.[63]

Vitamin E is a phenolic compound and the most significant antioxidant in the lipid phase, functioning as an inhibitor of lipid peroxidation mediated by free radicals in the membranes. This action of vitamin E has been linked to the suppression of activation of protein kinase C which is responsible for triggering NF-κB, the transcription factor that drives HIV expression. During this process vitamin E is oxidized to the tocopheryl radical from which it can be regenerated by vitamin C or GSH. In addition to its antioxidant function, vitamin E has been shown to exert immmune-stimulating effects in experimental animals and humans.[64-66] Vitamin E supplementation was shown to increase erythrocyte survival and granulocyte function in patients with an inborn GSH synthetase deficiency.[67,68] When used in combination with AZT in HIV-infected persons, it was shown to confer increased efficacy.[69]

β-carotene has shown clinical efficacy in small studies when tested in the dosage range of 60–180 mg/d (reviewed in Reference 47). A daily intake of 180 mg was found to elevate CD4 number, total white blood cell count, and CD4/CD8 ratios in HIV-infected patients, but not in those receiving a placebo.

Trace elements

The metallic antioxidants selenium, copper, zinc, and manganese are primarily components of antioxidant enzymes. Selenium is an essential constituent of GSH peroxidase, copper and zinc constitute the cytosolic Cu.Zn superoxide dismutase (SOD), and manganese is the component of the mitochondrial MnSOD. The levels of these trace elements and their respective enzymes are altered in HIV infection. Selenium deficiency is quite widespread and shown to have profound effects on the levels of GSH peroxidase in HIV-infected persons.[70] This can lead to accumulation of toxic peroxides, depletion of intracellular GSH, and enhancement of HIV activity. As discussed above, addition of selenium to HIV-infected cell lines resulted in increase of intracellular GSH peroxidase activity with concomitant suppression of NF-κB activation and HIV expression induced by PMA, TNF, or oxidative stress.

Low levels of selenium in plasma of HIV-infected persons were linked to impairment of natural killer-cell activity.[71] On the other hand, high plasma selenium levels were associated with decreased levels of IgG and IgM compared to those seen in persons with normal or low selenium levels. Thus, selenium supplementation needs to be approached with caution as both low and high levels are undesirable. Approaches aimed at restoring SOD activity also need to be experimentally explored.

Impact of nutrient status on HIV progression

In 1993, two prospective studies evaluating the impact of dietary intake on HIV progresion were published. Both studies assessed the relationship of dietary intake at baseline to the rate of disease progression in cohorts of asymptomatic HIV-infected men. One study tracked 296 HIV-seropositive persons enrolled in the San Francisco Men's Health Study[72] and the other followed 281 seropositive men in the Baltimore/Washington, D.C. site of the Multicenter AIDS Cohort Study.[73] Both studies reached similar conclusions (reviewed in Reference 2). In the San Francisco study, micronutrient consumption was correlated with a reduced incidence of AIDS. The intake of iron, vitamin E, riboflavin, and a daily multivitamin supplement were statistically significantly related to a reduced risk of AIDS development. Vitamin C, thiamine, and niacin showed a relationship that approached significance. In the Baltimore study, results from single nutrient analysis revealed that the highest intake of vitamins C, B_1, and niacin and median intake (between 9,000 and 20,000 IU) of vitamin A were associated with a significantly lowered rate of AIDS progression. Most unexpectedly, a low (<9,000 IU) and a high (>20, 000 IU) daily intake of vitamin A and 10–15 mg/d of zinc were linked to an increased risk of AIDS development. Aside from the latter result, the general conclusion from these studies is that micronutrient consumption early in HIV infection has a positive influence on retarding HIV progression to full-blown AIDS. Since these studies correlated dietary intake at baseline to AIDS development, further studies are required to evaluate the impact of subsequent dietary intervention on the rate of HIV progression. Also, it would be desirable to evaluate this impact in randomized arms within the study so that the influence of other factor(s) associated with increased micronutrient consumption is minimized.

Other antioxidants

Flavonoids

Flavonoids are phenolic compounds that form an important component of the antioxidant system of plants. They act as strong inhibitors of lipid peroxidation through their ability to scavenge directly peroxy radicals and chelate transition metal ions involved in Fenton reactions that generate reactive hydroxyl radicals.[74,75] They have been shown to inhibit the activity of enzymes such as protein kinase C, phospholipase A2, and other oxygenases involved in metabolism of arachidonic acid, which is linked to the production of inflammatory prostaglandins and leukotrienes.[74]

Certain flavonoids manifest strong antiviral activity. Among these, the compounds quercitin, hesperitin, and catechin were found to display a broad antiviral spectrum. Two classes were identified, one capable of virus inhibition through a selective effect on virus replication and another preventing virus uncoating through an interaction with the viral capsid protein.[76] The catechins were shown to inhibit the activities of various retroviral reverse transcriptases and cellular DNA/RNA polymerases.[77] In a recent study evaluating the activity of various flavonoids against HIV, the flavans (catechin derivatives) were shown to be highly effective in inhibiting infection by HIV-1, HIV-2, or SIV.[76] The mechanism of virus inhibition involved binding of the flavan with the surface glycoprotein gp120 resulting in prevention of virus interaction with the CD4 receptor.

Ubiquinones

These are phenolic fat-soluble antioxidants of which the protype member is Coenzyme Q_{10} (CoQ_{10}). The latter is an important component of the electron transport chain within the mitochondria involved in cellular respiration and

ATP generation. Its reduced form (ubiquinol 10) is a powerful membrane antioxidant that can scavenge peroxyl radicals after lipid peroxidation has been initiated. In the inner mitochondrial membrane, Coenzyme Q_{10} and vitamin E function in a complementary fashion to reduce free radical production.[78] Coenzyme Q_{10} has been extensively studied in patients with heart disease and shown to have benefits in improving cardiac function and survival.[79,80] It has been reported by Folkers and colleagues that patients with HIV infection, ARC, and AIDS have decreased levels of CoQ_{10} in blood compared to healthy subjects.[81] The same research group published findings from a small study in healthy volunteers showing improvement in T4/T8 ratios following supplementation with 100 mg/d of CoQ_{10} over a 2-month period.[78] Based on these observations it has been postulated that CoQ_{10} may have value in ARC or AIDS patients with low T4/T8 ratios. This proposal needs to be put to experimental test.

Synthetic Antioxidants

Several synthetic compounds with antioxidant activity including thiols such as dithiocarbamates (e.g., PDTC), thiocytic and lipoic acids, nordihydroquaretic acid, vitamin E derivatives (alpha tocopherol succinate and acetate), butylated hydroxyanisole (BHA), and butylated hydroxytoluene (BHT) have been shown to inhibit activation of NF-κB, the key enzyme regulating expression of HIV provirus in infected cells.[56,82-84] Because latent HIV is the reservoir for new virus production, NF-κB-inhibiting compounds with limited toxicity offer potential for development of anti-HIV therapy targeted at a different step from that inhibited by nucleoside analogs and protease inhibitors.

Conclusion

Epidemiologic and laboratory studies have unraveled evidence for the prevalence of oxidative stress and micronutrient imbalance in HIV-infected and AIDS patients. This has provided a compelling rationale for evaluating the effectiveness of antioxidant substances in HIV/AIDS. Experimental studies with biological and synthetic antioxidants have revealed promising results indicating multiple targets of action. In HIV-infected cells, antioxidant thiols and vitamin E derivatives were shown to block NF-κB transcription factor activation, HIV replicative expression, and cellular apoptosis. Trace elements such as selenium augmented intracellular GSH peroxidase with subsequent inhibition of NF-κB and HIV activities. Other physiological antioxidants such as ascorbic acid (vitamin C) and flavonoids efficiently suppressed HIV by inhibiting different steps in the viral life cycle. The broad-spectrum inhibitory effects of antioxidants targeted against HIV and infected cells offer promising possibilities for developing novel complementary therapies whose clinical efficacy needs to be tested promptly in controlled trials.

Acknowledgment

The outline of this article was prepared while the author was at the Linus Pauling Institute of Science and Medicine in Palo Alto. The author would like to acknowledge the assistance of Sonal Jariwalla with the preparation of the manuscript.

References

1. Greenspan, H.C. and Aruoma, O.I., Oxidative stress and apoptosis in HIV infection: a role for plant-derived metabolites with synergistic antioxidant activity, *Immunol. Today*, 15, 209, 1994.
2. Jariwalla, R.J., Micronutrient imbalance in HIV infection and AIDS: relevance to pathogenesis and therapy, *J. Nutr. Environ. Med.*, 5, 297, 1995.
3. Jarstrand, C., Akerlund, B., and Lindeke, B., Glutathione and HIV infection, *Lancet*, 1, 235, 1990.
4. Vaudercam B. et al., Resting energy expenditure (REE) in HIV-infected patients, *VIIIth International Conference on AIDS*, PuB7569, Amsterdam, 1992.
5. Martensson, J. and Meister, A., Glutathione deficiency decreases tissue ascorbate levels in newborn rats: ascorbate spares glutathione and protects, *Proc. Natl. Acad. Sci. U.S.A.*, 88, 4656, 1991.
6. Staal, F.J.T., Ela, S.W., Roederer, M., Anderson, M.T., Herzenberg, L.A., and Herzenberg, L.A., Glutathione deficiency and human immunodeficiency virus infection, *Lancet*, 339, 909, 1992.
7. Buhl, R. et al., Systemic glutathione deficiency in symptom-free HIV-seropositive individuals, *Lancet*, 2, 1294, 1989.
8. Staal, F.J.T., Roederer, M., Israelski, D.M. et al., Intracellular glutathione levels in T cell subsets decrease in HIV-infected individuals, *AIDS Res. Hum. Retrovirus.*, 8, 305, 1992.
9. Akerboom, T. and Sies, H., Glutathione transport and its significance in oxidative stress, in *Glutathione Metabolism and Physiological Functions*, Viña J., Ed., CRC Press, Boca Raton, FL, pp. 45, 1990.
10. Bauman, P.F. et al., The effect of dietary protein and sulfur amino acids on hepatic glutathione concentration and glutathione-dependent enzyme activities in the rat, *Can. J. Physiol. Pharmacol.*, 66, 1048, 1988.
11. Eck, H.-P. et al., Low concentrations of acid-soluble thiol (cysteine) in the blood plasma of HIV-infected patients, *Biol. Chem. Hoppe-Seyler*, 370, 101, 1989.
12. Kavanagh, T.J. et al., Proliferative capacity of human peripheral blood lymphocytes sorted on the basis of glutathione content, *J. Cell Physiol.*, 145, 472, 1990.
13. Dröge, W., Eck, H.P., and Mihm, S., HIV-induced cysteine deficiency and T-cell dysfunction — a rationale for treatment with N-acetylcysteine, *Immunol. Today*, 13(6), 211, 1992.
14. Staal, F.J., Roederer, M., and Herzenberg, L., Intracellular thiols regulate activation of nuclear factor kappa-β and transcription of human immunodeficiency virus, *Proc. Natl. Acad. Sci. U.S.A.*, 87, 9943, 1990.
15. Kalebic, T., Kinter, A., Guide, P., Anderson, M.E., and Fauci, A.S., Suppression of human immunodeficiency virus expression in chronically infected monocytic cells by glutathione ester, and N-acetyl cysteine, *Proc. Natl. Acad. Sci. U.S.A.*, 88, 986, 1991.

16. Sappey, C., Legrand-Poels, S., Best-Belpomme, M., Favier, A., Rentier, B., and Piette, J., Stimulation of glutathione peroxidase activity decreases HIV type 1 activation after oxidative stress, *AIDS Res. Hum. Retrovirus.*, 10(11), 1451, 1994.

17. Harakeh, S. and Jariwalla, R.J., Comparative study of the anti-HIV activities of ascorbate and thiol-containing reducing agents in chronically HIV-infected cells, *Am. J. Clin. Nutr.*, 54, 1231S, 1991.

18. Dethmers, J.K. and Meister, A., Glutathione export by human lymphoid cells: depletion of glutathione by inhibition of its synthesis decreases export and increases sensitivity to irradiation, *Proc. Natl. Acad. Sci. U.S.A.*, 78, 7492, 1981.

19. Kane, D.J. et al., Bcl-2 inhibition of neural death: decreased generation of reactive oxygen species, *Science*, 262, 1274, 1993.

20. Hockenberry, D.M. et al., Bcl-2 functions in an antioxidant pathway to prevent apoptosis, *Cell*, 75, 241, 1993.

21. Martensson, J., Han, J., Griffith, O.W., and Meister, A., Glutathione ester delays the onset of scurvy in ascorbate-deficient guinea pigs, *Proc. Natl. Acad. Sci. U.S.A.*, 90, 317, 1993.

22. Eck, H.P. and Dröge, W., Influence of the extracellular glutamate concentration on the intracellular cyst(e)ine concentration in macrophages and on the capacity to release cysteine, *Biol. Chem. Hoppe Seyler*, 370, 109, 1989.

23. Baum, M. et al., Association of vitamin B status with parameters of immune function in early HIV-1 infection, *J. AIDS*, 4, 1122, 1991.

24. Mihm, S., Ennen, J., Pessara, U., Kurth, R. and Dröge, W., Inhibition of HIV-1 replication and NF-κB by cysteine and cysteine derivatives, *AIDS*, 497, 503, 1991.

25. Waterson, S.K., Glutathione deficiency: therapeutic target in human immunodeficiency virus infection, *J. Orthomolec. Med.*, 7, 104, 1992.

26. Estrela, J.M. et al., The effect of cysteine and N-acetylcysteine on rat liver glutathione, *Biochem. Pharmacol.*, 32, 3483, 1983.

27. Burgunder, J.M. et al., Effect of N-acetylcysteine on plasma cysteine and glutathione following paracetemol administration, *Eur. J. Clin. Pharmacol.*, 36, 127, 1989.

28. Roederer, M., Staal, F.I., Raju, P.A., Ela, S.W., Herzenberg, L.A., and Herzenberg, L.A., Cytokine-stimulated human immunodeficiency virus replication is inhibited by N-acetyl-L-cysteine, *Proc. Natl. Acad. Sci. U.S.A.*, 87, 4884, 1990.

29. Clotet et al., Effects on surrogate markers of intravenous N-acetylcysteine in AIDS patients, *8th International Conference on AIDS*, POB3013, Amsterdam, 1992.

30. van Ashbeck, B.S. et al., Increased oxidant concentration in lymphocytes of patients with AIDS: ratio and effects of treatment with N-acetylcysteine, in *Oxidative Stress, Cell Activation and Viral Infection*, Pasquier, C. et al., Eds., Birkhauser Verlag, Basel/Switzerland, 1994.

31. Nottet, H.S.L.M. et al., Role for oxygen radicals in the self-sustained HIV-1 replication in monocyte-derived macrophages: enhanced HIV-1 replication by N-acetylcysteine, *9th International Conference on AIDS*, PO-A12-0199, Berlin, 1992.

32. Witschi, A. et al., Supplementation of N-acetylcysteine fails to increase glutathione in lymphocytes and plasma of patients with AIDS, *AIDS Res. Hum. Retrovirus.*, 11, 141, 1995.

33. Malorni, W., Rivabene, R., Santini, M.T., and Donelli, G., N-Acetylcysteine inhibits apoptosis and decreases viral particles in HIV-chronically infected U937 cells, *FEBS Lett.*, 327(1), 75, 1993.

34. Rene, O. et al., An antioxidant prevents apoptosis and early cell death in lymphocytes from HIV infected individuals, *8th International Conference on AIDS*, Po A2376, Amsterdam, 1992.
35. Chen, P. et al., Procysteine inhibits TNF-induced HIV production in U1 cells, *9th International Conference on AIDS*, Po-A13-0248, Berlin, 1993.
36. Josephs, S. et al., Procysteine (L-2-oxothiazolidine-4-carboxylic acid) reduces the toxicity of AZT and enhances the antiviral activity of AZT in cultured peripheral blood mononuclear cells (PBMC), *9th International Conference on AIDS*, PO-A25-0574, Berlin, 1993.
37. Skowron, G. et al., A phase 1 trial of oral procysteine (L-2-oxothiazolidine-4-carboxylic acid) in early HIV infection, *9th International Conference on AIDS*, PO-B29-2177, Berlin, 1993.
38. Kalaviian, R., A phasetrial of intravenous procysteine in HIV infected subjects, *8th International Conference on AIDS*, PoB3455, Amsterdam, 1992.
39. Picardo, M. et al., Vitamin E, polyunsaturated fatty acids of phospholipids, lipoperoxides and glutathione peroxidase status in HIV sero-positive patients, *7th International Conference on AIDS*, W.B. 2421, Florence, 1991.
40. Wong, G. et al., MnSOD is essential for cellular resistance to cytotoxicity of TNF, *Cell* 58, 923, 1989.
41. Flores, S.C. et al., Tat protein of human immunodeficiency virus type 1 represses expression of MnSOD dismutase in HeLa cells, *Proc. Natl. Acad. Sci. U.S.A.*, 90, 7632, 1993.
42. Sandstrom, P.A., Lipid hydroperoxides induce apoptosis in T cells displaying a HIV-associated glutathion peroxidase deficiency, *J. Biol. Chem.*, 269, 798, 1994.
43. Sandstrom, P.A., Inhibition of activation-induced death in T cell hybridomas by thiol antioxidants: oxidative stress as a mediator of apoptosis, *J. Leukoc. Biol.*, 55, 221, 1995.
44. Bogden, J.D., Baker, H., Frank, O., Perez, G., Kemp, F., Breuning, K., and Louria, D., Micronutrient status and human immunodeficiency virus (HIV) infection, *Ann. N.Y. Acad. Sci.*, U.S.A., 587, 189, 1990.
45. Baum, M.K. et al., Inadequate dietary intake and altered nutrient status in early HIV infection, *Nutrition*, 10, 16, 1994.
46. Graham, N.M.H., On specific nutrient abnormalities in asymptomatic HIV infection, *AIDS*, 6, 1552, 1992.
47. Coodley, G.O., Vitamins in HIV infection, in *Nutrition and AIDS*, Watson R.R., Ed., CRC Press, Boca Raton, FL., 89, 1994.
48. Jariwalla, R.J., and Harakeh, S., Antiviral and immunomodulatory activities of ascorbic acid, in *Subcellular Biochemistry. Vol. 25: Ascorbic Acid: Biochemistry and Biomedical Cell Biology*, Harris, J.R., Ed., Plenum Press, New York, 215, 1995.
49. Wayner, D.D.M. et al., The relative contributions of vitamin E, urate, ascorbate and proteins to the total peroxy radical-trapping antioxidant activity of human blood plasma, *Biochim Biophys. Acta*, 924, 408, 1987.
50. Frei, B., England, L., and Ames, B.N., Ascorbate is an outstanding antioxidant in blood plasma, *Proc. Natl. Acad. Sci. U.S.A.*, 86, 6377, 1989.
51. Yagi, K., Assay for serum lipid peroxide level and its clinical significance, in *Lipid Peroxides in Biology and Medicine*, Yagi, K., Ed., Academic Press, Orlando, FL, 223, 1982.
52. Sonnerborg, A., Increased production of malondialdehyde in patients with HIV infection, *Scand. J. Infect. Dis.*, 20, 287, 1988.

53. Henning, S.M. et al., Glutathione blood levels and other oxidant defense indices in men fed diets low in vitamin C, *J. Nutr.*, 121, 1969, 1991.
54. Johnston, C.S., Meyer, C.G., and Srilakshmi, J.C., Vitamin C elevates red blood cell glutathione in healthy adults, *Am. J. Clin. Nutr.*, 58, 103, 1993.
55. Harakeh, S., Jariwalla, R.J., and Pauling, L., Suppression of human immuno-deficiency virus replication by ascorbate in chronically and acutely infected cells, *Proc. Natl. Acad. Sci. U.S.A.*, 87, 7245, 1990.
56. Staal, F.J.T., Roederer, M., Raju, P.A., Anderson, M.T., Ela, S.W., Herzenberg, L.A., and Herzenberg, L.A., Antioxidants inhibit stimulation of HIV transcrip-tion, *AIDS Res. Hum. Retrovirus.*, 9, 299, 1993.
57. Harakeh, S. and Jariwalla, R.J., Comparative analysis of ascorbate and AZT effects on HIV production in persistently infected cell lines, *J. Nutr. Med.*, 4, 393, 1994.
58. Harakeh, S. and Jariwalla, R.J., Ascorbate effect on cytokine stimulation of HIV production, Supplement to *Nutrition*, 11, 684, 1995.
59. Harakeh, S. and Jariwalla, R.J., NF-κB-independent suppression of HIV ex-pression by ascorbic acid, *AIDS Res. Hum. Retrovirus.*, 13, 235, 1997.
60. Harakeh, S., Niedzwiecki, A., and Jariwalla, R.J., Mechanistic aspects of ascor-bate inhibition of human immunodeficiency virus, *Chem. Biol. Interact.*, 91, 207, 1994.
61. Jariwalla, R.J. and Harakeh, S., Ascorbic acid and AIDS: strategic functions and therapeutic possibilities, in *Nutrition and AIDS*, Watson, R., Ed., CRC Press, Boca Raton, FL, 117, 1994.
62. McGowan, J. et al., Cytokine profiles in HIV infected intestinal mucosa, *9th International Conference on AIDS*, PO-A13-0213, Berlin, 1993.
63. Scevola, D. et al., Lipolysis and liposynthesis in AIDS patients, *9th International Conference on AIDS*, PO-A13-0236, Berlin, 1993.
64. Reddy, P.G. et al., Effect of supplemental vitamin E on the immune system of calves, *J. Dairy Sci.*, 69, 164, 1986.
65. Benedich, A. et al., Dietary vitamin E requirement for optimum immune re-sponses in the rat, *J. Nutr.*, 116, 675, 1986.
66. Watson, R.R., Immunological enhancement by fat-soluble vitamins, minerals and trace metals: a factor in cancer prevention, *Cancer Detect. Prev.*, 9, 67, 1986.
67. Boxer, L.A. et al., Protection of granulocytes by vitamin E in glutathione synthetase deficiency, *NEJM*, 301, 901, 1979.
68. Spielberg, S.P. et al., Improved erythrocyte survival with high-dose vitamin E in chronic hemolyzing G6PD and glutathione synthetase deficiencies, *Ann. Int. Med.*, 90, 53, 1979.
69. Coodley, G.O. et al., Beta-carotene in HIV infection, *J. AIDS*, 6, 272, 1991.
70. Dworkin, B. et al., Selenium deficiency in the acquired immune deficiency syndrome, *J. Parent. Enter. Nutr.*, 10, 405, 1986.
71. Mantero-Atienza, E. et al., Selenium status and immune function in early HIV infection, *7th International Conference on AIDS.*, M.C. 3126, Florence, 1991.
72. Abrams, B. et al., A prospective study of dietary intake and acquired immune deficiency syndrome in HIV-seropositive homosexual men, *J. AIDS*, 6, 949, 1993.
73. Tang, A.M. et al., Dietary micronutrient intake and risk of progression to AIDS in human immunodeficiency virus type 1 (HIV-1)-infected homosexual men, *Am J Epidemiol.*, 138, 937, 1993.
74. Middleton, E., The flavonoids, *TIPS*, 5, 335, 1984.

75. Afanas'ev, I.B. et al., Chelating and free radical scavenging mechanisms of inhibitory action of rutin and quercitin in lipid peroxidation, *Biochem. Pharmacolog.*, 38, 1763, 1989.
76. Mahmood, N. et al., Inhibition of HIV infection by caffeoyl-quinic acid derivatives, *Antiviral Chem. Chemother.*, 4(4) 235, 1993.
77. Nakaul, H. et al., Differential inhibition of HIV-reverse transcriptase and various DNA and RNA polymerase by some catechin derivatives, *Nucleic Acid Res. Symp.*, Series 21, 1989.
78. Folkers, K. et al., Coenzyme Q_{10} increases T4/T8 ratio of lymphocytes in ordinary subjects and relevance to patients having the AIDS-related complex, *Biochem. Biophys. Res. Commun.*, 176, 786, 1991.
79. Mortensen, S.A. et al., Coenzyme Q_{10}: clinical benefits with biochemical correlates suggesting a scientific breakthrough in the management of chronic heart failure, *Int. J. Tissue React.*, 12, 155, 1990.
80. Langsjoen, P.H. et al., A six-year clinical study of the therapy of cardiomyopathy with coenzyme Q_{10}, *Int. J. Tissue React.*, 12, 169, 1990.
81. Folkers, K. et al., Biochemical deficiencies of coenzyme Q_{10} in HIV infection and the exploratory treatment, *Biochem. Biophys. Res. Commun.*, 153, 888, 1988.
82. Schreck, R., Rieber, P., and Bauerele, P.A., Reactive oxygen intermediates as apparently widely used messengers in the activation of the NF-κB transcription factor and HIV-1, *EMBO J.*, 10, 2247, 1991.
83. Israel, N., Gougerot-Pocidalo, M.-A., Aillet, F., and Virelizier, J.-L., Redox status of cells influences constitutive or induced NF-translocation and HIV long terminal repeat activity in human T and monocytic cell lines, *J. Immunol.*, 149, 3386, 1992.
84. Suzuki, Y.J. and Packer, L., Inhibition of NF- kappaB DNA binding activity by alpha-tocopheryl succinate, *Biochem. Mol. Biol. Int.*, 31, 693, 1993.

section two

Absorption and AIDS

chapter seven

Appetite and energy intake in human immunodeficiency virus (HIV) infection and AIDS

Carolyn D. Summerbell

Introduction

Weight loss is one of the most important clinical and psychological symptoms associated with HIV infection and AIDS and is caused by altered metabolism due to cytokine activity, malabsorption, and/or a reduction in energy intake. Each of these causes of weight loss is important, but a reduction in energy intake appears to be responsible for the greatest losses in weight in individuals with HIV infection at all stages of disease.[9] A loss of appetite or anorexia is one of the inevitable consequences of cytokine activity which is increased in response to opportunistic infections such as those seen in AIDS. However, loss of appetite associated with HIV infection can be caused by a number of other factors listed below and result in episodic weight loss during the course of the infection. Indeed, cross-sectional data suggest that significant amounts of weight are lost during the asymptomatic and symptomatic stages of HIV disease.[10,16] Therefore, it is important to understand the etiology of reduced energy intake if nutrition-based interventions are to succeed.

The major cause of a reduced energy intake is loss of appetite. Anorexia is one of the inevitable consequences of cytokine activity, which is increased in response to opportunistic infections such as those seen in AIDS, but its mechanisms are poorly understood. Cytokines such as tumor necrosis factor may play a part, particularly in hypothalamic centers regulating food intake, although plasma concentrations of tumor necrosis factor are not consistently increased in patients with HIV infection.[5] However, there are a number of

0-8493-8561-X/98/$0.00+$.50
© 1998 by CRC Press LLC

other factors which can depress appetite and / or reduce energy intake during all stages of HIV disease.

Causes of loss of appetite

Anxiety and depression

A variety of psychological factors can occur during HIV infection and inter-fere with food intake; anxiety and depression are often cited by patients as the cause of their reduced appetite. There may be many different causes of anxiety and depression in individuals with HIV disease, but more obvious causes for the HIV-positive individual include the shock following initial knowledge of their positive HIV status, informing close family and friends that they are HIV positive (and for some individuals informing their close family and friends that they are also gay), where appropriate tracing previ-ous partners, and also coming to terms with their terminal illness. The mechanisms responsible for the effect of anxiety and depression on appetite are unclear and difficult to identify since some individuals, particularly the obese, report overconsumption of food when anxious or depressed. Clearly, anxiety and depression do not affect appetite in a fixed direction, and a greater understanding of this relationship should be a priority for future research.

Fatigue

Individuals with HIV infection may experience profound fatigue and extreme tiredness, even during the early stages of disease. Because of this individuals with HIV infection are less able to cater to themselves following diagnosis; consequently, people with HIV infection eat out more often and have more meals prepared for them at home.[15] Support for these individuals via volunteers, meals on wheels, and day centers should be utilized together with energy-saving appliances, convenience and snack foods.[13] However, take-out meals should be avoided since there is a small risk of food poisoning associated with these types of meals. Intestinal infectious diseases and result-ing systemic infections such as *salmonella* can be threatening to people with HIV disease because of their already suppressed immune function.

Economic factors

Many individuals with HIV infection can find their financial resources dra-matically reduced. Some may be too ill, physically or psychologically, to work. Others may suffer prejudice at work and are forced to resign or have their contract terminated, even though this is illegal practice. Community-based nutrition programs can help individuals increase their energy intake and offer psychological support.

Mechanical problems

Oral and/or esophageal conditions or lesions are commonly associated with HIV infection and can make eating difficult, unpleasant, or painful, and result in voluntary food restriction. Oral and esophageal candida is probably the most common cause of dysphagia seen in HIV disease. (There is a line of thought that *Lactobacillus bifidus* in unpasteurized natural yogurt may help to prevent the colonization of this organism). However, the use of prescribable drugs can, in most instances, resolve the symptoms of candida extremely quickly. Kaposi's sarcoma is also commonly associated with HIV infection, and when it occurs on the palate it can cause an exceptionally sore mouth and swallowing difficulties.

Occasionally, difficulty in eating can occur as a side effect of some of the prescribed drugs used in the management of this disease. For example, the use of DDI (Dideoxyinosine), an antiretroviral, can cause a dry, sore mouth.

Dementia

Problems encountered by individuals with HIV infection who also have dementia may involve feeding and swallowing difficulties and an inability to remain self-caring with respect to nutritional needs. There is a planning requirement for the nutritional care of these individuals both in the hospital and in the community.

Altered taste sensation and food aversion

Individuals with HIV infection often report changes in taste sensation, particularly in association with oral candidiasis or chemotherapy, which reduce the palatability of certain foods. Food aversions are also occasionally reported. However, little research has been carried out to quantify the impact of these factors on food intake.

Nausea and vomiting

Nausea and vomiting, which can also cause food avoidance, may result from infectious complications, obstructions caused by tumors, or drug therapy. A common side effect of many drugs is nausea. Septrin (co-trimoxazole), which is commonly used as a prophylaxis against pneumocystis carinii pneumonia (PCP), frequently causes nausea, and patients taking this drug should be reviewed regularly for any changes in appetite and body weight. Chemotherapy for Kaposi's sarcoma can also cause severe nausea and vomiting.

The use of recreational drugs appears more common in gay men, regardless of their HIV status, compared with the general public, and some of these drugs may depress appetite.[11] On the other hand, some patients report using marijuana as an appetite stimulant, and, indeed, a prescribable drug based on the famous weed (Dronabinol) is now available.

Early satiety

Early satiety may occur with massive hepatomegaly or splenomegaly caused by several complications of AIDS or by infiltrative diseases of the stomach and small bowel. Food intake may also be reduced by dyspnea associated with respiratory complications and by adrenal insufficiency.

Diarrhea

Diarrhea may depress food intake, either because patients attempt to reduce fecal output by restricting food consumption or because of specific suppression of appetite as a response to the presence of unabsorbed nutrients in the lower intestine.[7] A mediator for the latter process has not been identified, but its existence has been thought to contribute to weight loss seen in other conditions of intestinal injury and disease. Such a process could provide the explanation for the clinical observation that food intake is often greatest in the morning in patients with AIDS and malabsorption.

Voluntary weight loss

Some newly diagnosed patients may voluntarily reduce energy intake in an attempt to lose weight because they see themselves as fat and believe that to be slim would be healthier. This misconception comes from their belief that if being slim is a healthy body weight for the general public, then it should also be healthy for them. However, this probably is not the case.[16] Maintenance of body weight and extra fat reserves may well serve as an insurance policy for inevitable episodes of weight loss associated with opportunist infections, even during the early stages of HIV disease. The health professional must try to deter the patient from losing excess body weight without inducing fear or anxiety.

Many patients also believe that they should be changing their diet along the lines of the healthy eating guidelines recommended for the general public.[15] However, this "healthy diet" is aimed at reducing avoidable mortality from coronary heart disease and stroke, and since this relatively young patient group is more likely to die of AIDS than any other cause of death, this "healthy diet" may be less appropriate for these individuals.

Other patients may try alternative diets, such as the anti-candida diet or a macrobiotic diet, and lose weight because these types of restrictive diets have a low energy density. Indeed, this is one of the main arguments against the use of such diets. However, the health professional should not appear negative about the use of such diets since they can offer psychological benefit, and a diet should be formulated which is both acceptable to the patient and provides an adequate energy intake.

Drug addicts

HIV-positive individuals who are also intravenous drug users tend to be malnourished compared with those who do not inject drugs.[3,17] The reasons for this are unclear, but it may be because this group of individuals gives eating and food a low priority compared with HIV-positive people who are not intravenous drug users. The consumption of heroin, cocaine, and other drugs is associated with anorexia[11] for the same reason. Drug consumers frequently change their eating habits and rarely eat more than once a day, losing interest in everything besides drugs. Furthermore, intravenous drug users are more prone to repeated infections which contribute to the development of undernutrition.

Hospitalization

Finally, hospital food, even if you feel well, can depress your appetite.

Appetite and energy intake

The exact impact of these factors has received little research activity, and there is a need for quantitative data to document these observations. Part of the reason for this lack of activity may be due to the fact that many cross-sectional studies which have assessed food intake during HIV infection have found that, in clinically and weight stable patients, energy intake does not differ with stage of HIV disease, body weight, nor when compared to seronegative controls.[1,2,6,7,8,14]

However, the dietary records of these patients do not tell us about energy intake during periods of weight loss and, as highlighted by Dworkin (1990),[1] food intake may have been reduced during periods of weight-loss prior to the time of study. Indeed, weight-losing patients with AIDS suffer a dramatic reduction in appetite and energy intake,[4] and the degree of weight loss is closely correlated with the reduction in energy intake.[9] Whether energy intake is reduced during periods of weight loss is not associated with opportunistic infections remains unknown. However, it is possible that energy intake, like body weight, fluctuates over the course of the disease, and that these fluctuations mirror one another.

To quantify the role which energy intake plays in the pathogenesis of weight loss a prospective study needs to be conducted. The methodology of such a study should involve the use of a simple technique to assess energy intake since patients who are losing weight are more likely to be feeling unwell and, therefore, less likely to complete a dietary record. For example, a simple diet diary or food frequency questionnaire may be more appropriate than a weighed dietary intake. Also, because of the potential for greater variation in energy intake between days due to sickness, food intake should be assessed over a longer period of time than that recommended for healthy individuals.[12]

Summary

In conclusion, loss of appetite (and thus decrease in energy intake) appears to be the most significant cause of weight loss associated with HIV disease. However, there is a lack of research in this area and more work needs to be done to clarify the impact of the various causes of appetite suppression discussed above on weight loss in HIV disease.

References

1. Dworkin, B.M., Wormser, G.P., Axelrod, F., Pierre, N., Schwarz, E., Schwartz, E., and Seaton, T., Dietary intake in patients with acquired immunodeficiency syndrome (AIDS), patients with AIDS-related complex, and serologically positive human immunodeficiency virus patients: correlations with nutritional status, *J. Parenter. Enter. Nutr.*, 14, 605, 1990.
2. Foskett, M., Kapembwa, M., Sedgwick, P., and Griffin, G.E., Prospective study of food intake and nutritional status in HIV infection, *J. Hum. Nutr. Dietetics*, 4, 149, 1991.
3. Gomez-Sirvent, J.L., Santolaria-Fernandez, F.J., Gonzalez-Reimers, C.E., Batista-Lopez, J.N., Jorge-Hernandez. J.A., Rodriguez-Moreno, F., Martinez-Riera, A., and Hernandez-Garcia, M.T., Nutritional assessment of drug addicts. Relation with HIV infection in early stages, *Clin. Nutr.*, 12, 75, 1993.
4. Grunfield, C., Pang, M., Shimizu, L., Shigenada, J.K., Jensen, P., and Feingold, K.R., Resting energy expenditure, caloric intake and weight in human immunodeficiency virus infection and the acquired immunodeficiency syndrome, *Am. J. Clin. Nutr.*, 55, 455, 1992.
5. Grunfield, C. and Feingold, K.R., Metabolic disturbances and wasting in the acquired immunodeficiency syndrome, *N. Engl. J. Med.*, 327, 329, 1992.
6. Hommes, M.J.T., Romijn, J.A., Godfried, M.H., Eeftinck Schattenkerk, J.K.M., Buurman, W.A., Endert, E., and Sauerwein, H.P., Increased resting energy expenditure in human immunodeficiency virus-infected men, *Metabolism*, 39, 1186, 1990.
7. Kotler, D.P., Tierney, A.R., Brenner, S.K., Couture, S., Wang, J., and Pierson, R., Preservation of short-term energy balance in clinically stable patients with AIDS, *Am. J. Clin. Nutr.*, 51, 7, 1990.
8. Luder, E., Godfrey, E., Godbold, J., and Simpson, D.M., Assessment of nutritional, clinical, and immunological status of HIV infected, inner-city patients with multiple risk factors, *J. Am. Diet. Assoc.*, 95, 655, 1995.
9. Macallan, D.C., Noble, C., Baldwin, C., Jebb, S.A., Prentice, A.M., Coward, W.A., Sawyer, M.B., McManus, T.J., and Griffin, G.E., Energy expenditure and wasting in human immunodeficiency virus infection, *N. Engl. J. Med.*, 333(2), 83, 1995.
10. McCorkindale, C., Dybevik, K., Coulston, A.M., and Sucher, K.P., Nutritional status of HIV-infected patients during the early disease stages, *J. Am. Diet. Assoc.*, 90(9), 1236, 1990.
11. Mohs, M.E., Watson, R.R., and Leonard-Green, T., Nutritional effects of marijuana, heroin, cocaine, and nicotine, *J. Am. Diet. Assoc.*, 90(9), 1261, 1990.

12. Nelson, M., Black, A.E., Morris, J.A., and Cole, T.J., Between- and within-subject variation in the nutrient intake from infancy to old age: estimating the number of days required to rank dietary intakes with desired precision, *Am. J. Clin. Nutr.*, 50, 155, 1989.

13. Peck, K. and Johnson, S., The role of nutrition in HIV infection, *J. Hum. Nutr. Diet.*, 3, 147, 1990.

14. Sharkey, S.J., Sharkey, K.A., Sutherland, L.R., Church, D.L., and GI/HIV study group. Nutritional status and food intake in human immunodeficiency virus infection, *J. Acquir. Immunodefic. Virus Syndrome*, 5(11), 1091, 1992.

15. Summerbell, C.D., Catalan, J., and Gazzard, B.G., A comparison of the nutritional beliefs of human immunodeficiency virus (HIV) seropositive and seronegative homosexual men, *J. Hum. Nutr. Diet.*, 6 (1), 23, 1993.

16. Summerbell, C.D., Appetite and nutrition in human immunodeficiency virus (HIV) infection and acquired immunodeficiency virus syndrome (AIDS), *Proc. Nutr. Soc.*, 53(1), 139, 1994.

17. Varela, P., Marcos, A., Ripoll, S., Requejo, A., Herrera, P., and Caas, A., Nutritional status assessment of HIV-positive drug addicts, *Eur. J. Clin. Nutr.*, 44, 415, 1990.

chapter eight

Assessing the role of intestinal absorption, permeability, and nutrition in AIDS patients

Michael Ott and Bernhard Lembcke

In at least 50% of North American and European patients with the acquired immunodeficiency syndrome (AIDS) and in nearly 90% of patients in developing countries diarrhea and other gastrointestinal symptoms develop at some time during the course of disease. These symptoms are often troublesome with a significant impact on the patient's quality of life.[52] Furthermore, impaired intestinal function is likely to contribute to weight loss, malnutrition, deterioration of the immune system and overall mortality in HIV-infected patients.

The rapid increase in the number of microbes identified as a source of intestinal infection has complicated the task of physicians to diagnose which cause is responsible for the symptoms of an individual patient. Today, our knowledge about the gastrointestinal tract as a target of HIV infection is still incomplete, but information derived from clinical and laboratory studies collected through the last decade can help in the clinical management of HIV-infected patients with intestinal dysfunction. Epidemiological surveys have provided insights into the prevalence of diarrhea, malabsorption, and other forms of intestinal dysfunction and its impact on malnutrition, immune function, and mortality in AIDS patients. Others have examined in detail the morphology, microbiology, and the functional capacity of the intestine at various stages of the HIV infection and in various subgroups of patients. A limited number of studies have investigated the upper gastrointestinal tract of a primate model infected with the simian immunodeficiency virus (SIV) and the effect of pathogens on intestinal morphology and function in other animal models, which may be relevant to HIV-induced intestinal disease.

0-8493-8561-X/98/$0.00+$.50
© 1998 by CRC Press LLC

Intestinal dysfunction in HIV-infected patients

The gastrointestinal tract is one of the organs most frequently affected in AIDS patients. Throughout the course of the disease inflammation, loss of water and nutrients, as well as abnormalities of the intestinal barrier function have been reported in HIV-infected patients, both with and without the presence of secondary opportunistic manifestations of the intestine. Early studies in AIDS patients[25,31,32] already indicated a high prevalence of malabsorption in a mixed patient population. In one of the most comprehensive studies so far, Keating et al.[3] established the incidence and severity of malabsorption and changes in intestinal permeability for small molecules as evidence for altered barrier function in patients with HIV infection at various stages of immune deficiency. They compared the intestinal function of HIV-positive male homosexual patients and healthy volunteers by using an oral absorption/permeability test containing the three monosaccharides 3-O-methyl-D-glucose, D-xylose, L-rhamnose, and the disaccharide lactulose. Active and passive carrier-mediated carbohydrate transport across the brush border membrane as indicated by decreased absorption of monosaccharides was significantly impaired in AIDS patients with severe immunodeficiency compared to healthy volunteers and HIV-positive patients with earlier stages of the disease. Malabsorption of monosaccharides ranged from 30% in stable AIDS patients without intestinal symptoms or wasting (D-xylose) to 89% of AIDS patients with one or more identifiable pathogens and diarrhea (L-rhamnose). Additionally, patients with diarrhea regardless of the presence of intestinal pathogens were more likely to present carbohydrate malabsorption than patients without diarrhea. Intestinal permeability in this study was assessed by the lactulose/rhamnose ratio (LL/R-r) and found to be increased in patients with mild as well as severe immunodeficiency. These data extended earlier observations by Ott and colleagues, who first described increased LL/R-r in AIDS patients with and without gastrointestinal symptoms. While the changes in intestinal permeability were comparable with results obtained in patients with celiac disease in both studies, Keating et al.[3] showed that jejunal morphology was far less affected in patients with HIV infection at any stage. Lim and coworkers[27] also demonstrated abnormal intestinal permeability at all stages of HIV-disease but not as profoundly abnormal as the changes seen in patients with untreated celiac disease. Kapembwa et al.[61] reported a high prevalence of abnormal intestinal lactulose/mannitol-permeability in Caucasians as well as Africans, predominantly in patients with advanced HIV disease and diarrhea, regardless of the presence of intestinal infections. Interestingly, the LL/M-r in Africans with AIDS and no gastrointestinal symptoms was significantly increased compared to control subjects, but not in Caucasians with asymptomatic AIDS. Aggravated malnutrition and the overall health status in African patients with AIDS may account for these differences.

Most of the studies provide strong evidence that nutrient malabsorption and abnormal intestinal permeability develop frequently in HIV-infected patients with gastrointestinal symptoms regardless of secondary intestinal infections present at the time of testing. More controversial data, however, are reported in HIV-infected patients at early stages of the disease and AIDS patients without gastrointestinal symptoms. Tepper et al.[29] did not find abnormal intestinal lactulose and mannitol uptake-ratio (LL/M-r) in asymptomatic HIV-infected patients compared to healthy control patients. AIDS patients without diarrhea had lactulose recovery similar to healthy controls, but reduced mannitol recoveries, whereas AIDS patients with diarrhea had increased lactulose recovery and decreased mannitol recovery.

Much has to be learned about the causes, confounding disease conditions, and time of onset of intestinal symptoms and dysfunction in HIV-infected patients. The role of some obligate and opportunistic pathogens, which frequently infest the intestine of late stage AIDS patients, in the pathogenesis of intestinal malabsorption and altered permeability has been clearly established in clinical studies as well as in animal models.

The pathogenesis of gastrointestinal dysfunction in "pathogen-negative" HIV patients, however, is less well established. No correlation of intestinal dysfunction with decreasing blood CD-4 cell counts, a marker of the worsening immune defect in HIV, was found. The immunohistochemical detection of HIV antigens in intestinal tissue has led to the assumption that HIV itself rather than the immune deficiency is responsible for some functional defects seen in "pathogen-negative" HIV patients.

A primate animal model has provided some insights about gastrointestinal disease associated with immunodeficiency viruses. The simian immunodeficiency virus (SIV) infection of rhesus macaques resembles HIV infection in humans with respect to the spectrum of immunological changes, some opportunistic disease manifestations, clinical symptoms, and specific morphological and functional abnormalities of various organs. Stone et al.[6] have used this model to study the pathology of the gastrointestinal tract at various times after inoculation of SIV. Eight out of nine SIV-infected monkeys exhibited malabsorption detected either by sucrose breath hydrogen (H_2) analysis and/or decreased blood D-xylose levels. D-xylose malabsorption occurred more frequently with disease progression and in the presence of enteropathogens. Bacterial overgrowth may also have caused malabsorption of D-xylose in some animals. However, no firm association was observed between abnormal D-xylose absorption and the presence or degree of bacterial overgrowth, and diarrhea and sucrase activities in homogenates of jejunal biopsies were significantly reduced throughout the course of SIV-infection indicating early functional abnormalities in animals without secondary intestinal infections. Based upon the clinical and experimental evidence of gastrointestinal disease in "pathogen-negative" HIV-infected patients several investigators have studied the underlying morphology and function of the intestine in these individuals.

Intestinal morphology and function in patients with "HIV enteropathy"

The term "HIV enteropathy" has been widely used to describe functional and morphological disease of the small intestine in the absence of secondary intestinal HIV manifestations. The diagnosis requires exclusion of pathogens other than HIV by adequate microscopic examination, culture, and special analytic methods of stool, intestinal fluids, biopsy materials, and aspirates. The term, however, is misleading, because no firm cause and effect relationship between the presence of HIV in mucosal cells and gastrointestinal symptoms or abnormal mucosal architecture has been established. In 1984, Kotler and co-workers[25] were the first to characterize the intestine in HIV-infected patients with chronic diarrhea and no identifiable pathogen. Since this intial report the intestinal morphology and function in a number of patients presenting with "HIV enteropathy" have been studied. Because of differences in histological methods and patient selection, however, the morphological features of "HIV enteropathy" remain controversial. Early studies reported both chronic, nonspecific inflammatory changes in the lamina propria of the intestine with crypt hyperplasia and villous atrophy[25,31,32] as well as normal findings. These studies most likely included a variable number of patients with, at that time, undescribed opportunistic pathogens and semi-quantitative histology, which may partly explain the discrepancies. In 1989, Ullrich et al.[20] described "low grade" small bowel atrophy with hyporegeneration and maturational defects in enterocytes as the predominant intestinal morphology in "pathogen-negative" patients. Analysis with three-dimensional morphometry revealed that HIV-infected patients without intestinal manifestation had reduced villus height and surface areas and a normal crypt depth with a lower number of mitotic figures in the crypts. The abnormal architecture was most pronounced in patients with the HIV antigen p24 in the intestinal mucosa and was seen in patients with and without gastrointestinal symptoms.

Several other studies[21,36,51] found villous atrophy with impaired crypt hyperplasia and crypt mitotic activity relative to the extent of villus blunting indicating an inadequate proliferative response of the intestinal mucosa to injury. The degree of mucosal damage measured in one of these studies did not correlate with the clinical stage of the disease.[21] Greenson et al.[36] showed that altered villus and crypt architecture and subnormal proliferative response in advanced HIV infection were independent of the presence of diarrhea or enteric infection. In contrast, others found morphological features resembling the histology, a celiac disease and other immune-mediated diseases of the intestine.[3]

Decreased active and passive transport of monosaccharides and increased intestinal permeability have been detected to variable degrees in patients with "HIV enteropathy", predominantly in patients presenting with chronic diarrhea. However, a correlation between the morphological architecture of the intestine and the severity of carbohydrate malabsorption is not firmly established. While ultrastructural analysis did not reveal abnormalities in the morphology of enterocytes in one study, Mathan et al.[62] showed jejunal enterocytes with proliferation of small endoplasmic reticulum, mitochondrial abnormalities, intracytoplasmatic vacuolization and intracellular deposition of fat. Additionally, Ullrich et al.[20] have detected lactase and alkaline phosphatase deficiencies in HIV-infected patients indicating incomplete maturation of the enterocyte lineage. Ileal malabsorption of vitamin B_{12}, but rarely vitamin B_{12} deficiency, has also been described in "pathogen negative" HIV-infected patients with chronic diarrhea.

The abnormal intestinal morphology and function observed in "pathogen-negative" HIV-infected patients is most likely caused by multiple pathogenetic factors. Cellular damage caused by direct intestinal infection with HIV or mediated by enhanced expression of proinflammatory cytokines released by activated mucosal lymphocytes or macrophages have been invoked as pathophysiological mechanisms. Other pathogenetic factors include mucosal depletion of CD-4 lymphocytes, abnormalities in T cell differentiation and loss of immunglobulin A-producing cells.[38] The roles of intestinal autonomic neuropathy, perturbations in the enteroendocrine system,[39] and small bowel bacterial overgrowth and enteropathy as etiologic or contributing factors remain to be determined. Finally, a partial loss of brush border disaccharide activities,[10] which may persist after small intestinal infection has been resolved, unrelated diseases such as inflammatory bowel disease or irritable bowel syndrome as well as side effects from numerous medications — probably a very significant contribution — must be considered in some patients.

The clinical consequences associated with "HIV enteropathy" are less obvious and morbidity is usually less compared to AIDS patients with opportunistic intestinal infections. The survival times of patients with AIDS and "pathogen-negative" diarrhea are considerably longer than those of patients with identifiable gut pathogens and are comparable to patients without diarrhea.[18,19,36] Wilcox et al.[18] calculated that patients with unexplained diarrhea had a median survival of 14.2 months compared with 8.3 months in those eventually found to have an enteric pathogen. Of 25 AIDS patients without a specific diagnosis, diarrhea improved or spontaneously resolved in 9 (38%). A recent British study reported a median survival of 49 months in 31 patients with AIDS and unexplained diarrhea, whereas the median survival of a matched control group with identified pathogens was only 10 months. Diarrhea resolved in the majority of these patients and was mild or intermittent in all but 3.

Absorption and permeability in AIDS patients with intestinal infections

HIV-infected patients are at risk for acquiring a variety of intestinal infections, which can impair the integrity of the intestinal mucosa and lead to the loss of specific functions. Prospective studies of chronic diarrhea in patients with AIDS suggest that identifiable enteric pathogens account for 75 to 85% of cases. Among opportunistic protozoal infections *Cryptosporidium parvum, Microsporidia, Isopora belli, Giardia lamblia,* and *Cyclospora* species can infect the small intestine of severely immunocompromised AIDS patients and are frequently diagnosed in patients with advanced HIV infection. *Salmonellae, Shigellae, Clostridium difficile, Campylobacter* species, *Mycobacterium avium,* and a number of viruses are more frequently found in the gastrointestinal tract of AIDS patients and may cause diarrhea and malabsorption. Organisms whose pathogenicity is inconsistent or uncertain (*Blastocystis hominis,* spirochaetes, some enteric viruses) are occasionally identified. Bacterial overgrowth of the upper gut has been documented in patients with AIDS with hypochlorhydria and diarrhea.

Protozoal infections

Cryptosporidium parvum

Infection with this protozoal parasite causes the initial AIDS defining manifestation in ~2% of patients with AIDS in the U.S. and in up to 50% of patients with AIDS and chronic diarrhea in developing countries. Cardinal features of the disease include chronic, persistent, large volume diarrhea that is often associated with localized abdominal pain, nausea, anorexia, hepatobiliary disease, and malabsorption of fat, D-xylose and, occasionally, vitamin B_{12}. In immune-competent hosts infection is self-limited and either remains unrecognized or causes only mild diarrhea. Although symptoms may be commonly intermittent, spontaneous cures in advanced stages of HIV infection are extremely rare.

Infection with *Cryptosporidium* occurs mainly in HIV-infected patients with severely compromised immune function (<200 CD4 cells/µl). *Cryptosporidium* can colonize the entire intestine and may extend to the biliary tree. The intensity of symptoms is determined by the extent of infection and directly correlates with the number of cysts excreted in stool. An autopsy study found that the terminal ileum was the preferred site of *Cryptosporidium* infection in AIDS patients and several studies describe a high prevalence of vitamin B_{12} malabsorption. Extension of infection to the duodenum and jejunum is associated with worse malabsorption. Five of 16 patients with *Cryptosporidium* infection had abnormal D-xylose tests in a study by Goodgame and coworkers. D-xylose absorption correlated with the number of cysts excreted in 24 hour stools as well as the duodenal extent of infection .

Microsporidia species

Microsporidia comprise a complex group of unicellular parasites that have only recently been recognized as human pathogens. Gastrointestinal microsporidiosis was first observed in humans in 1985 in electron microscope studies of the the small-bowel biopsy specimens from two patients with AIDS. The most common species implicated in diarrhea is *Enterozytozoon bieneusi*. Recent work indicates that *Microsporidia* may be the most common enteric pathogen responsible for chronic diarrhea during the advanced stages of AIDS. With various diagnostic techniques, *Microsporidia* have been detected in up to 30% of patients with AIDS and chronic unexplained diarrhea. The organism is found mostly in patients with severe immunodeficiency with CD-4 cell counts <100 cells/mm. The role of *Microsporidia* in the pathogenesis of HIV-related chronic diarrhea and intestinal malabsorption remains controversial. Eeftinck Schattenkerk et al.[55] reported microsporidiosis in 27% of AIDS patients with unexplained diarrhea compared to 3% in a matched group of AIDS patients without diarrhea. In all patients with microsporidiosis the median CD-4 cell count was ≥100 CD-4 cells/mm. Lambl et al.[73] recently found severe malabsorption and nutritional deficiencies in patients with microsporidiosis. Fecal fat and fecal weight were significantly increased in these patients compared to normal controls and patients with unexplained, pathogen-negative diarrhea. D-xylose and Schilling tests were abnormal, concomitant with reduced RBC folate and serum vitamin B_{12} levels, indicating global nutrient malabsorption. While several studies provide strong evidence that *Microsporidia* can cause diarrhea, malabsorption, and wasting, Rabeneck et al.[65] did not find a positive association between the presence of *Microsporidia* and gastrointestinal symptoms. Infection of the biliary tract by *E. bieneusi* has also been associated with AIDS-related cholangitis.The currently available data emphasize the pathogenetic role of microsporidiosis in HIV-associated gastrointestinal disease with a clinical disease spectrum ranging from asymptomatic carrier status to severe diarrhea, malabsorption, wasting, and cholangitis.

Isospora belli

Infection with *Isospora belli* may also cause severe and protracted diarrhea in patients with AIDS. The parasite is the cause of gastrointestinal infection in approximately 1 to 3% of patients with AIDS and diarrhea in the U.S. but in 15 to 19% of patients in developing countries. Clinically, isosporiasis resembles cryptosporidiosis. Watery diarrhea without blood or inflammatory cells, cramping, abdominal pain, weight loss, anorexia, malaise, and fever are usually present. Laboratory findings in isosporiasis may include steatorrhea and, in contrast to cryptosporidiosis, eosinophilia. Although heavily concentrated in the small intestine, *Isospora belli* can be identified throughout the entire gastrointestinal tract and in other organs.

Giardia lamblia

Giardia lamblia is a common source of diarrhea worldwide both in normal as well as in immunodeficient hosts. Despite the prevalence of this pathogen, the pathophysiology of *Giardia* infections is not fully understood. Clinical malabsorption in giardiasis has been associated with severe villous atrophy and crypt hyperplasia in some cases and with normal histology in others. Infection of Mongolian gerbils with a *Giardia lamblia* strain pathogenic to humans results in crypt hyperplasia and villous atrophy with electrolyte and fluid malabsorption associated with decreased absorptive surface.

Bacterial infections

Mycobacterium avium-intracellulare

It is estimated that ~40% of patients with AIDS have disseminated infections due to *M. avium-intracellulare*. Infection of the gastrointestinal tract is most often manifested as chronic diarrhea, abdominal pain, malabsorption, and wasting. Biopsy specimens of the small intestine usually show changes similar to those seen in Whipple's disease, with wide villi, dilated lacteals, and infiltration of the lamina propria with macrophages that are positive for the PAS reaction. The prevalence of *M. avium-intracellulare* enteritis among AIDS patients with chronic diarrhea is variably reported at 5 to 23%.

Clostridium difficile and other bacteria

Patients with HIV infection are subject to the same types of enteric pathogens that are encountered in the healthy population; however, their infections may be unusually severe or prolonged, and some pathogens may assume unusual virulence in the presence of immunodeficiency. Because of the frequent use of antibiotics AIDS patients are at high risk of developing diarrhea associated with *Clostridium difficile* infection. The frequency of salmonellosis among patients with HIV infection is increased approximately 20-fold over that observed for the general observation. The most common isolate is *S. typhimurium*. Patients with HIV infection also have increased rates of infection with *Shigella* species, non-jejuni strains of *Campylobacter* and possibly *Campylobacter* jejuni.

Enteric viral infections

Cytomegalovirus infects the entire gastrointestinal tract and in some patients causes severe small intestinal inflammation. Malabsorption of nutrients may result from small intestinal disease or as a complication of pancreatitis, cholangitis, and papillary stenosis. Several other viruses have been implicated as enteric pathogens in HIV-infected patients. In a study by Grohmann et al.,[26] viruses were detected in 35% of 109 fecal specimens from patients with diarrhea but in only 12% of 113 specimens from those without diarrhea. Specimens from patients with diarrhea were more likely than those from patients without diarrhea to have astrovirus, picobirnavirus, caliciviruses, including small round structured viruses, and adenoviruses as well as a mixed viral infection. These results suggest that intestinal virus infections may be more common agents of diarrhea in HIV-infected patients than bacterial and parasitic pathogens. An earlier report by Kaljot et al.[71] found that enteric viruses were more prevalent in HIV-infected patients, but not associated with diarrhea. No systematic studies are available that have investigated the importance of enteral viruses in the development of malabsorption or other signs of small intestinal dysfunction.

Intestinal malabsorption and malnutrition

Weight loss and "wasting" are hallmarks of "end stage" HIV disease and have been included as a diagnostic criterion for AIDS by the Centers for Disease Control. The development of weight loss, changes in body composition, and intestinal malabsorption predict survival in HIV-infected patients. However, the pathogenetic role and the impact of intestinal malabsorption on malnutrition and "wasting" syndrome of AIDS patients are not well defined. Several clinical and animal studies suggest that nutrient malabsorption plays an important role in the development of malnutrition and "wasting". The presence of malabsorption is negatively correlated with body weight, the mass of body compartments, and serum nutrional parameters. Carbohydrate malabsorption significantly correlated with the "body mass index",[3] and D-xylose is more pronounced in patients with AIDS and "wasting syndrome" than in patients with only minor changes in body weight.[4] Furthermore, in AIDS patients with abnormal D-xylose tests body weight, body mass index, body cell mass, and the serum nutrition parameters (LDL, albumin, etc.) are significantly reduced.

Whether or not the correlation of malabsorption with the extent of malnutrition in HIV-infected patients implies a pathogenetic role for the intestine or rather reflects a consequence of the "wasting syndrome" cannot be answered by these studies. It is, however, obvious that other pathogenetic factors, i.e., reduced food intake and hypermetabolism, participate in the development of HIV-related malnutrition and "wasting" as changes in body composition, weight loss, and imbalances in the vitamin and micronutrient levels also occur in patients without clinical intestinal disease.

Clinical diagnosis of intestinal malabsorption

Malabsorption in HIV-infected patients may significantly contribute to weight loss, malaise, morbidity, and to uncertainties about the bioavailability of medical therapy as well as to diminished success and reduced tolerance of nutritional support. Regarding all these aspects, malabsorption correlates to both a reduced quality of life and diminished survival. Therefore, symptoms of malabsorption such as diarrhea, steatorrhea, weight loss, or signs of nutritional deficiencies should initiate a careful workup for treatable etiologies of malabsorption. In the first step this requires performing stool cultures for identifiable bacteria, ELISA or microscopy for giardiasis, and specific staining for *Cryptosporidia*. With a positive pathogen identified, this should be treated before further diagnostic tests are performed.

Although fecal fat analysis forms part of our daily routine in patients with malabsorption, we do not collect feces of HIV-infected patients for the analysis of fecal fat. Similarly, we do not recommend (or use) $^{13}CO_2$- or $^{14}CO_2$-breath tests for assessing fat absorption in AIDS patients because endogenous CO_2 production cannot be anticipated to be normal. Usually, serum levels of β-carotene may serve as an indicator for the malabsorption of fat, and in case of steatorrhea (mean fecal fat >7gm/d) serum β-carotene concentration is <47 µg/100 ml).

Small intestinal absorptive capacity may be assessed by the 25gm D-xylose test which is considered abnormal if urinary excretion is <4 gm (26.6 mmol)/5 h. after xylose ingestion. Serum D-xylose concentrations after the administration of 25 gm of the pentose (in 600 ml of weak tea or water) normally exceed 10 mg/100 ml at 15 min and 30 mg (2 mmol/l)/100 ml at 1 and 2 h. An abnormal D-xylose test not only indicates a significant intestinal pathology but also may be considered a limiting factor for enteral nutrition strategies and will require further investigation. Because mucosal atrophy, small bowel bacterial overgrowth, and motility disturbance (markedly delayed transit as well as intestinal hurry) may contribute to an abnormal D-xylose test, diagnostic tests for these conditions should be used. These include primarily upper gastrointestinal endoscopy including an adequate number of duodenal biopsies (at least 3 specimens for histology), specific staining for *Microsporidia* (or even asservation for electron microscopy), search for *Cryptosporidia* and lambliasis). In the same endoscopy it is wise to look for gastric pH in addition to other gastric and esophageal pathologies.

Diagnosis of small bowel bacterial overgrowth is difficult because established diagnostic tests such as the H_2 breath test, after (80 gm) glucose usually have only about 60–70% sensitivity, and the frequent use of antibiotics in HIV-infected and AIDS patients will further deteriorate their utility. However, this test is both rapid and convenient, and while there is no really superior test at hand, a positive test may guide therapeutic decisions.

The same holds true for lactose tolerance testing with the H_2 breath test after administration of 50 gm of lactose. We perform this test on HIV-infected and AIDS patients for the detection of lactose malabsorption, which is much more frequently a significant etiology of bloating than of diarrhea. Antibiotics do not *a priori* preclude the use of H_2 breath tests, but some interference has to be taken into account. The simultaneous analysis of blood glucose increments may be helpful (to some extent) in reducing the number of false negative results with the H_2 breath test.

While a number of subtle motility tests are among the armamentarium of contemporary gastroenterology, they are not of substantial clinical value in decision making, i.e., establishing the cause of malabsorption in HIV-infected or AIDS patients. Instead, we prefer to perform an enteroclysma of the small bowel (Sellink) which not only gives valuable information about delayed or accelerated transit, but additionally discloses mucosal edema, ulcerations, evidence for intestinal Kaposi's sarcoma, or lymphoma and fistula.

References

1. Süttmann, U., Ockenga, J., Selberg, O., Hoogestraat, L., Deicher, H., and Müller M.J., Incidence and prognostic value of malnutrition and wasting in human immunodeficiency virus-infected outpatients, *J. Acquir. Immune Defic. Syndr.*, 8, 239, 1995.
2. Goodgame, R.W., Kimball, K., Ou, C.-N., Clinton White, A., Genta, R.M., Lifschitz, C.H., and Chappell, C.L., Intestinal function and injury in acquired immunodeficiency syndrome-related cryptosporidiosis, *Gastroenterology*, 108, 1075, 1995.
3. Keating, J., Bjarnason, I., Somasundaram, S., Mcpherson, A., Francis, N., Price, A.B., Sharpstone, D., Smithson, J., Menzies, I.S., and Gazzard, B.G., Intestinal absorptive capacity, intestinal permeability and jejunal histology in HIV and their relation to diarrhea, *Gut*, 37, 623, 1995.
4. Ehrenpreis, E.D., Ganger, D.R., Kochvar, G.T., Patterson, B.K., and Craig, R.M., D-xylose malabsorption: characteristic finding in patients with AIDS wasting syndrome and chronic diarrhea, *J. Acquir. Immune Defic. Syndr.*, 5, 1047, 1992.
5. Ehrenpreis, E.D., Patterson, B.K., Brainer, J.A., Yokoo, H., Rademaker, A.W., Glogowski, W., Noskin, G.A., and Craig, R.M., Histopathological findings of duodenal biopsy specimens in HIV-infected patients with and without diarrhea and malabsorption, *Am. J. Clin. Pathol.*, 97, 21, 1992.
6. Stone, J.D., Heise, C.C., Miller, Ch. J., Halsted, C.H., and Dandekar, S., Development of malabsorption and nutritional complications in simian immunodeficiency virus-infected rhesus macaques, *AIDS*, 8, 1245, 1994.
7. Ott, M., Lembcke, B., and Caspary, W.F., Intestinale Permeabilität von niedermolekularen Zuckern bei chronisch-endzündlichen Darmerkrankungen, Ökosystem Darm II, Ottenjann, R., Müller, J., Seifert, J. (Hrsg.), 23, 1990.
8. Ott, M., Lembcke, B., Staszewski, S., Helm, E.B., and Caspary, W.F., Intestinale Permeabilität bei Patienten mit erworbenem Immundefekt-Syndrom (AIDS), *Klin. Wochenschr.* 69, 715, 1991.
9. Lembcke, B. and Ott, M., Intestinale Permeabilitätsstörungen als ätiologischer Faktor bei M. Crohn — F(r)iktionen und Fakten, *Z. Gastroenterol.*, 29, 407, 1991.
10. Ott, M., Lembcke, B., Herrmann, G., Windmann, A., Dillmann, E., and Caspary, W.F., Intestinal polyamine metabolism and disaccharidases in AIDS — influence of intestinal cytomegalovirus infection. Polyamines in the gastrointestinal tract: proceedings of the 62nd Falk Symposium (Titisee/Black Forest, Germany), Dowling, R.H., Fölsch, U.R., and Löser, C., Eds., 263, 1991.
11. Ott, M., Lembcke, B., Fischer, H., Jaeger, R., Polat, H., Geier, H., Rech, M., Staszewski, S., and Caspary, W.F., Early changes of body composition in human immunodeficiency virus-infected patients: tetrapolar impedance analysis indicates significant malnutrition, *Am. J. Clin. Nutr.*, 57, 15, 1993.
12. Ott, M., Wegner, A., Caspary, W.F., and Lembcke, B., Intestinal absorption and malnutrition in patients with the acquired immunodeficiency syndrome (AIDS), *Z. Gastroenterol.*, 31, 661, 1993.

13. Lembcke, B., Schulte Bockholt, A., Wehrmann, T., Ott, M., and Caspary, W.F., Ernährungsstatus und Ernährungstherapie bei HIV-Infizierten, Ökosystem Darm VI, Caspary, W.F. et al. (Hrsg.), 47, 1994.

14. Ott, M., Fischer, H., Polat, H., Helm, E.B., Frenz, M., Caspary, W.F., Lembcke, B., Bioelectrical impedance analysis as a predictor of survival in patients with human immunodeficiency virus infection, *J. Acquir. Immune Defic. Syndr.*, 9, 20, 1995.

15. Heise, C., Vogel, P., Halsted, CH., and Dandekar, S., Simian immunodeficiency virus infection of the gastrointestinal tract: functional, pathological and morphological changes, *Am. J. Pathol.*, 142, 1759, 1993.

16. Schneider, T., Jahn, H.-U., Schmidt, W., Riecken, E.-O., Zeitz, M., Ullrich, U., and the Berlin Diarrhea/Wasting Study Group, Loss of CD4 T lymphocytes in patients infected with human immunodeficiency virus type 1 is more pronounced in the duodenal mucosa than in peripheral blood, *Gut*, 37, 524, 1995.

17. McGowan, I., Radford-Smith, G., and Jewell, D.P., Cytokine gene expression in HIV-infected intestinal mucosa, *AIDS*, 8, 1569, 1994.

18. Wilcox, C.M., Schwartz, D.A., Cotsonis, G., and Thompson, S.E., III, Chronic unexplained diarrhea in human immunodeficiency virus infection: determination of the best diagnostic approach, *Gastroenterology*, 110, 30, 1996.

19. Connolly, G.M., Forbes, A., and Gazzard, B.G., Investigation of seemingly pathogen-negative diarrhoea in patients with HIV1, *Gut*, 31, 886, 1990.

20. Ullrich, R., Zeitz, M., Heise, W., L`age, M., Hoffken, G., and Riecken, E.O., Small intestinal structure and function in patients infected with human immunodeficiency virus infection (HIV): evidence for HIV-induced enteropathy, *Ann. Intern. Med.*, 111, 15, 1989.

21. Batman, P.A., Miller A.R.O, Forster, S.M., Harris, J.R.W., and Pinching, A.J., Jejunal enteropathy associated with human immunodeficiency virus infection: quantitative histology, *J., Clin., Pathol.*, 42, 275, 1989.

22. Carlson, S., Yokoo, H., and Craig, R.M., Small intestinal HIV-associated enteropathy: evidence for panintestinal enterocyte dysfunction, *J. Lab. Clin. Med.*, 124, 652, 1994.

23. Blanshard, C. and Gazzard, B.G., Natural history and prognosis of diarrhoea of unknown cause in patients with acquired immunodeficiency syndrome, *Gut*, 36, 283, 1995.

24. Bartlett, J.G., Belitsos, P.C., and Sears, C.L., AIDS enteropathy, *Clin. Infect. Dis.*, 15, 726, 1992.

25. Kotler, D.P., Gaetz, H.P., and Lang, M., Enteropathy associated with the acquired immunodeficiency syndrome, *Ann. Intern. Med.*, 101, 421, 1984.

26. Grohmann, G.S., Glass, R.I., Pereira, H.G., Monroe, S.S., Hightower, A.W., Weber, R., and Bryan, R.T., Enteric viruses and diarrhea in HIV-infected patients, *N. Engl. J. Med.*, 329, 14, 1993.

27. Lim, S.G., Menzies, I.S., Lee, C.A., Johnson, M.A., and Pounder, R.E., Intestinal permeability and function in patients infected with human immunodeficiency virus, *Scand. J. Gastroenterol.*, 28, 573, 1993.

28. Pignata, C., Budillon, G., Monaco, G., Nani, E., Cuomo, R., Parilli, G., and Ciccimara, F., Jejunal bacterial overgrowth and intestinal permeability in children with immunodeficiency syndromes, *Gut*, 31, 879, 1990.

29. Tepper, R.E., Simon, D., Brandt, L.J., Nutovits, R., and Lee, M.J., Intestinal permeability in patients infected with the human immunodeficiency virus, *Am. J. Gastroenterol.*, 89, 878, 1994.

30. Heise, C., Miller, C.J., Lackner, A., and Dandekar, S., Primary acute SIV-infection of intestinal lymphoid tissue is associated with gastrointestinal dysfunction, *J. Infect. Dis.*, 169, 1116, 1994.

31. Gillin, J.S., Shike, M., Alcock, N., et al., Malabsorption and mucosal abnormalities in of the small intestine in the acquired immunodeficiency syndrome, *Ann. Intern. Med.*, 102, 619, 1985.

32. Dworkin, B., Wormser, G.P., Rosenthal, W.S., et al., Gastrointestinal manifestations of the acquired immunodeficiency syndrome: a review of 22 cases, *Am. J. Gastroenterol.*, 80, 774, 1985.

33. Buret, A., Hardin, J.A., Olson, M., E., and Gall, D.G., Pathophysiology of small intestinal malabsorption in gerbils infected with Giardia lamblia, *Gastroenterology*, 103, 506, 1992.

34. Cotte, L., Rabodonirina, M., Piens, M.A., Perreard, M., Mojon, M., and Trepo, C., Prevalence of intestinal protozoans in French patients infected with HIV, *J. Acquir. Immune Defic. Syndr.*, 6, 1024, 1993.

35. Yolken, R.H., Hart, W., Oung, I., Shiff, C., Greenson, J., and Perman, J.A., Gastrointestinal dysfunction and disaccharide intolerance in children infected with human immunodeficiency virus, *J. Pediatrics*, 118, 359, 1991.

36. Greenson, J.K., Belitsos, P.C., Yardley, J.H., and Bartlett, J.G., AIDS enteropathy: occult enteric infections and duodenal mucosal alterations in chronic diarrhea, *Ann. Intern. Med.*, 114, 366, 1991.

37. Ullrich, R., Heise, W., Bergs, C., L`age, M., Riecken, E.O., and Zeitz, M., Effects of zidovudine treatment on the small intestinal mucosa in patients infected with the human immunodeficiency virus, *Gastroenterology*, 102, 1483, 1992.

38. Janoff, E.N., Jackson, S., Wahl, S.M., Thomas, K., Petermann, J.H., and Smith, P.D., Intestinal mucosal immunoglobulins during human immunodeficiency virus type 1 infection, *J. Infect. Dis.*, 170, 299, 1994.

39. Sharkey, K.A., Sutherland, L.R., Davison, J.S., Zwiers, H., Gill, M.J., and Church, D.L., Peptides in the gastrointestinal tract in human immunodeficiency virus infection, The GI/HIV Study Group of the University of Calgary, *Gastroenterology*, 103, 18, 1992.

40. Genta, R.M., Chapell, C.L., White, A.C., Kimball, K.T., and Goodgame, R.W., Duodenal morphology and intensity of infection in AIDS-related intestinal cryptosporidiosis, *Gastroenterology*, 105, 1769, 1993.

41. Benhamou, Y., Kapel, N., Hoang, C., Matta, H., Meillet, D., Magne, D., Raphael, M., Gentilini, M., Opolon, P., and Gobert, J G., Inefficacy of intestinal secretory immune reponse to Cryptosporidium in acquired immunodeficiency syndrome, *Gastroenterology*, 108, 627, 1995.

42. Laine, L, Garcia, F., McGilligan, K., Malinko, A., Sinatra, F.R., and Thomas, D.W., Protein loosing enteropathy and hypalbuminemia in AIDS, *AIDS*, 7, 837, 1993.

43. Pol, S., Romana, C.A., Richard, S., Amouyal, P., Desportes-Livage, I., Carnot, F., Pays, J.S., and Berthelot, P., Microsporidia infection in patients with the human immunodeficiency virus and unexplained cholangitis, *N. Engl. J. Med.*, 328, 95, 1993.

44. Smith, P.D., Quinn, T.C., Strober, W., Janoff, E.N., and Masur, H., NIH Conference. Gastrointestinal infections in AIDS, *Ann. Int. Med.*, 116, 63, 1992.

45. Kotler, D.R. and Orenstein, J.M., Chronic diarrhea and malabsorption associated with enteropathogenic bacterial infection in a patient with AIDS, *Ann. Int. Med.*, 119, 127, 1993.

46. Kotler, D.P., Reka, S., and Clayton, F., Intestinal mucosal inflammation associated with human immunodeficiency virus infection, *Dig. Dis. Sci.*, 38, 1119, 1993.
47. Smith, G.H., Treatment of infections in the patient with acquired immunodeficiency syndrome, *Arch. Int. Med.*, 154, 949, 1994.
48. Budhraja, M.D., Levendoglu, H., Kocka, F., Mangkornkanok, M., and Sherer, M., Duodenal mucosal T-cell subpopulation and bacterial cultures in acquired immunodeficiency syndrome, *Am. J. Gastroenterol.*, 82, 427, 1987.
49. Belitsos, P.C., Greenson, J.K., Yardley, J.H., Sisler, J., and Bartlett, J.G., Association of gastric hypoacidity with opportunistic enteric infections in patients with AIDS, *J. Infect. Dis.*, 166, 277, 1992.
50. Batman, P.A., Miller, A.R.O., Sedgwick, P.M., and Griffin, G.E., Autonomic denervation of jejunal mucosa of homosexual men with HIV, *AIDS*, 5, 1247, 1991.
51. Cummins, A.G., Labrooy, J.T., Stanley, D.P., Rowland, R., and Shearman, D.J.C., Quantitative histological study of enteropathy associated with HIV infection, *Gut*, 31, 317, 1990.
52. Lubeck, D.P., Bennett, C.L., Mazonson, P.D., Fifer, S.K., and Fries, J.F., Quality of life and health service use among HIV-infected patients with chronic diarrhea, *J. Acquir. Immune Defic. Syndr.*, 6, 478, 1993.
53. Pape, J.W., Verdier, R.I., Boncy, M., Boncy, J., and Johnson, W.D., Cyclospora infection in adults infected with HIV; clinical manifestations, treatment and prophylaxis, *Ann. Int. Med.*, 121, 654, 1994.
54. Kotler, D.P. and Orenstein, J.M., Prevalence of intestinal microsporidiosis in HIV-infected individuals referred for gastroenterological diagnosis, *Am. J. Gastroenterol.*, 89, 1998, 1994.
55. Eeftinck Schattenkerk, J.K.M., Van Gool, V., Van Ketel, R.J., Bartelsman, J.F.W.M., Kuiken, C.L., Terpstra, W.J., and Reiss, P., Clinical significance of small intestinal microsporidiosis in HIV-infected individuals, *Lancet*, 337, 895, 1991.
56. Simon, D. and Brandt, L.J., Diarrhea in patients with the acquired immunodeficiency syndrome, *Gastroenterology*, 105, 1238, 1993.
57. Orenstein, J.M., Tenner, M., and Kotler, D.P., Localization of infection by microsporidian Enterocytozoon bieneusi in the gastrointestinal tract of AIDS patients with diarrhea, *AIDS*, 6, 195, 1992.
58. Ortega, Y.R., Sterling C.R., Gilman, R.H. et al., Cyclospora species: a new protozoan pathogen in humans, *N. Engl. J. Med.*, 328, 1308, 1993.
59. Editorial, HIV enteropathy, *Lancet*, 777, 1989.
60. Kapembwa, M.S., Batman, P.A., Fleming, S.C., and Griffin, G.E., HIV-enteropathy (letter), *Lancet*, 2, 1521, 1989.
61. Kapembwa, M.S., Fleming, S.C., Sewankambo, N. et al., Altered small intestinal permeability associated with diarrhoea in human immunodeficiency virus infected Caucasian and African subjects, *Clin. Sci.*, 81, 327, 1991.
62. Mathan, M.M., Griffin, G.E., Miller A. et al., Ultrastructure of the jejunal mucosa in human immunodeficiency virus infection, *J. Pathol.*, 161, 119, 1990.
63. Harriman, G.R., Smith, P.D., Horne, N.K., et al., Vitamin B_{12} malabsorption in patients with acquired immunodeficiency syndrome, *Arch. Int. Med.*, 149, 2039, 1989.
64. Smith, P.D., Lane, C., Gill, V.J., et al., Intestinal infections in patients with the acquired immunodeficiency syndrome (AIDS), *Ann. Int. Med.*, 108, 328, 1988.

65. Rabeneck, L., Gyorkey, F., Genta, R.M., Gyorkey, P., Foote, L.W., and Risser, J.M.H., The role of Microsporidia in the pathogenesis of HIV-related chronic diarrhea, *Ann. Int. Med.*, 119, 895, 1993.
66. DeHovitz, J.A., Pape, J.W., Boncy, M. et al., Clinical manifestations and therapy of Isospora belli infection in patients with the acquired immunodeficiency syndrome, *N. Engl. J. Med.*, 315, 87, 1986.
67. Greenson, J.K., Belitsos, P.C., and Bartlett, J.G., AIDS enteropathy (letter), *Ann. Int. Med.*, 115, 328, 1991.
68. Soave, R. and Johnson, W.D., *Cryptosporidium* and *Isospora belli* infections, *J. Infect. Dis.*, 157, 225, 1988.
69. Payne, P., Lancaster, L.A., Heinzman, M., and McCutchan, J.A., Identification of Cryptosporidium in patients with acquired immunodeficiency syndrome (letter), *N. Engl. J. Med.*, 309, 613, 1984.
70. Levine, W.C., Buehler, J.W., Bean, N.H., and Tauxe, R.V., Epidemiology of non-typhoidal *Salmonella bacteremia* during the human immunodeficiency virus epidemic, *J. Infect. Dis.*, 164, 81, 1981.
71. Kaljot, K.T., Ling, J.P., Gold, J.W. M., et al., Prevalence of acute enteric viral pathogens in acquired immunodeficiency syndrome, *Gastroenterology*, 97, 1031, 1989.
72. Miller, R.F. and Semple, S.J.G., Autonomic neuropathy in AIDS, *Lancet*, 2, 343, 1987.
73. Lambl, B.B., Federman, M., Pleskow, D., and Wanke, C.A., Malabsorption and wasting in AIDS patients with *Microsporidia* and pathogen-negative diarrhea, *AIDS*, 10, 739, 1996.

chapter nine

Malabsorption of nutrients and drugs in patients with AIDS and mycobacteriosis and their obviation by parenteral therapy

Lawrence A. Cone

Mycobacteria have in the past been known to infect the gastrointestinal tract. These infections involving *Mycobacterium tuberculosis* and *Mycobacterium bovis* gradually all but vanished in the developed nations of the world with the use of effective chemotherapy, public health measures, and tuberculin testing of dairy herds. Since 1982 a dramatic recurrence of mycobacterial infections of the gastrointestinal tract became apparent due to a hitherto unknown gastrointestinal pathogen, *Mycobacterium avium-intracellulare*. This unusual pulmonary pathogen, well-recognized in the southeastern U.S., had previously been recorded to have caused only 24 cases of disseminated mycobacterial disease.[1] Within five years of the onset of the human immunodeficiency virus (HIV) pandemic, *M. avium-intracellulare* (MAI) was noted to be the most common bacterial infection in this population of patients,[2] and is now the third most common opportunistic disease in the U.S. associated with the acquired immunodeficiency syndrome (AIDS).[3] Simultaneously, evidence for extrapulmonary tuberculosis has also increased in HIV+ individuals, being higher among parenteral substance abusers and persons born in Haiti, the Phillipines, Mexico, Central America, and Africa.[4]

Epidemiology

MAI is an ubiquitous, environmental organism that can be isolated from numerous sources including water, dust, aerosols, soil, mud, plants, poultry and livestock, and their products.[5] Although MAI has worldwide distribution,[6] overall isolation rates are higher in developed vs. developing countries principally because piped water systems have higher isolation rates compared to rivers and lakes. In Finland, where nontuberculous mycobacteria were recovered from 100% of brook water samples, it would appear that high organic content and low pH favor mycobacterial isolation.[7] For the same reasons river and streams appear to supply higher yields of MAI than lakes.

The *M. avium-intracellulare* complex is divided into many serotypes, with serovars 1,4, and 8 predominating in patients with AIDS. Restriction fragment length polymorphism studies show that most are identical at the molecular level and distinct from the mycobacteria isolated from the stools of healthy subjects. The close identity of these strains suggests that they are clonal in origin.[8]

Skin testing with *M. avium* sensitin in the U.S., Finland, Kenya, and Trinidad demonstrate similar, low levels of positivity in healthy persons indicating that the high frequency of disease in the U.S. and the low incidence in Africa does not relate to reactivation.[6] In all likelihood the high frequency of disseminated MAI in developed nations depends upon a total lower CD4+ cell count and reinfection due to exposure to mycobacterial contamination of residential and hospital water supply systems.

Another nontuberculous mycobacterium, *M. xenopi*, which was originally isolated from a cutaneous lesion of a laboratory frog used for pregnancy testing,[9] is also an enviromental organism present in cats, swine, and hospital hot-water taps.[10] Found considerably more often in France, England, and Canada[11] than the U.S., disseminated disease has now been reported in patients with AIDS.[12-14] In three patients seen at the Eisenhower Medical Center with clinical *M. xenopi* infections, two had gastrointestinal involvement.[15]

Pathogenesis

MAI displays little virulence in the normal host and asymptomatic colonization of the respiratory or gastrointestinal tract can occur.[16] In contrast HIV+ persons, particularly those with <50 CD4+/mm³ cell counts, dissemination may ensue. Chin et al.[17] noted a substantial risk for developing MAI bacteremia when CD4 cells were <50/mm³ — 45% within one year and 60% when the organism was isolated from sputum or stool. The portal of entry of the organism is either the respiratory or gastrointestinal tract. Histopathologic studies by Klatt et al.[18] and Wallace and Hannah[19] indicate that the latter is twice as common as the former. Once disseminated disease is established, then both organ systems may be secondarily involved.

Studies with mice would indicate that the ability of the host to resist infection with mycobacteria is strongly dependent upon expression of a single gene, *Bcg*. Expression of these alleles influences the priming of host macrophages for bactericidal function.[20,21] Ultrastructural analyses reveal that phagosome-lysosome fusion is enhanced in *Bcg*-resistant mouse cells leading to restricted growth and degradation of *M. avium*.[22] Adverse direct or indirect influences upon this macrophage function in patients with AIDS allows survival and proliferation of *M. avium* in macrophages. Consequently, the histiocytes are engorged with acid-fast bacilli resulting in tissue burdens of nearly 10 billion colony forming units per gram.[23] Given the known impairment in cell-mediated immunity with HIV+ infection, it appears logical to assume that certain cytokines other than gamma interferon[24] play significant roles. These include migration inhibition factor, tumor necrosis factor, interleukin-2 and granulocyte-macrophage colony-stimulating factor.[24-27] When macrophages are doubly infected *in vitro* with both HIV and *M. avium*, then decreased macrophage survival is noted as well as protracted cytokine production especially tumor necrosis factor alpha and interleukins-6 and 1-beta.[28]

With progression and subsequent hematogenous dissemination of the *M. avium* many organs may be involved. Aside from both small and large intestine and lung we have observed brain abscessses, thyroiditis, esophageal and gastric ulcerations, liver and splenic involvement, lymphadenopathy and buboes, and skin nodules. Others have also described meningeal disease and ocular, tongue, breast, parathyroid, adrenal, kidney, pancreas, prostate, and testicular involvement.[25]

Clinical studies

Sooner or later the patient develops symptoms associated with disseminated mycobacteriosis. These include fever, night sweats, abdominal pain, fatigue, weight loss, and diarrhea. In 1982 gastrointestinal involvement by MAI was first reported by Zakowski et al.[29] Since then considerable clinical and pathologic data have accumulated with regard to the cause and results of the symptomatology of intestinal mycobacterial infection.

Clinical intestinal mycobacteriosis results from direct invasion of the lamina propria of the intestine by infected macrophages in addition to Peyer's patches, and mesenteric and retroperitoneal lymph nodes. Furthermore, it is likely that several cytokines including tumor necrosis factor alpha and interleukins-1 and 6 may alter the growth of MAI and play significant roles in the development of diarrhea and weight loss.[30] Massive thickening of the proximal intestine may result.[31]

The overlying villi may be deformed in patients with extensive disease. As a result of lymphatic infiltration and an intramucosal block in lymphatic flow, the pathophysiology of gastrointestinal dysfunction is similar to Whipple's disease,[32] resulting in malabsorption and an exudative enteropathy.[31] The duodenum is usually most extensively involved. Figure 9.1 depicts the endoscopic appearance of small, white tubercles extensively studding the duodenal mucosa in a patient with *M. avium* infection. Figure 9.2 demonstrates the dense infection of the macrophages by acid fast bacilli.

We have investigated a number of patients with histologically and bacteriologically confirmed *M. avium* infection of the small bowel. Most patients present with positive blood cultures for MAI, but in some the diagnosis can

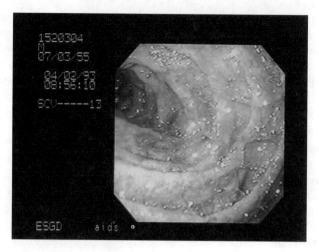

Figure 9.1 Endoscopic appearance of small, white tubercles extensively studding the duodenal mucosa in patient with *M. avium* infection.

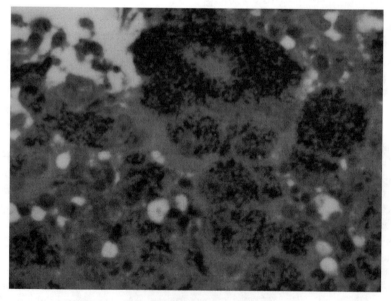

Figure 9.2 Dense infection of macrophages by acid fast bacilli.

only be established by small bowel biopsy even in the face of a relatively normal appearing duodenum. The mean patient age was 38 years and all but one (a parenteral substance abuser) were gay males. All expressed less than 50 CD4+ cells/mm^3. When HIV viral levels were measured, they were significantly elevated in all patients. The time interval from the discovery of HIV+ to the diagnosis of MAI enterocolitis ranged between 3 months and 9 years.

Laboratory studies invariably revealed an anemia, which was often recalcitrant despite successful antimycobacterial therapy. Neutropenia and thrombocytopenia were not uncommon. Platelet bound antibodies were studied in some patients but never identified. In two patients cardiolipin antibodies were identified in moderate titer, principally in the IgG class. Liver function studies were often abnormal, particularly the alkaline phosphatase and gamma glutamyl transpeptidase reflecting probable hepatic infection by *M. avium*. In four individuals concommitant chronic hepatitis B was also identified, but in these individuals the transaminases were also elevated. The serum carotene was uniformly depressed. In two patients a persistent elevation of thyroid T4 was noted, an important consideration in a patient with weight loss. Further testing failed to demonstrate hyperthyroidism, but did reveal an elevation of thyroid-binding globulin, which is likely responsible for the spurious elevation of the T4. Hypercalcemia, leading to transient azotemia, was also noted in two patients, probably secondary to an elevation of calcitriol known to accompany granulomatous mycobacterial disease.[33] Hypercalcemia has also been attributed to T-cell lymphoma and cytomegalovirus infection as well as HIV.[34,35]

Computerized tomography (CT) of the abdomen often reveals a marked enlargement of both the mesenteric and retroperitoneal lymph nodes. When indicated these abdominal nodes have been aspirated using a fine needle technique and generally yield large numbers of acid-fast bacilli that grow MAI.

Malabsorption is known to occur in patients with AIDS-related enteropathy where no offending pathogen is identified in the gastrointestinal tract. In such individuals DNA hybridization studies have demonstrated HIV in mononuclear cells in the lamina propria.[36] More often however, a variety of bacterial, fungal and parasitic organisms invade the intestinal mucosa leading to chronic infection and malabsorption. A companion paper in this volume deals with microsporidiosis and malabsorption.[37]

We have studied ten patients with small intestinal MAI infection with regard to both macronutrient and drug malabsorption. On a hospital diet, stool studies for fat done over 24 hours for 2 consecutive days revealed greater than 10 grams of fat/24 hours in all but one patient. Similarly D-xylose studies revealed less than 20 mg/ml in serum at 2 hours and less than 5 gms in urine at 5 hours in all patients. These findings are indicative of both fat and carbohydrate malabsorption and undoubtedly lead to wasting — defined as an involuntary weight loss of >10% body weight plus chronic diarrhea or chronic weakness and fever for >30 days. Although wasting appears to be more related to loss of lean body mass rather than fat, as seen in starvation, measuring weight remains much easier on a practical basis.[38]

We have utilized parenteral nutrition to counteract weight loss associated with malabsorption in patients with intestinal MAI. Previous studies by Kotler et al.[39] indicated that patients with AIDS and decreased intake or malabsorption gained weight with parenteral nutrition, while those without these characteristics but with systemic infection did not. In our patient population weight gain was nearly always associated with the use of parenteral nutrition both in hospital and as outpatients. Additionally in those with poor appetites, megesterol acetate was prescribed as well.[40,41]

The treatment of *M. avium* infection has improved significantly since the introduction of the newer macrolides, clarithromycin and azithromycin. Our most recent preferred regimen includes azithromycin, ethambutal, and rifabutin in accordance with a recent study by Shafran and colleagues.[42] Yet, our greatest experience is with clarithromycin, ethambutal, and clofazimine. The observation that single drug therapy[43] is ineffective in treating MAI infection consequently necessitates the use of a combined drug regimen. Our studies with oral therapy with clofazimine and ethambutal indicate poor absorption of both drugs with conventional drug dosing. Therapeutic blood levels of 0.5 to 2 μg/ml and 2 to 5 μg/ml respectively are rarely achieved. As a result it is usually necessary to increase the dosage of both drugs in order to achieve therapeutic values. In some instances visual difficulties develop since either drug may cause optic neuritis or a retinopathy.[44] In addition to increasing oral dosages, we have used intravenous therapy to obviate drug malabsorption. Amikacin, intravenous rifampin, and ciprofloxacin are often effective agents with good *in vitro* activity against *M. avium*.

As a consequence of these therapeutic manipulations we have been able to significantly prolong survival in this group of patients with advanced intestinal mycobacteriosis. Indeed, no patient appears to have succumbed to MAI infection alone, but rather from unrelated bacterial and fungal pneumonia, lactic acidosis, lymphoma, endocarditis, and effects of widespread Kaposi's sarcoma. Since we first presented our data on the treatment of *M. avium*-related enterocolitis in 1989,[45] survival has improved from a median of 6 to 17 months. With the use of newer combinations of effective antimycobacterial agents, and adjustments made for decreased absorption as well as the selective need for parenteral therapy, survival times should continue to improve. There is recent experimental and clinical evidence to show that liposomal encapsulation may serve to augment drug efficacy and reduce toxicity.

Finally, the issue of the development of antimicrobial resistant strains of *M. avium* needs to be addressed in addition to the clinical value of *in vitro* antimycobacterial testing. We continue to use these sensitivity studies to guide our therapy and make necessary changes in the therapeutic regimen based upon those results. We have also noted the development of mycobacterial resistance during therapy and alter the drug regimen accordingly.

Summary

Intestinal infection by *M. avium-intracellulare* complex has evolved into a very common complication of HIV infection. It is currently the third most common opportunistic disease in patients with AIDS. The disorder is most commonly encountered in developed countries, probably secondary to lower CD4 cell counts and contamination of residential and hospital water supply systems. With advanced disease patients develop weakness, weight loss, fever, and diarrhea. Blood cultures and CT abdominal scans usually confirm the diagnosis, although endoscopy with biopsy is sometimes required for confirmation of the diagnosis. Most patients develop a wasting syndrome due to malabsorption. Additionally, drug therapy may be ineffective due to poor absorption. We have attempted to obviate these absorptive problems by parenteral hyperalimentation and increasing oral drug dosing or by intravenous administration of antimycobacterial drugs. In our experience, survival of patients with this disorder has, consequently, significantly improved. New drug regimens and liposomal encapsulation will add increased efficacy to the management of mycobacterial infections of the gastrointestinal tract in the future.

References

1. Horsburgh, C.R. Jr., Mason, U.G., III, Farhi, D.C., and Iseman, M.D., Disseminated infection with *Mycobacterium avium-intracellulare, Medicine* (Baltimore), 64, 36, 1985.
2. Hawkins, C.C., Gold, J.W.M., Whimbey, E., Kiehn, T.E., Brannon, P., Cammarata, R., Brown, A.E., and Armstrong, D., *Mycobacterium avium* complex infections in patients with the acquired immunodeficiency syndrome, *Ann. Intern. Med.*, 105, 184, 1986.
3. Horsburgh, C.R. Jr., Advances in the prevention and treatment of *Mycobacterium avium* disease (editorial), *N. Engl. J. Med.*, 335, 428, 1996.
4. Slutsker, L., Castro, K.G., Ward, J.W., and Dooley, S.W. Jr., Epidemiology of extrapulmonary tuberculosis among persons with AIDS in the United States., *Clin. Infect. Dis.*, 16, 513, 1993.
5. Grange, J.M., Yates, M.D., and Broughton, E., The avian tubercle bacillus and its relatives, *J. Appl. Bacteriol.*, 68, 411, 1990.
6. von Reyn, C.F., Waddell, R.D., Eaton, T. et al., Isolation of *Mycobacterium avium* complex from water in the United States, Finland, Zaire, and Kenya, *J. Clin. Microbiol.*, 31, 3227, 1993.
7. Iivanainen, E.K., Martikainen, P.J., Vaananen, P.K., and Katila, M.L., Environmental factors affecting the occurrence of mycobacteria in brook waters, *Appl. Environ. Microbiol.*, 59, 398, 1993.
8. Hampson, S.J., Thompson, J., Moss, M.I., Portaels, F., Green, E.P., Herman-Taylor, J., and McFadden, J.J., DNA probes demonstrate a single highly conserved strain of Mycobacterium avium infecting AIDS patients, *Lancet*, 1, 65, 1989.
9. Schwabacher, H., A strain of Mycobacterium isolated from skin lesions of a cold-blooded animal, *Xenopus laevis*, and its relation to atypical acid-fast bacilli occurring in man, *J. Hyg.* (London), 57, 56, 1959.
10. Sniadack, D.H., Ostroff, S.M., Karlix, M.A., Smithwick, R.W., Schwartz, B., Sprauer, M.A., Silcox, V.A., and Good, R.C., A nosocomial pseudo-outbreak of *Mycobacterium xenopi* due to a contaminated potable water supply:lessons in prevention, *Infect. Control Hosp. Epidemiol.*, 14, 636, 1993.

11. Simor, A.E., Salit, I.E., and Vellend, H., The role of *Mycobacterium xenopi* in human disease, *Am. Rev. Respir. Dis.*, 129, 435, 1984.

12. Eng, R.H.K., Forrester, C., Smith, S.M., and Sobel, H., *Mycobacterium xenopi* infection in a patient with acquired immunodeficiency syndrome, *Chest*, 86, 145, 1984.

13. Tecson-Tumang, F.T., and Bright, J.L., *Mycobacterium xenopi* and the acquired immunodeficiency syndrome (letter), *Ann. Intern. Med.*, 100, 461, 1984.

14. Shafer, R.W. and Sierra, M.F., *Mycobacterium xenopi*, *Mycobacterium fortuitum*, *Mycobacterium kansasii*, and other nontuberculous mycobacteria in an area of endemicity for AIDS, *Clin. Infect. Dis.*, 15, 161, 1992.

15. Cone, L.A., Byrd, R.G., and Greenwald, G., *Mycobacterium xenopi* infections in patients with AIDS, in *4th Conf. Retroviruses and Opportunistic Infections*, Washington, D.C., Jan 28–Feb 2, 1997 (submitted).

16. Mills, C.C., Occurrence of Mycobacteria other than *Mycobacterium tuberculosis* in the oral cavity and sputum, *Appl. Microbiol.*, 24, 307, 1972.

17. Chin, D.P., Hopewell, P.C., Yajko, D.M. et al., *Mycobacterium avium* complex in the respiratory or gastrointestinal tract and the risk of *M. avium* complex bacteremia in patients with human immunodeficiency virus infection, *J. Infect. Dis.*, 169, 289, 1994.

18. Klatt, E.C., Jensen, D.F., and Meyer, P.R., Pathology of *Mycobacterium avium-intracellulare* infection in acquired immunodeficiency syndrome, *Hum. Pathol.*, 18, 709, 1987.

19. Wallace, J.M. and Hannah, J.B., *Mycobacterium avium* complex infection in patients with the acquired immunodeficiency syndrome, *Chest*, 93, 926, 1988.

20. Stach, J.L., Gros, P., Forget, A., and Skamene, E., Phenotypic expression of genetically controlled natural resistance to *Mycobacterium bovis* (BCG), *J. Immunol.*, 132, 888, 1989.

21. Appelberg, R. and Sarmento, A.M., The role of macrophage activation of *Bcg*-encoded macrophage function(s) in control of *Mycobacterium avium* infection in mice, *Clin. Exp. Immunol.*, 80, 324, 1990.

22. de Chastellier, C., Frehel, C., Offredo, C., and Skamene, E., Implication of phagosome-lysosome fusion in restriction of *Mycobacterium avium* growth in bone marrow macrophages from genetically resistant mice, *Infect. Immun.*, 61, 3775, 1993.

23. Wong, B., Edwards, F.F., Kiehn, T.E., Whimbey, E., Donnelly, H., Bernard, E.M., Gold, J.W.M., and Armstrong, D., Continuous high-grade *Mycobacterium avium-intracellulare* bacteremia in patients with the acquired immune deficiency syndrome, *Am. J. Med.*, 78, 35, 1985.

24. Bermudez, L.E.M. and Young, L.S., Tumor necrosis factor, alone or in combination with IL-2 but not IFN-gamma, is associated with macrophage killing of *Mycobacterium avium* complex, *J. Immunol.*, 140, 3006, 1988.

25. Orme, I.M., Furney, S.K., Skinner, P.S., Roberts, A.D., Brennan, P.J., Russell, D.G., Shiratsuchi, H., Ellner, J.J., and Weiser, W.Y., Inhibition of growth of *Mycobacterium avium* in murine and human mononuclear phagocytes by migration inhibition factor, *Infect. Immun.*, 61, 338, 1993.

26. Horsburgh, C.R. Jr., *Mycobacterium avium* complex infection in the acquired immunodeficiency syndrome, *N. Engl. J. Med.*, 324, 1332, 1991.

27. Bermudez, L.E.M. and Young, L.S., Recombinant granulocyte-macrophage colony-stimulating factor activates human macrophages to inhibit growth or kill *Mycobacterium avium* complex, *J. Leuk. Biol.*, 48, 67, 1990.

28. Newman, G.W., Kelley, T.G., Gan, H., Kandil, O., Newman, M.J., Pinkston, P., Rose, R.M., and Remold, H.G., Concurrent infection of human macrophages with HIV-1 and *Mycobacterium avium* results in decreased cell viability, increased *M. avium* multiplication and altered cytokine production, *J. Immunol.,* 151, 2261, 1993.

29. Zakowski, P., Fligiel, S., Berlin, G.W., and Johnson, B.L. Jr., Disseminated *Mycobacterium avium-intracellulare* infection in homosexual men dying of acquired immunodeficiency, *JAMA,* 248, 2980, 1982.

30. Coodley, G.O., Loveless, M.O., and Merrill, T.M., The HIV wasting syndrome: a review, *J. Acquir. Immune Def. Syndr.,* 7, 681, 1994.

31. Kotler, D.P., Gastrointestinal manifestations of human immunodeficincy virus infection, *Adv. Intern. Med.,* 40, 197, 1995.

32. Roth, R.I., Owen, R.L., Keren, D.F. et al., Intestinal infection with *Mycobacterium avium* in acquired immunodeficiency syndrome (AIDS): histological and clinical comparison with Whipple's disease, *Dig. Dis. Sci.,* 30, 497, 1985.

33. Lemann, J. and Gray, R.W., Calcitriol, calcium and granulomatous disease (Editorial), *N. Engl. J. Med.,* 311, 1115, 1984.

34. Zaloga, G.P., Chernow, B., and Eil, C., Hypercalcemia and disseminated cytomegalovirus infection in the acquired immunodeficiency syndrome, *Ann. Intern. Med.,* 92, 331, 1985.

35. Jacobs, M.B., The acquired immunodeficiency syndrome and hypercalcemia, *West J Med.,* 144, 469, 1986.

36. Fox, C.H., Kotler, D.P., Tierney, A.R. et al., Detection of HIV-1 RNA in intestinal lamina propria of patients with AIDS and gastrointestinal disease, *J. Infect. Dis.,* 159, 467, 1989.

37. Cone, L.A., Intestinal microsporidiosis, in *Nutrients, Foods and Alternative Medicines for AIDS,* CRC Press, Boca Raton, FL, 1998 (in press).

38. World Health Organization, Acquired immunodeficiency syndrome (AIDS): WHO/CDC case definition for AIDS, *Weekly Epidemiol. Rec.,* 61, 69, 1986.

39. Kotler, D.P., Tierney, A.R., Culpepper-Morgan, J.A., Wang, J., and Pierson, R.N. Jr., Effect of home total parenteral nutrition on body composition in patients with acquired immunodeficiency syndrome, *J. Parent. Enter. Nutr.,* 14, 454, 1990.

40. von Roenn, J.H., Armstrong, D., Kotler, D.P., Cohn, D.L., Klimas, N.G., Tchekmedyian, N.S., Cone, L.A., Brennen, P.J., and Weizman, S.A., A placebo-controlled trial of megesterol acetate in patients with AIDS-related anorexia and cachexia, *Ann. Intern. Med.,* 121, 393, 1994.

41. Oster, M.H., Enders, S.R., Samuels, S.J., Cone, L.A., Hooten, T.M., Broder, H.P., and Flynn, N.M., Multicenter clinical trial comparing high-dose megesterol acetate and placebo in cachectic patients with acquired immunodeficiency syndrome (AIDS), *Ann. Intern. Med.,* 121, 400, 1994.

42. Shafran, S.D., Singer, J., Zarowny, D.P. et al., A comparison of two regimens for the treatment of *Mycobacterium avium* complex in AIDS: rifabitin, ethambutol, and clarithromycin vs. rifampin, ethambutol, clofazimine, and ciprofloxacin, *N. Engl. J. Med.,* 335, 377, 1996.

43. Heifets, L., Mor, N., Vanderkolk, J., *Mycobacterium avium* strains resistant to clarithromycin and azithromycin, *Antimicrob. Agents Chemother.,* 37, 2364, 1993.

44. Heufelder, A.E., Leinung, M.C., and Northcutt, R.C., Bull's eye retinopathy and clofazimine (letter), *Ann. Intern. Med.,* 116, 876, 1992.

45. Cone, L.A., Woodard, D.R., Wade, D., Curry, N., Boughton, W., and Fiala, M., Fever, weight loss, anemia, splenomegaly and abdominal lymphadenopathy are highly predictive of disseminated mycobacteriosis in patients who are HIV antibody positive, *5th International Conference on AIDS*, Florence, Italy, THBP53, 424, 1989.

chapter ten

Malabsorption and microsporidia

Lawrence A. Cone

Introduction

Microsporidia comprise an order of phylogenetically ancient organisms that belong to the subkingdom Protozoa and the phylum Microspora. They are unicellular parasites and are considered to be eukaryotes because they possess a nucleus and nuclear membrane, but resemble prokaryotes in that they lack mitochondria, peroxisomes, and Golgi membranes. The phylum consists of over 100 genera and almost 1000 species.[1] First identified in 1857,[2] these organisms have caused serious economic problems for the silkworm, honeybee, and commercial fishing industries.[3] They are obligate intracellular spore-forming protozoa and are found in many invertebrate and all vertebrate species. Along with members of the phylum Sporozoa including Isospora, Cryptosporidia, and Cyclospora, they constitute the four intestinal spore-forming protozoa of humans.[4]

The organisms

Five genera of microsporidia are known to cause disease in humans, and include *Enterocytozoon bieneusi* and *Septata intestinalis,* which are intestinal pathogens, and *Encephalitozoon* spp., *Nosema* spp., and *Pleistophora* sp. which are rare and nonintestinal and may cause keratitis, myositis, encephalitis, sinusitis, bronchitis, pneumonitis, hepatitis, and nephritis.[5-8] Recently, genetic studies of the *S. intestinalis rrs* gene encoding small subunit ribosomal RNA (srRNA)[9] indicates that this protozoan is more closely related to *Encephalitozoon* and should be reclassified *Encephalitozoon intestinalis.*

The typical mammalian microsporidian spore measures 1.5 μm to 5 μm and is ordinarily ovoid in shape with a thick wall consisting of an exospore, a chitinous endospore, and a plasma membrane rendering the spores environmentally resistant.[1] The nucleus is either single or binucleate, varying

0-8493-8561-X/98/$0.00+$.50
© 1998 by CRC Press LLC

dependent upon the genus and the phase of the life cycle. The spores have a complex tubular extrusion consisting of coiled polar tubule for injecting the infecting agent or sporoplasm into the host cell.[1]

The life cycle of microsporidia include three distinct phases. After the spore is released into the environment, it is, in the case of intestinal microsporidia, probably transmitted by the fecal-oral route. Upon ingestion by the host, the spore is stimulated in the small intestine by changes in the pH and ionic concentrations to evert its coiled tubule. Thereafter, the tubule penetrates the host cells and injects the sporoplasm which initiates a proliferative meragonic or binary fission and schizonic or multiple fission phase. When meronts develop into sporonts, sporogeny is initiated and completed when sporoblasts mature into spores. Microsporidia have great reproductive potential, being capable of multiplying within cells and spreading from cell to cell, filling the enterocytes with their progeny.

Epidemiology

The epidemiology of intestinal microsporidiosis is under intensive study but still remains somewhat obscure. Transmission of the parasite is thought to occur primarily by the fecal-oral route, but transovarial and transplacental infection also occurs in animal species. Since there is no known nonhuman source of the intestinal microsporidia, *E. bienuesi* and *S. intestinalis*, the worldwide presence of these protozoa in patients with the acquired immunodeficiency syndrome (AIDS) is compelling evidence that human-to-human transmission via the fecal route is likely. Neither animal reservoirs nor intermediate hosts nor invertebrate vectors have been discovered. Moreover, fecal-oral transmission is also encountered with the other spore-forming intestinal protozoan infections in humans.

In patients with human immunodeficiency virus infection (HIV) over 400 cases of microsporidiosis have been documented,[10] the majority due to *E. bieneusi*. First reported in France in 1985 by Modigliani et al.[11] and named by Desportes and coworkers,[12] it was characterized at the ultrastructural level. Although previously experienced only in HIV+ persons, a self-limited infection has recently been reported in an immunocompetent medical student who had traveled to the Middle East.[13]

Diagnosis

Whereas in the past a diagnosis of intestinal microsporidiosis was established by electron microscopy and considered difficult in paraffin- or epoxy-embedded sections of tissues examined by light microscopy,[14] more current studies have indicated that diagnosis by light microscopy can be made accurately either by gram or Giemas-stained smears of duodenal/jejunal biopsies.[11,15] A Warthin-Starry silver stain for the visualization of both intermediate stages and spores is also acceptable. Routine hematoxylin-eosin stained sections often fail to reveal the parasites even in experienced hands.

Most recently, *E. bieneusi*-infected duodenal biopsy material has been subjected to DNA amplification by PCR[16] with successful identification not only of microsporidia but also with speciation of the parasite.

A coprodiagnostic technique recently described by Weber et al.[17] has significantly enhanced the ease by which the diagnosis of intestinal microsporidiosis can be made. The chromotrope-based staining technique uses a procedure that is similar to the trichrome method. The chromototrope concentration in the new stain is higher and includes chromotrope 2R, fast green, and phosphotungstic acid. Identification of microsporidia spores by this coprodiagnostic technique is as sensitive and as specific as light and electron microscopy.[17,18] At our institution we currently rely upon this method to identify intestinal microsporidia. Other techniques that may be useful in the coprodiagnosis are Giemsa staining of stool specimens which stain microsporidia blue, but so are other fecal elements stained with the same color and chemifluorescent agents such as calcofluor white, which require fluorescent microscopy, and are not truly specific. Several serologic assays have been described for the detection of *Encephalitozoon cuniculi*, a rare cause of encephalitis in humans[7,19] and able to cause disseminated microsporidiosis in a number of animal species.[3,20,21] These include the enzyme-linked immunosorbent assay and an indirect immunofluorescent test. Cross-reaction with sporozoa (e.g., malaria) detracts from the reliability of such serologic assays and their value as screening tests for the prevalence of microsporidial infection.[22]

Pathology

Both *E. bieneusi* and *S. intestinalis* infection appear to be limited to the small intestinal enterocytes and biliary epithelium. As a result and depending upon the intensity of infection, degeneration, necrosis, and sloughing of these enterocytes occurs. Additionally, villous atrophy and a variable inflammatory response of mononuclear cells is seen in the lamina propria. Goblet cell depletion and crypt elongation are also noted.[23-25] Decreased brush border disaccharidase activities has also been observed.[26]

Clinical manifestations

The clinical result of intestinal microsporidial infestation is usually chronic diarrhea and wasting. It is probably responsible for 30% of such symptoms in patients with AIDS when no other cause is identified.[27] Symptoms are most common when the CD4 cell counts fall below $100/mm^3$ and are characterized by three to ten watery, large volume bowel movements that are not bloody. There is abdominal cramping in some and bloating in most. Appetite is ordinarily preserved but weight loss averaging 2 kg/month[1] is frequent. Fever is absent unless simultaneous infection with other agents such as cytomegalovirus, *Mycobacterium avium-intracellare,* or enteric pathogens occurs.[28] When infection spreads to contiguous organs such as the biliary tree or pancreatic ducts, cholangitis, cholecystitis, and pancreatitis may ensue.[29] In patients infected by *S. intestinalis* dissemination to the urinary tract may result in cystitis, interstitial nephritis, hematuria, and progressive renal failure.[1,30] These microsporidia have also on rare occasions been identified in sinonasal and lower respiratory infections in HIV infected persons.[31]

Intestinal malabsorption

Since 1990, 14 patients with intestinal microsporidiosis and one with microsporidial keratitis have been diagnosed at the Eisenhower Medical Center (E.M.C.) in Southern California, which serves as a community hospital and referral center for a population of over 250,000 inhabitants and over a million visitors annually. The facility is situated in the arid Coachella Valley in the Desert Southwest, and nearly 1000 persons with AIDS have been treated at E.M.C. from 1981 through 1995.

All 14 patients had large volume diarrhea (more than 500cc stool/24h). Thirteen of the 14 were studied with regard to malabsorption utilizing D-xylose absorption testing, a 72-hour collection of stool for fat, and a serum carotene determination. The diagnosis of microsporidiosis was established in 7 patients by small bowel biopsy and electron microscopy and in the remainder by stool examination using the chromotrope stain. All patients were homosexual males and in none was another simultaneous intestinal infection detected. All patients had negative stools for enteric pathogens, *Clostridium difficile*, cryptosporidium, ova and parasites, and mycobacteria. None was febrile, and all patients complained of diarrhea for at least 30 days.

All 13 patients revealed a serum carotene level that was significantly depressed, and 10 of 13 patients manifested increased fat in stool in at least two of three 24-hour collections. Eleven of 13 revealed a decreased excretion of D-xylose in the urine 5 hours after ingestion. These data demonstrate that at least 75% of patients with intestinal microsporidiosis manifest malabsorption for fat and carbohydrate. It would appear likely that weight loss in this group of patients can be related directly to malabsorption since their energy intake appears to be adequate in most instances.

Therapy

Several drugs are available for the treatment of microsporidiosis in invertebrate and vertebrate hosts including humans. Control of the microsporidia *Nosema* in the honeybee by fumagilin has been known since 1952,[32] and *E. cuniculi* in rabbits since 1980,[33] yet a durable elimination of these protozoa is difficult to achieve.

In patients with AIDS the imidazole, metronidazole, was shown be somewhat effective against 10 of 13 individuals with mild microsporidial diarrhea.[23] More recently,[34-36] the benzimidazole, albendazole, has been shown to be effective therapy in reducing diarrhea and weight loss in patients with intestinal microsporidiosis. In particular *S. intestinalis* appears to respond better than *E. bieneusi* infections. At E.M.C. 14 patients with intestinal microsporidiosis were treated with 400 to 800 mg albendazole twice daily from 4 weeks to 5 months. Albendazole, currently an investigational drug in the U.S., was provided by Smith-Kline Beecham, Welwyn Garden City, Hertfordshire, U.K., and Conshohocken, PA, U.S., and informed consent was obtained from all patients in accordance with regulations established by a central Institutional Review Board.

Following the institution of albendazole therapy 12 of 14 patients noted a decrease in stool volume and frequency. Weight loss ceased in 3 patients and they gained between 2 and 12 lb (0.91 to 5.5 kg), while the remainder continued to lose weight despite continued treatment with albendazole.[36] In the 3 patients who gained weight, microsporidia were no longer identified in the stool while the remainder continued to excrete microsporidial spores in their feces. Unfortunately, no effort was made to distinguish between *E. bieneusi* and *S. intestinalis* by transmission electron microscopy[37] in these patients, which could have demonstrated a difference in clinical responsiveness to albendazole.

Albendazole is a broad-spectrum antiparasitic drug that displays activity against protozoa, cestodes, and nematodes.[38-40] Albendazole binds to the colchicine-sensitive sight of tubulin, inhibiting its polymerization into microtubules,[41] thus interfering with nutrient uptake and cell division which takes place at both the meront and sporont stages. The two metabolites of the drug, a sulphoxide and a sulphone, are also active and are excreted in the urine. Although in previous reports and in the E.M.C. experience most patients become transiently less symptomatic when initiating albendazole, relapse occurs when the drug is discontinued or even while on therapy. Long-term treatment with higher dosage may obviate these unsatisfactory results. Adverse effects of the drug appear to be unusual.

None of our patients with microsporidiosis survived more than 15 months following diagnosis. However, death was never attributable directly to the protozoan infection, although in one individual death was due to undiagnosed renal failure, a known sequel to *S. intestinalis* infection. The remainder expired secondary to other AIDS-related opportunistic infections or neoplasms although malnutrition due to microsporidiosis may have contributed to their demise.

Ancillary therapy used by us to treat patients with intestinal microsporidiosis included octreotide[42] when oral antidiarrhetics failed, megesterol acetate[43,44] to stimulate appetite, and parenteral nutrition.

Summary

Intestinal microsporidiosis is a common cause of wasting due to diarrhea and malabsorption in patients with HIV and a CD4 cell count below 100/mm^3. The protozoan can be isolated in up to 30% of patients with AIDS and diarrhea in whom no other cause is identified. Two parasites have been identified in humans as responsible for the infection: *Enterocytozoon bieneusi* and *Septata intestinalis*. As the infection progresses due to the high proliferative activity of microsporidia, enterocyte loss and villous atrophy ensue resulting in diarrhea and wasting.

Recently, a new benzimidazole, albendazole, has been made available to treat patients with microsporidiosis. It appears to show more efficacy than previous antiparasitic drugs, and perhaps with longer periods of treatment and higher dosing will bring this worldwide protozoal infection under control. When a precise understanding of the transmission of microsporia is known, then preventive measures can be introduced. Meanwhile attempts to prevent fecal-oral spread of the parasite appear prudent.

References

1. Weber, R., Bryan, R.T., Schwartz, D.A., and Owen, R.L., Human microsporidial infections, *Clin. Microbiol. Rev.*, 7, 426, 1994.
2. Naegeli, K.W., Ueber die neue Krankheit der Seidenraupe und verwandte Organismen, *Z. Bot.*, 15, 760, 1857.
3. Canning, E.U., Lom, J., and Dykova, I., *The Microsporidia of Vertebrates*, Academic Press, NY, 1986.
4. Goodgame, R.W., Understanding intestinal spore-forming protozoa: cryptosporidia, microsporidia isospora, and cyclospora, *Ann. Intern. Med.*, 124, 429, 1996.
5. Davis, R.M., Font, R.L., Keisler, M.S., and Shadduck, J.A., Corneal microsporidiosis. A case report including ultrastructural observations, *Ophthalmology*, 97, 953, 1990.
6. Chupp, G.L., Alroy, J., Adelman, L.S., Breen, J.C., and Skolnick, P.R., Myositis due to *Pleistophora* (Microsporidia) in a patient with AIDS, *Clin. Infect. Dis.*, 16, 15, 1993.
7. Bergquist, N.R., Stintzing, G., Smedman, L., Waller, T., and Andersson, T., Diagnosis of encephalitozoonosis in man by serologic tests, *Br. Med. J.*, 288, 902, 1984
8. Lacey, C.J.N., Clark, A., Frazer, P., Metcalfe, T., and Curry, A., Chronic microsporidian infection in the nasal mucosae, sinuses and conjunctivae in HIV disease, *Genitourin. Med.*, 68, 179, 1992.
9. Bryan, R.T. and Weber, R., Microsporidia: emerging pathogens in immunodeficient persons, *Arch. Pathol. Lab. Med.*, 117, 1243, 1993.
10. Hartskeerl, R.A., Van Gool, T., Schuitema, A.R.J., Didier, E.S., and Terpstra, W.J., Genetic and immunological characterization of the microsporidian *Septata intestinalis* Cali, Kotler and Orenstein,1993: reclassification to *Encephalitozoon intestinalis*. *Parasitology*, 110, 277, 1995.
11. Modigliani, R., Bories, C., le Charpentier, Y., Salmeron, M., Messing, R., Galian, A., Rambaud, J.C., Lavergne, A., Cochand-Priollet, B., and Desportes, I., Diarrhoea and malabsorption in acquired immune deficiency syndrome: a study of four cases with special emphasis on opportunistic protozoan infections, *Gut*, 26, 179, 1985.

12. Desportes, I., le Charpentier, Y., Galian, A., Bernard, F., Cochand-Priollet, B., Lavergne, A., Ravisse, P., and Modigliani, R., Occurrence of a new microsporidian: *Enterocytozoon bieneusi* n.g.,n.sp., in the enterocytes of a human patient with AIDS, *J. Protozool.*, 32, 250, 1985.
13. Sandfort, J., Hannemann, A., Gelderblom, H., Stark, D., Owen, R.L., and Ruf, B., *Enterocytozoon bieneusi* infection in an immunocompetent patient who had acute diarrhea and who was not infected with the human immunodeficiency virus, *Clin. Infect. Dis.*, 19, 514, 1994.
14. Rabeneck, L., Gyorkey, F., Genta, R.M., Gyorkey, P., Foote, L.W., and Risser, J.M.H., The role of *Microsporidia* in the pathogenesis of HIV-related chronic diarrhea, *Ann. Intern., Med.*, 119, 895, 1993.
15. Rijpstra, A.C., Canning, E.U., van Ketel, R.J., Eeftinck Schattenkerk, J.K.M., and Laarman, J.J.., Use of light microscopy to diagnose small intestinal microsporidiosis in patients with AIDS, *J. Infect. Dis.*, 157, 827, 1988.
16. Franzen, C., Mueller, A., Hegener, P., Salzberger, B., Hartmann, P., Faetkenheuer, G., Diehl, V., and Schrappe, M., Detection of microsporidia (*Enterocytozoon bieneusi*) in intestinal biopsy specimens from human immunodeficiency virus-infected patients by PCR, *J. Clin. Microbiol.*, 33, 2294, 1995.
17. Weber, R., Bryan, R.T., Owen, R.L., Wilcox, C.M., Gorelkin, L., Visvesvara, G.S., Improved light-microscopical detection of microsporidia spores in stool and duodenal aspirates, *N. Engl. J. Med.*, 326, 161, 1992.
18. Svenson, J., MacLean, J.D., Kokoskin-Nelson, E., Szabo, J., Lough, J., and Gill, M.J., Microsporidiosis in AIDS patients, *Can. Commun. Dis. Rep.*, 19, 13, 1993.
19. Matsubayashi, H., Koike, T., Mikata, T., and Hagiwara, S., A case of *Encephalitozoon*-like body infection in man, *Arch. Pathol.*, 67, 181, 1959.
20. Nelson, J.B., An intracellular parasite resembling a microsporidian, associated with ascites in Swiss mice, *Proc. Soc. Exp. Biol. Med.*, 109, 714, 1962.
21. Weiser, J., On the taxonomic position of the genus *Encephalitozoon* Levaditi, Nicolau & Schoen, 1923 (Protozoa, *Microsporidia*), *Parasitology*, 54, 749, 1964.
22. Singh, M., Kane, G.J., Mackinley, L., Quaki, I., Yap, E.H., Ho, B.C., Ho, L.C., and Kim, L.C., Detection of antibodies to *Nosema caniculi* (Protozoa: *Microsporidia*) in human and animal sera by the indirect fluorescent antibody technique, *Southeast Asian J. Trop. Med. Public Health*, 13, 110, 1982.
23. Eeftinck Schattenkerk, J.K.M., van Gool, T., van Ketel, R.J., Bartelsman, J.M., Kuiken, C.L., Terpstra, W.J., and Reiss, P., Clinical significance of small-intestinal microsporidiosis in HIV-1-infected individuals, *Lancet*, 337, 895, 1991.
24. Greenson, J.K., Belistos, P.C., Yardley, J.H., and Bartlett, J.G., AIDS enteropathy: occult enteric infections and duodenal mucosal alterations in chronic diarrhea, *Ann. Intern. Med.*, 114, 366, 1991.
25. Molina, J.M., Sarfati, C., Beauvais, B., Lemann, M., Lesourd, A., Ferchal, F., Casin, I., Lagrange, P., Modigliani, R., Derouin, F., and Modai, J., Intestinal microsporidiosis in human immunodeficiency virus-infected patients with chronic unexplained diarrhea: prevalence and clinical and biologic features, *J., Infect., Dis.*, 167, 217, 1993.
26. Kotler, D.P., Reka, S., Chow, K., and Orenstein, J.M., Effects of enteric parasitoses and HIV infection upon small intestinal structure and function in patients with AIDS, *J. Clin. Gastroenterol.*, 16, 10, 1993.
27. Sharpstone, D. and Gazzard, B., Gastrointestinal manifestations of HIV infection, *Lancet*, 348, 379, 1996.

28. Weber, R., Sauer, B., Luethy, R., and Nadal, D., Intestinal coinfection with *Enterocytozoon bieneusi* and *Cryptosporidium* in a human immunodeficiency virus-infected child with chronic diarrhea, *Clin. Infect. Dis.*, 17, 480, 1993.

29. Pol, S., Romania, C., Richard, S.R., Amouyal, P., Desportes-Livage, I., Carnot, F., Pays, J.F., and Berthelot, P., Microsporidia infection in patients with the human immunodeficiency virus and unexplained cholangitis, *N. Engl. J. Med.*, 328, 95, 1993.

30. Schwartz, D.A., Bryan, R.T., Hewan-Lowe, K.O., Visvesvara, G.S., Weber, R., Cali, A., and Angritt, P., Disseminated microsporidiosis (*Encephalitozoon hellem*) and acquired immunodeficiency syndrome, *Arch. Pathol. Lab. Med.*, 116, 660, 1992.

31. Hartskeerl, R.A., Schuitema, A.R.J., van Gool, T., and Terpstra, J., Genetic evidence for the occurrence of extra-intestinal *Enterocytozoon bieneusi* infections, *Nucleic Acids Res.*, 21, 4150, 1993.

32. Ketznelson, H. and Jamieson, C.A., Control of *Nosema* disease of honey bees with fumagillin, *Science*, 115, 70, 1952.

33. Shadduck, J.A., Effect of fumagillin on *in vitro* multiplication of *Encephalitozoon cuniculi*, *J. Protozool.*, 27, 202, 1980.

34. Blanshard, C., Ellis, D.S., Tovey, D.G., Dowell, S., and Gazzard, B.G., Treatment of intestinal microsporidiosis in patients with AIDS, *AIDS*, 6, 311, 1992.

35. Dieterich, D.T., Lew, E.A., Kotler, D.P., Poles, M.A., and Orenstein, J.M., Treatment with albendazole for intestinal disease due to *Enterocytozoon bieneusi* in patients with AIDS, *J. Infect. Dis.*, 169, 178, 1994.

36. Cone, L.A., Dzekov, C.I., and Merickel, R.A., Use of albendazole in certain parasitic infections, *Recent Research Developments in Antimicrobial Agents and Chemotherapy*, Research Sign Post, Kerala State, India, 1996.

37. Cali, A., Orenstein, J.M., Kotler, D.P., and Owen, R., A comparison of two microsporidian parasites in enterocytes of AIDS patients with chronic diarrhea, *J. Protozool.*, 38, 96S, 1991.

38. Horton, R.J., Chemotherapy of *Echinococcus* infection in man with albendazole, *Trans. R. Soc. Trop. Med. Hyg.*, 83, 97, 1989.

39. Edind, T.D., Hang, T.L., and Chakraborty, P.R., Activity of antihelminthic benzimidazoles against *Giardia lamblia in vitro*, *J. Infect. Dis.*, 162, 1408, 1990.

40. Chine, B.L., Little, M.D., Bartholomew, R.K., and Halsey, N.A., Larvical activity in albendazole against *Necator americanus* in human volunteers, *Am. J. Trop. Med. Hyg.*, 33, 387, 1984.

41. Lacey, E., Mode of action of benzimidazoles, *Parasitol Today*, 6, 112, 1990.

42. Cello, J.P., Grendell, J.H., Basuk, P., Simon, D., Weiss, L., Wittner, M., Rood, R.P., Wilcox, M., Forsmark, C.E., Read, A.E., Satow, J.A., Weikel, C.S., and Beaumont, C., Effect of octreotide on refractory AIDS-associated diarrhea. A prospective, multicenter clinical trial, *Ann. Intern. Med.*, 115, 705, 1991.

43. Von Roenn, J.H., Armstrong, D., Kotler, D.P., Cohn, D.L., Klimas, N.G., Tchekmedyian, N.S., Cone, L.A., Brennen, P.J., and Weitzman, S.A., A placebo-controlled trial of megesterol acetate in patients with AIDS-related anorexia and cachexia, *Ann. Intern. Med.*, 121, 393, 1994.

44. Oster, M.H., Enders, S.R., Samuels, S.J., Cone, L.A., Hooten, T.M., Broder, H.P., and Flynn, N.M., Multicenter clinical trial comparing high-dose megesterol acetate and placebo in cachectic patients with acquired immunodeficiency syndrome (AIDS), *Ann. Intern. Med.*, 121, 400, 1994.

chapter eleven

The role of home delivered meals and community-based medical nutrition therapy in HIV care

Dorothy C. Humm and Bruce C. Oliver

Background

Food assistance is one of the most critical needs of people living with HIV disease.[1] In an assessment of essential needs conducted in the major urban epicenter of the AIDS epidemic, New York City, food and nutrition were ranked as second by HIV+ clients and third by HIV/AIDS service providers.[2] Community food programs for people living with HIV/AIDS are becoming more common and are welcome sights to those in need. Some of these programs provide home delivery.[3] By 1995 in the U.S., there were 17 formally structured HIV-home delivered meals (HIV-HDM) programs which were within AIDS case management agencies.[2] In New York state, there are other formal HIV-HDM programs which were built upon already established home delivered meals programs.[4]

Without adequate intake of energy, protein, and micronutrients, people with HIV/AIDS are at substantial risk for muscle wasting, weight loss, and micronutrient depletion.[5,6] Decreases in lean body mass has been shown to be correlated with decreased survival in people with HIV/AIDS.[7] Death occurs when their body mass approaches 66% of ideal body mass or when body cell mass approaches 54% of normal. The degree of wasting is similar to that seen during starvation. This suggests that the *amount* of wasting, rather than the specific *cause*, is the major determinant of death.[8] Thus, this chapter will address methods to decrease that wasting through interventions provided by cost effective medical nutrition therapy in a home and community based setting.

The program from which this chapter is written is a part of a long established (1958) HDM program located in an upstate New York community. It is a strategic partnership of a not-for-profit certified home health agency (under which the HDM program falls), a nonprofit agency which provides the food, and a for-profit nutrition education firm which provides the registered dietitians to do the home visiting to provide medical nutrition therapy. The program has active networking ties with the community's HIV-AIDS case management agencies and their staff. The beginning of the formal HIV-HDM program was March, 1993 and by August, 1993 the program was serving 50 to 60 participants daily. That level of service has been maintained for 3 years. In 1996, 10 meal offerings were converted to traditional Latino foods and are delivered by a bilingual driver.

Criteria for service

To qualify to receive the HIV-HDM a person must:

- live in the county served,
- have an HIV+ diagnosis (although it is not confirmed with their physician),
- be willing to be at home to receive the meals and the dietetic professional visits (unless a call is made to the meals office 24 hours in advance),
- be frail and unable to get out easily (homebound), and
- have no more than 18 hours per day of home health aide assistance.

If there is a waiting list for start of service, prioritization is made by giving various weights to the following:

- type of referral source
- family/social setting
- symptoms/co-morbidities
- weight loss
- food security
- amount of home health aide service.

A written agreement clarifies and acknowledges the responsibilities of the person with HIV disease with the meal program.[2]

Meal program description

The kitchen which serves the 50 people with HIV/AIDS also serves about 950 additional people (96% of whom are elders over 60 years of age.) The HIV-HDM participant receives 1 or 2 meals for 5 to 7 days per week and 1 or 2 weekly snack packs. This combination provides a high calorie, high biological protein base which should meet two-thirds of the daily food needs of the people with HIV/AIDS or about two-thirds of a 3,000-kcalorie diet with 22% protein, 37% carbohydrate, and 40% fat. The meals are individualized to the extent that there are 9 therapeutic diets served, a choice of type of routine beverage they receive, and choice of up to 3 standing food preferences they wish not to receive.

Meals

Typically, participants receive 2 meals on each of the 7 days. If the meal recipient lives in the more rural sections of our service area, they receive the frozen weekend meals on the 2 days before the weekend; otherwise, meals are delivered hot each day. The daily calorie level for 2 meals is approximately 1,800 to 2,000 kilocalories and about 104 grams of protein. Menus are analyzed to provide two-thirds of most needed vitamin and mineral requirements. The meals are modified from the standard elder home delivered meals (one-third of daily nutrient needs per meal) by doubling the entree portion in the hot noon-time meal and in the cold sandwich protein portion in the evening meal. To date, this HIV-HDM program has not done formal studies on how much of the meals are eaten. However, there are studies such as the one done by Hannema, et al. which look at the amount eaten and the reasons for incomplete meal consumption. [9]

Snack pack

In addition to the daily meals, the participants have the option of receiving 1 or 2 shelf stable "snack packs." The purpose of the snack pack is to both supplement meals to meet two-thirds of a 3000 kcalorie diet and to educate participants on how to deal with symptoms when they arise. One snack pack provides a weekly additional 1400 kcalories and 45 gm protein. It consists of canned and dried foods that are in individual size servings. Included are items such as single service juice, single serving cereal, can of soda pop, pack of chewing gum, protein-fortified cookies or candy, simple candy, simple sugar, and more. Each item in the pack has a specific reason for its inclusion. For example, the chewing gum is there to stimulate moisture in the mouth when a participant has dry mouth. Only non-citrus juices are included so that the participant who has thrush has a substitute on a day when we serve a citrus juice.

Medical nutrition therapy and food safety education

Since the role of nutrition is one which enhances the quality of life and maintains nutritional homeostasis to delay disease progression[10,11] as well as to decrease nutritional deficiencies which may exacerbate clinical immune deficiency[12,13,14,15,16,17] the HDM program focuses on giving complete nutritional care. Efficacy of the program is enhanced by providing medical nutrition therapy and food safety education at regular intervals by registered dietitians. The screening, assessing, intervening, counseling, and education of a full medical nutrition therapy program[18] are essential necessities along the entire continuum of HIV disease management. Medical nutrition therapy provided by registered dietitians helps to reduce barriers to meal consumption such as low nutrition knowledge or special food preferences. It replaces them with knowledge of how to consume nutrient dense foods, how to treat foods in a safe and sanitary manner to eliminate food-borne infections, and what to do when symptoms occur which discourage eating. By receiving, and acting upon, medical nutrition therapy provided by a qualified nutrition professional, the people with HIV/AIDS can maintain overall weight, sustain body cell mass and adequate micronutrient stores, and manage symptoms related to opportunistic infections and side effects of medications.[19,20,21] As a part of the overall meals program, registered dietitians provide in-depth nutritional assessment, a nutritional plan of care, and individualized nutritional counseling specifically modified for people living with HIV/AIDS at each visit. Visits are at 1 month, 3 months, and every 6 months thereafter, as long as the participant is active with the HDM program. Coupled with the medical nutrition therapy, the registered dietitian takes out a medical nutritional supplement "sampler" package at the first 3 visits. These "sampler" packages contain 1 to one and 1½ calories per cc supplements from various pharmaceutical companies. There are a variety of flavors in the "sampler" packages. The purpose of the "sampler" packages is to educate the participant on the various liquid medical food products. It also allows the people with HIV/AIDS the opportunity to taste-test them prior to actually purchasing a case of them.

Outcome measures

Quality of life outcomes

Satisfaction surveys mailed to participants show that they are 98% satisfied or completely satisfied with the food, the service and the program. (The participants receiving the Latino style meals are 100% completely satisfied.) Surveys administered by the registered dietitians show that participants feel that the program has helped to improve their quality of life.

Clinical outcomes

It is a struggle to measure outcomes in a free living population. The outcome that we are able to measure is the change in total body weight over the period that a person with HIV/AIDS is receiving HIV-HDM. A baseline weight is obtained by a dietetic technician on the initial assessment visit prior to admission to the program and every 6 months thereafter. In addition to these weights, a registered dietitian weighs the participant at 1 month and 3 months and every 6 months thereafter. See Table 1.

Table 1 Weight Changes While on HIV-HDM

	Number of Months				
	3	9	15	21	27
Gained weight	86 (48%)	27 (40%)	15 (41%)	8 (40%)	3 (38%)
Stable	18 (10%)	1 (<1%)	4 (10%)	—	—
Lost weight	75 (41%)	39 (60%)	18 (49%)	12 (60%)	5 (62%)
Total	179 (100%)	67 (100%)	37 (100%)	20 (100%)	8 (100%)

Thus, every 3 months, there are weights taken on the participant to measure status. Of the participants' weights, 50% improve during the first 6 months. From 9 months and beyond, that percent fluctuates between 50% and 40% gaining or maintaining weight. It is hoped that this is because of the well-balanced meals that are regularly eaten coupled with the food safety education and medical nutrition therapy provided by the registered dietitians. Since we know from the registered dietitian reports that many of the participants had not previously developed regular eating patterns nor adequate intake of daily food prior to starting on the HDM program, there is high probability that these two factors play an important part in the initial weight gain. In 1995, one registered dietitian began to use a bioimpedance monitor with participants who would allow it. The preliminary data are showing that although the participants generally maintain or gain weight,[4] they are losing muscle mass. This HDM program does not yet include any type of exercise or physical therapy component to build muscle mass.

Problems

Problems that are encountered include:

- Not home — Participants are not consistently homebound and, thus, are not at home for meal delivery at a rate of 4%, which is twice as frequent as the elders whom we serve on the same routes.
- Substance use — This program accepts active substance users. At times, due to their substance use, they are unable, or unavailable, to receive their meals.
- Unseen need — Some participants don't see the value of the information that the dietetic professional provides. This includes help in alleviating AIDS-related complications or symptoms such as dry mouth, mouth sores, chewing difficulties, taste changes, dysphagia, nausea or vomiting, constipation or diarrhea, and most often, poor appetite.
- Large portions — By doubling the protein portions, the participant, who may have a poor appetite, is faced with a 6-oz cooked portion (equal to ½ lb a of meat) in the hot tray and a 4-oz portion in the cold tray. This has caused some participants to temporarily lose their appetite. It also creates a concern related to food safety and how the part of the meal not eaten is saved until it is eaten.

- Education sampler — The supplement "sampler" packages are not individualized for the participant's flavor preference, for stage of the disease process, nor for any therapeutic diet modifications which may be needed.
- Communication — It is difficult to develop a communication mechanism which connects all service providers (medical, social, other.)
- Screening — It is difficult to screen for quality of telephone referrals. In other words, a person may appear to be eligible for the program when a telephone referral is made, but then the dietetic technician discovers on the initial visit that the person does not meet all of the criteria for service.

Recommendations

People or programs considering instituting a HDM program for people with HIV/AIDS will find the following section helpful in setting up a well-accepted program.

- Build the meals service program in cooperation with Area Agencies for the Aging, which provide home delivered meals for elders. Encourage that program to provide high biological vegetarian meals if they are not already being offered.
- Modify the meal plan offerings to provide cold plate meals as a regular option.
- Hire a registered dietitian who is knowledgeable in HIV/AIDS care (preferably with experience in home care) to work with them to plan the meals, analyze the nutrients provided, and visit the recipients to provide food and food safety education along with medical nutrition therapy (screening, assessing, intervening, and counseling related to nutritional needs of the individual.)
- Consider requiring that the person be referred, or at least active with, an AIDS case management program.
- Consider working with an exercise physiologist to develop exercise regimens that not only build lean body mass, but are "user friendly" so that the meal recipient will do them.
- Consider strategic partnerships with HIV disease researchers who are studying HIV related weight loss and wasting.
- Network with other local providers of HIV/AIDS care in the community you will be serving.
- Learn sources of funding for the HIV/AIDS community and what they require. These may be federal, state, and/or local.
- Consider staging the dietetic professional visits differently or restructuring what is done at the visits by the dietetic technicians.
- Determine a system for periodic reevaluation of eligibility.
- Contact several HIV-HDM programs to learn various ways of providing adequate food and medical nutrition therapy.

- Contact God's Love We Deliver for their technical assistance manual.[22]
- Subscribe to "Positive Nutrition: A Newsletter for People with HIV and AIDS and Health Care Professionals" [23].

References

1. Hall, C.S., Food Programs: Assessing and Developing Community-Based Nutritional Support Programs for People with HIV-Related Illness. National AIDS Network, Washington, D.C., 1989.
2. Kraak, V., Home-delivered meal programs for homebound people with HIV/AIDS, *J. Am. Diet. Assoc.,* 95, 476, 1995.
3. Goldner, D., Delivering God's Love, Abundantly, New York Times, Dec. 15, 1993, C-1.
4. Topping, C., Humm, D., Fischer, R., and Brayer, K., A community-based, interagency approach by dietitians to provide meals, medical nutrition therapy, and education to clients with HIV/AIDS, *J. Am. Diet. Assoc.,* 95, 6, 683, June, 1995.
5. Grunfeld, C. and Kotler, D.P., Pathophysiology of AIDS wasting syndrome, in *AIDS Clinical Reviews 1992,* Volberding, P. and Jacobson, M.A., Eds., Marcel Dekker, New York, 191, 1992.
6. Abrams, B., Duncan, D., and Hertz-Picciotto, I., A prospective study of dietary intake and acquired immune deficiency syndrome in HIV-seropositive homosexual men, *J. Acquir. Immune Defic. Syndr.,* 6, 949, 1993.
7. Codley, G.O., Loveless, M.O., and Merrill, T.M., The HIV wasting syndrome: a review, *J. Aquir. Immune Defic. Syndr.,* 7, 681, 1994.
8. Kotler, D.P., Tierney, A.R., Wang, J., and Pierson, R.N., Magnitude of body cell mass depletion and timing of death from wasting in AIDS, *Am. J. Clin. Nutr.,* 50, 444, 1989.
9. Hannema, C., Chan, M.M., and Canty, D.J.., Meal consumption of AIDS patients and home delivered meals, *AIDS Patient Care,* 9, 290, Dec., 1995.
10. Turner, J., Muurahuinen, N., and Terrel, C., Nutritional status and quality of life, *10th Intl. Conf. AIDS,* 431B, 1994.
11. Grunfeld, C. and Feingold, K.R., Metabolic disturbances and wasting in the acquired immunodeficiency syndrome, *N. Engl. J. Med.,* 327, 329, 1992.
12. Chelbowski, R.T., Significance of altered nutritional status in acquired immunodeficiency syndrome (AIDS), *Nutr. Cancer,* 7, 85, 1985.
13. Chandra, R.K., Nutrition, immunity and infection: present knowledge and future directions, *Lancet,* 1, 688, 1983.
14. Beach, R.S. and Laura, P.F., Nutrition and the acquired immunodeficiency syndrome, Ann. Intern. Med., 99, 565, 1983.
15. Gray, R.H., Similarities between AIDS and PCM, *Am. J. Public Health,* 73, 1332, 1983.
16. Beach, R.S., Mantero-Atienza, E., Van Riel, F., and Fordyce-Baum, M., Potential implications of nutritional deficiencies in early HIV-1 infected patients, *Arch. AIDS Res.,* 3, 225, 1989.
17. Moseson, M., Zelenicuch-Jacquotte, A., Belsito, D.V., Shore, R.E., Marmor, M., and Pasternack, B., The potential role of nutritional factors in the induction of immunologic abnormalities in HIV-positive homosexual men, *J. Acquir. Immune Defic. Syndr.,* 2, 235, 1989.

18. *Nutrition Interventions Manual for Professionals Caring for Older Americans*, A publication of the Nutrition Screening Initiative (a project of the Am. Acad. Family Physicians, Am. Dietetic Assoc., and Natl. Council on Aging; partially funded by Ross Products Div., Abbott Laboratories).

19. Newman, C.F., The role of nutritional assessments and nutritional plans in the management of HIV/AIDS: an overview of the PAAC nutrition initiative, in *Nutrition and HIV/AIDS:* Proc. 1992 Int. Symp. Nutrition and HIV/AIDS, Nary, G., Ed. PAAC Publishing, Chicago, IL, 57, 1992.

20. Hyman, C. and Kaufman, S., Nutritional impact of acquired immune deficiency syndrome: a unique counseling opportunity, *J. Am. Diet. Assoc.*, 89, 520, 1989.

21. Resler, S.S., Nutrition care of AIDS patients, *J. Am. Diet. Assoc.*, 88, 828, 1988.

22. Abdale, F., *Community-Based Nutrition Support for People Living with HIV and AIDS: A Technical Assistance Manual*, published by God's Love We Deliver, New York, 1995.

23. "Positive Nutrition: A Newsletter for People with HIV and AIDS and for Health Care Professionals", A quarterly newsletter from Project Open Hand, 2720 17th Street, San Francisco, CA 94110-1405.

Animal models for nutrition and AIDS

chapter twelve

T cell receptor peptide and immune modulation

Bailin Liang, James Y. Wang, and Ronald R. Watson

Introduction

The immunopathogenic mechanisms underlying HIV infection and disease are not unidimensional, but rather are extremely complex.[1] Preferential expansion, deletion, and activation of some CD4+ αβT cells induced by retroviral super or chronic antigen exposure in human and murine acquired immune deficiency syndrome (AIDS) may be important immunopathogenic mechanisms.[3-4] Selective antigen activation of CD4+ αβT cells may lead to polyclonal stimulation of T and B cells at early stages, with subsequent aberrant cytokine production and CD4+ T cell depletion. Eventually, these abnormalities lead to profound immununosuppression of cell-mediated immunity and immunodeficiency.[1]

T cell receptor peptide and autoantibodies

Autoantibodies (AAbs) binding peptide determinants corresponding to the CDR1 of the T cell receptor (TCR) Vβ domain were elevated early in murine retrovirus infection.[5] The elevation of the levels of these AAbs is an early event following retroviral infection which corresponds in part to the general polyclonal activation of the B cells with selectivity for particular Vβ sequences occurring later. The production of high levels of anti-TCR AAbs early in this disease with continued production of some suggests that the latter might be involved in retrovirus immunopathogenesis. The AAbs directed against CDR1 determinants can be considered natural antibodies against public or regulatory idiotypes[6] since this region is the least variable of the CDRs and is completely specified by the Vβ gene sequence.

A set of overlapping 16-mer peptides that duplicate covalent structure of the VBDBJBCB protein[7-8] predicted from a human TCR Vβ gene sequence has been produced.[9] The complete range of peptide sequences is published in detail elsewhere.[10] Here, we focus on the sequence C K P I S G H N S L F W Y R Q T that corresponds to the completed CDR1 and N-terminal five residues of Fr2[7,10] of the human Vβ8. 1 gene product.[9] As a control peptide we used a 16-mer corresponding to the CDR1 of the light chain MCG[11] because the LP-BM5 infected mice did not produce AAbs to this peptide. Its sequence is as follows: T G T S S D V G G Y N X V S W Y. The peptide preparations were free of endotoxin. We have shown elsewhere that normal polyclonal IgG pools contain natural AAbs against peptide segments corresponding to CDR1, Fr3, and to a constant region "loop" peptide of the TCR β chain.[7] Untreated mice also have natural IgG antibodies directed against the same peptide segments; in particular, there is strong reactivity to the human CDR1 test peptides. A computer comparison of human and murine Vβ sequences (Schluter, S.F. and Marchalonis, J.J., unpublished analysis) using the progressive alignment algorithm of Feng and Doolittle[12] showed that certain human and murine Vβ sequences could be grouped into families; e.g., human Vβ6 and Vβ8 correspond to murine Vβll, and human and murine Vβ5 are in the same clusters.

T cell receptor peptide and immune modulation in AIDS

Administration of a TCR Vβ CDR1 peptide prior to infection significantly prevented retrovirus-induced suppression of immune responses. When administered shortly after LP-BM5 infection, normal cytokine production was largely maintained. Preservation of immune function occurred similarly in mice injected with the peptide prior- as well as post-retrovirus infection. The greater the elapsed time post infection before Vβ peptide treatment the greater the immune dysfunction that developed. Thus, TCR Vβ peptide treatment prevented immune dysfunction rather than restoring it. However, a control peptide from a lambda light chain CDR1 had no effect on preventing retrovirus-induced immune deficiency. These results indicate that TCR Vβ peptide could be considered as an immunoregulatory element in the complex network of interactions between the components of the immune response. They provide an insight not only to the pathogenesis of AAbs production during the progression to murine AIDS,[5,13] but also to possible functioning of idiotypic networks involving AAbs and autoreactive T cells as regulatory elements.

Most antigens are recognized through their interaction with the variable V portions of the TCR α and β chains. However, T cells recognize another category of ligands, the superantigens, on the basis of the expressed Vβ region alone, independently from the other variable TCR segments. The progression of CD4+ T cell expansion/depletion requires stimulation of T cell clones or subgroups with retroviral chronic or superantigen exposure, resulting over time in excessive activation followed by energy of CD4+ T

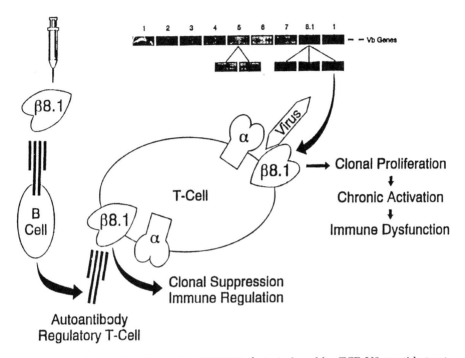

Figure 12.1 Autoantibodies against TCR Vβ chain induced by TCR Vβ peptide treatment may slow the selective deletion/expansion of T cell clones by cytolysis or other inhibitory mechanisms, including obstructed binding of the antigen to TCR Vβ chain.

cell bearing antigen selected Vβs. AAb against peptide defined epitopes of T cell receptors that were used to select the peptide treatment studies here were also found in high levels in HIV+ patients.[14] Since there is no detectable homology between these peptides and the sequences of the two retroviruses, it is reasonable to hypothesize that this overproduction results from a failure in regulation.

Possible mechanisms of T cell receptor peptide on immune modulation

Two potential mechanisms could be hypothesized for prevention of immune dysfunction during murine retrovirus infection and concomitant Vβ peptide treatment — first, treatment against specific regulatory determinants on the products of individual Vβ genes (Figure 12.1 and second, the possibility that peptides corresponding to the CDR1 and Fr2 segment of the Vβ chain could interact with MHC molecules necessary for the presentation of peptide antigen, altering this process (Figure 12.2).[13] We believe that a general mechanism of this nature is required because the effective peptide corresponds to only one of a possible set of >30 peptides, and it is unlikely that any single one would have an overall regulating effect based upon its idiotype specificity.

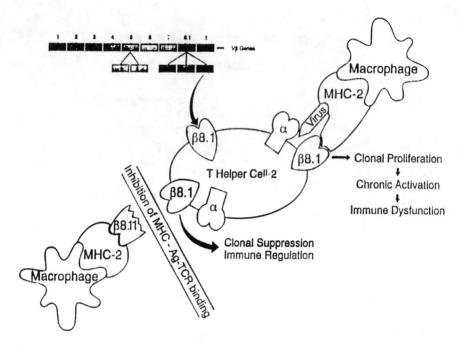

Figure 12.2   TCR peptides corresponding to the CDR1 and Fr2 segment of the Vβ chain of TCR could interact with MHC molecules necessary for the presentation of antigen, altering the antigen presentation process.

AAbs to TCR Vβ induced by treatment of TCR Vβ CDR1 may slow the selective deletion/expansion of some Vβ T cells by cytolysis or other inhibitory mechanisms, including obstructed binding of the antigen to TCR Vβ chains. The increased production of AAbs to the TCR Vβ peptides alone during murine AIDS may not be enough to alter the TCR Vβ expression profiles induced by retroviral super or chronic antigen exposure. While the murine retrovirus infection caused selective induction of high levels of AAbs against the TCR Vβ CDR1 peptide, presumably due to increased TCR Vβ T cell expression, it is unclear why TCR Vβ can prevent retrovirus-induced immunosuppression and cytokine dysregulation. It is possibly caused by a difference in the affinity of the different Vβ for the superantigen after specific AAbs interference. The presence of a dose-response relationship, as well as significant immune preservation in the presence of low doses of peptide in combination with two adjuvants, further suggests an immunoregulatory mechanism. Vβ peptide treatment prior to or early in the retrovirus infection could slow activation of T-cells as we found a smaller increase in IL-2r+ activated cells in treated, infected animals than in the infected, untreated mice. Thus, during Vβ peptide treatment, fewer cells may be activated to become Th2 or permitted to remain as immature Th0 cells with their high production of IL-4 and IL-10. This would preserve but not restore normal function in most bystander cells that were close enough to be affected by cytokines produced by T cell clones stimulated by super or chronic retroviral antigen exposure, without the increased IL-4 production by Th2 cells. In this situation more cells would remain as Th1 cells, producing IFN-γ and IL-2 during retrovirus antigen exposure. They would also suppress Th2 cytokine production in neighboring cells. Progression to severe pathology due to murine retrovirus infection may be dependent on a switch from Th1 subset to Th2 subset dominated responses.[15] It is characterized by loss of Th1-cytokine (IL-2 and IFN-γ) production concomitant with increases in Th2-cytokine (IL-5 and IL-10) production.[6-7,15] Th1 and Th2 cytokine profiles in murine retrovirus infection are in accordance with this hypothesis.[6-7] Recent studies have demonstrated in C57BL/6 mice that the stimulation of a strong Th1 immune response via Leishmania major infection before the onset of or early in the progression of LP-BM5 infection inhibits the development of murine AIDS symptoms.[16] Administration of TCR Vβ CDR1 peptide both prior and post infection significantly prevented the murine retrovirus-induced suppression of IL-2 and IFN-γ secretion, while the control peptide, MCG3, from the lambda light chain V region of immunoglobulins did not. Increased IL-2 release by TCR Vβ administration is in accordance with increased T cell proliferation as was the loss of IL-2 secretion by cells from mice that were progressing to severe pathology during murine retrovirus infection.[6-7] IFN-γ also has multiple distinct biological activities including anti-viral activity, activating phagocytosis of macrophages and neutrophil cells, cytotoxicity of NK cells, and cytotoxic T lymphocytes.[17] Thus, increased IFN-γ by TCR Vβ CDR1 peptide would be expected to prevent development of suppressed cell-mediated immunity in murine AIDS. On the other hand, IFN-γ inhibits Th2 cytokine secretion, which usually is elevated during the progression of the murine retrovirus infection. This notion is supported by our findings that administration of TCR Vβ CDR1 peptide in murine AIDS significantly reduced retrovirus-induced elevation of IL-5, IL-10, and IgG production, while a control peptide did not. Increased production of IFN-γ by TCR Vβ peptide after retrovirus infection is also in agreement with the enhancement of NK cell activity by the peptide. Taken together, the prevention of imbalanced Th1 and Th2 cytokine production by TCR Vβ CDR1 peptide administration could contribute to the normalization of the entire immune response, thereby retarding development of immune dysfunction during murine retrovirus infection. The dose of peptide which produced optimal slowing of development of immune dysfunction during murine retrovirus infection, 200 μg, was the same dose found optimal in humans with an autoimmune disease.[18] The two adjuvants tested enhanced the effectiveness of low doses of a TCR Vβ peptide. This treatment may be involved with production of AAbs[13] or cellular immunity.

In vivo activated B cells and macrophages from HIV patents produce a high level of TNF-α,[1] as we found with LPS-stimulated splenocytes for LP-BM5 retrovirus-infected mice.[6] An elevated level of TNF-α may be involved with lipid metabolism, inducing hypertriglyceridemia,[17] and loss of vitamin E,[19] and increased lipid peroxidation[17] during development of murine AIDS.

An elevated level of TNF-α has also been associated with the stimulation of HIV replication in macrophages/monocytes and T cells.[20] Thus, reduction by TCR Vβ peptide treatment of elevated levels of TNF-α in murine retrovirus infection should ameliorate pathological symptoms of the host initiated by retrovirus infection. Peptide treatment also largely prevented loss of tissue vitamin E (unpublished data). Surprisingly, peptide treatment did not prevent lymphadenopathy and splenectomy, although there was a tendency toward less splenectomy in some experiments. So it does not ameliorate all symptoms of retrovirus infection and may not prevent deaths due to asphyxiation from enlarged lymph nodes. In addition, treatment with a single Vβ TCR peptide did not totally prevent immune dysfunction. AAbs were maintained in high levels in two of seven Vβ peptide families tested,[13] suggesting that several T cell families or clones were stimulated by the retrovirus infection. Complete maintenance of normal immune function may be possible by preventing stimulation of all clones induced by the murine retrovirus antigen by treatment with the Vβ peptides from the several TCR clones stimulated by murine retrovirus infection.

Conclusion

In summary, a TCR Vβ CDR1 peptide is a potentially immunomodulating agent that achieves its immune-enhancing effects through indirect mechanisms, possibly by preventing selective expansion of TCR Vβ T cells induced by the chronic retroviral antigen exposure. These findings help evaluate the mechanisms contributing to retrovirus-caused immunodeficiency and aid in preventing their functioning. TCR peptide treatment to produce AAbs could provide long-term prevention of retrovirus-induced immune dysfunction. In addition, the use of TCR Vβ CDR1 may be important in forestalling initial episodes of general immune disorders in some patients by extending the period between retrovirus infection and the appearance of immune deficiencies.

References

1. Fauci, A.S. Multifactorial nature of human immunodeficiency virus disease: implications for therapy, *Science*, 262, 1011. 1993.
2. Selvey, L.A., Morse, H.C., III, Granger, L.G., and Hodes, R.J., Preferential expansion and activation of VB5+ CD4+ T cells in murine acquired immunodeficiency syndrome, *J. Immunol.*, 151, 1712. 1993.
3. Soudeyns, H., Rebai, N., Pantaleo, G.P., Ciurli, C., Boghossian, T., Sekaly, P.P., and Fauci, A.S., The T cell receptor V beta repertoire in HIV-1 infection and disease, *Semin. Immunol.*, 5, 175. 1993.
4. Imberti, L., Sottini, A., Bettinardi, A., Puoti, M., and Primi, D., Selective depletion in HIV infection of T cells that bear specific T cell receptor VB sequences, *Science*, 254, 860. 1991.
5. Marchalonis, J.J., Deghanpisheh, K., Huang, D., Schluter, S.F., and Watson, R.R., Autoantibodies to T-cell receptors following infection by murine retrovirus, *Lymphology*, 27S, 853. 1994.

6. Victor-Kobrin, C., Bonilla, F.A., Barak, Z., and Bona, C., Structural correlates of a regulatory idiotype, *Immunol. Rev.,* 110, 151. 1989.
7. Marchalonis, J.J., Kaymaz, H., Dedeoglu, F., Schluter, S.F., Yocum, D.E., and Edmundson, A.B., Human autoantibodies reactive with synthetic autoantigens from T-cell receptor B chain, *Proc. Natl. Acad. Sci. U.S.A.,* 89, 332. 1992.
8. Dedeoglu, F., Hubbard, R.A., Schluter, S.F., and Marchalonis, J.J., T-cell 23 receptors of man and mouse studied with antibodies against synthetic peptides, *Exp. Clin. Immunogenet.,* 9, 95. 1991.
9. Toyonaga, B. and Mak, T.W., Genes of the T-cell antigen receptor in normal and malignant T-cells, *Ann. Rev. Immunol.* 5, 585. 1987.
10. Kaymaz, H., Dedeoglu, F., Schluter, S.F., Edmundson, A.B., and Marchalonis, J.J., Reactions of anti-immunoglobulin sera with synthetic T-cell receptor peptides: implications for the three-dimensional structure and function of the TCRB chain, *Int. Immunol.,* 5, 941. 1993.
11. Marchalonis, J.J., Kaymaz, H., Dedeoglu, F., Schluter, S.F., and Edmundson, A.B., Antigenic mapping of a human light chain: correlation with 3-dimensional structure, *J. Protein Chem.,* 11, 129. 1992.
12. Feng, D.F. and Doolittle, R.F., Progressive sequence alignment as a prerequisite to correct phylogenetic trees, *J. Mol. Evol.,* 25, 351. 1987.
13. Dehghanpisheh, K., Huang, D.S., Schuter, S.F., Watson, R.R., and Marchalonis, J.J., Production of IGG autoantibodies to T-cell receptors in mice infected with the retrovirus LP-BM5, *Int. Immunol.,* 7, 31. 1995.
14. Wang, Y., Ardestani, S.K., Liang, B., Beckham, L., and Watson, R.R., Anti-IL-4 monoclonal antibody and interferon-my administration retards development of immune dysfunction and cytokine dysregulation during murine AIDS, *Immunology,* 83, 384, 1994.
15. Wang, Y., Huang, D.S., Giger, P.T., and Watson, R.R., The kinetics of imbalanced cytokine production by T cells and macrophages during the murine AIDS, *Adv. Biosci.,* 86, 335, 1993.
16. Doherty, T.M., Morse, H.C., III, and Coffman, R.L., Modulation of specific T cell responses by concurrent infection with Leishmania major and LP-BM5 murine leukemia viruses, *Int. Immunol.,* 7, 131. 1995.
17. Odeleye, O.E., Eskelson, C.D., and Watson, R.R., Changes in hepatic lipid composition after infection by LP-BM5 causing murine AIDS, *Life Sci.* 51, 129. 1992.
18. Boardette, D.N., Whitman, R.H., Chou, Y.K., Morrison, W.J., Atherton, J., Kenny, C., Liefeld, D., Hashim, G.A., Offner, H., and Vandenbark, A.A., Immunity to TCR peptides in multiple sclerosis. I. Successful immunization of patients with synthetic VB 5.1 and VB 6.1 CDR2 peptides, *J. Irnmunol.,* 152, 2510. 1994.
19. Wang, Y., Liang, B. and Watson, R.R., Suppression of tissue levels of vitamin A, E, zinc and copper in murine AIDS, *Nutr. Res.,* 14, 1031. 1994.
20. Mellors, J.W., Griffith, B.P., Ortiz, M.A., Landry, M.L., and Ryan, J.L., Tumor necrosis factor-alpha/cachectin enhances human immunodeficiency virus type 1 replication in primary macrophages, *J. Infect. Dis.,* 163, 78. 1991.

chapter thirteen

Antioxidants and AIDS

Zhen Zhang, Paula Inserra, Bailin Liang,
and Ronald R. Watson

Introduction

Acquired immunodeficiency syndrome (AIDS) is a result of infection with human immunodeficiency virus (HIV-1 or HIV-2) which eventually destroys subset CD4+ helper T lymphocytes. This results in enhanced susceptibility to opportunistic infection and neoplasms.[1] Oxidative stress plays a major role in the progression of HIV infection to AIDS and has been suggested to contribute to the decline in CD4+ lymphocytes.[2] The existence of oxidative stress in HIV infection and AIDS is exemplified by the excess production of reactive oxygen species (ROS) and a general loss of antioxidant defenses in HIV-infected patients.[3] Therefore, the reduction of oxidative stress by antioxidant treatment may be a desirable therapy during the asymptotic HIV infection as well as advanced AIDS.[4]

Oxidative stress and HIV infection

Oxidative stress is a pathologic phenomenon resulting from an imbalance between the system producing ROS and the antioxidant defense systems which function synergistically to prevent or destroy ROS.[5] An increased production of ROS is caused by infecting agents in neutrophils and macrophages[6] as well as by abnormal production of TNF-α in HIV-infected patients.[7,8] Increased secretion of TNF-α results from direct stimulation by free radicals and the antigens of opportunistic bacteria only in AIDS when severe immunedysfunction permits persistent infection. In the asymptomatic stage, activation of the TNF gene occurs by the viral replication machinery.[5] TNF may play an important role in causing a further increase in the levels of oxidants by providing an "amplification loop" that feeds back to excite further production of ROS from macrophages and neutrophils.[9] It may also

0-8493-8561-X/98/$0.00+$.50
© 1998 by CRC Press LLC

react with T cells to enhance expression of autocrine cell activators, such as IL-2, and receptors, thereby promoting activation of T cell respiratory activity for greater intracellular ROS.[10,11] The excessive production of oxygen-free-radicals causes the oxidation of circulating or membrane lipids, proteins, and DNA, and functions as a potent inducer of viral activation, DNA damage, and immunosuppression.[12]

Apoptosis, programmed cell death of CD4+ lymphocytes, is of fundamental importance in progression towards AIDS.[3] The cascade of events that results from oxidative stress can initiate apoptosis, a possible pathway of immune cell loss in patients with HIV infection.[3] It includes oxidation of cellular membranes, alteration in metabolic pathways, disruption of electron transport systems, depletion of cellular ATP production, loss of Ca^{2+} homeostasis, endonuclease activation, and DNA/chromatin fragmentation. The DNA damage caused by oxidative stress may be related to HIV-associated malignancies and disease progression.[13] Downstream events secondary to these effects may also play a role in activation of the latent virus and subsequent viral replication.[3] Oxidative stress is a known activator of HIV replication *in vitro* through the activation of a nuclear factor κB (NF-κB). NF-κB in turn stimulates HIV gene expression by acting on the promoter region of the viral long terminal repeat (LTR), a critical region for transcription in the integrated virus.[13] TNF-α is an important activator of HIV by generating ROS which activates NF-κB.[14]

Antioxidants and AIDS

The suggestion that oxidative stress is a feature of HIV infection and AIDS is also supported by multiple nutritional deficiencies and increased metabolism of antioxidants in HIV-infected patients.[3] This results from malabsorption of nutrients, hypermetabolism, and drug-nutrient interactions.[15] The antioxidant status of lymphocytes is important for their functioning, which is closely linked to their redox potential, particularly to their cysteine and glutathione levels.[5] In a weakened antioxidant system, DNA repair capacity of the cells may be altered and lymphocytes may be killed or impaired.[16-18] Since ROS is involved in the signal transduction mechanisms for HIV activation, a possible therapeutic use of antioxidants in preventing HIV activation has been suggested.[19-23]

Glutathione and N-acetylcysteine

Glutathione (GSH), a thiol derived from cysteine, is important in scavenging reactive oxygen intermediates released by activated neutrophils and monocytes.[24] It regulates many lymphocyte functions including their proliferative response to mitogens, responsiveness of cytotoxic T cells to IL-2, and cytotoxicity of lymphokine-activated killer cells.[25-29] Depletion of GSH inhibits proliferation of T lymphocytes, particularly those from HIV-infected patients.[30] Another important effect of GSH is its ability to inhibit HIV replication when stimulated by TNF or phorbol myristate acetate (PMA) in infected macrophages and lymphoid cells.[31]

HIV-infected patients have greatly decreased levels of GSH in their plasma and peripheral blood lymphocytes.[32,33] The decreased levels of GSH are highly correlated with depressed numbers of CD4+ cells.[24] GSH is a good candidate for clinical investigation, as flow cytometry can measure glutathione levels in T cell subsets and has been used to show GSH changes in such subsets following HIV infection.[18] Since GSH and vitamin E spare each other, vitamin E appears to prevent the drop in GSH levels and thus TNF-α-induced HIV replication.[34]

N-acetylcysteine (NAC) has both a direct and indirect antioxidant role. It is a cysteine precursor which is converted intracellularly into GSH and can also act directly as an antioxidant.[4] By increasing cellular GSH levels and decreasing TNF-α, it can also inhibit TNF-α-induced HIV replication and prevent TNF-α-induced apoptosis of T lymphocytes and other cells in HIV-infected people.[35,36] NAC has been reported to increase antibody-dependent cell mediated cytotoxitity of neutrophils.[35] Early clinical trials have shown that NAC prevents the decline in CD4+ cells in GSH-deficient individuals.[37] Unfortunately, oral and intravenous GSH do not effectively enhance cellular GSH stores.[38] Although aerosolized GSH does increase cellular stores, the most effective means for raising cellular GSH levels is oral or intravenous administration of the GSH precursor NAC.[34,38] Therefore, treating patients with NAC may be a useful strategy in slowing the progression of the disease.

L-2-oxothiazolidine 4-carboxylate (OTC) is another pro-GSH drug that has been proposed for AIDS therapy. Although both NAC and OTC were shown to block cytokine induction of HIV *in vitro*, NAC was far more effective than OTC.[4] In isolated peripheral blood mononuclear cells, NAC fully replenishes depleted intracellular GSH whereas OCT only minimally replenishes GSH.[4] Although NAC is markedly more effective at blocking HIV expression than OCT *in vitro*, both drugs could prove equally effective in the clinical setting.[4] A report studying rats noted that procysteine, also a pro-drug for glutathione, effectively reduced ischemia-induced heart damage by increasing levels of cellular GSH.[39] In what manner procysteine will be effective in people with AIDS remains to be determined.

Vitamin E (tocopherol)

Vitamin E, a fat soluble vitamin, is also a well-known natural antioxidant. It attaches to free radicals and prevents the further generation of free radicals which ultimately prevents membrane lipid peroxidation.[40] Vitamin E functions as an immune enhancer by its antioxidant activity. Deficiencies in vitamin E lead to prooxidant status and have detrimental effects on the immune system.[15]

Plasma vitamin E levels were demonstrated to be lower in HIV-infected patients than in controls.[41] Vitamin E derivatives such as vitamin E acetate, α-tocopheryl succinate and 2,2,5,7,8-Pentamethyl-6-hydroxychromane (PMC) exhibited a concentration dependent inhibition of NF-κB activation by TNF-α.[1] Thus, vitamin E acetate which is a natural, safe compound, and PMC which was demonstrated to be very effective in blocking NF-κB activation, should be considered for possible inclusion in combination therapies for AIDS.[1] The intake of supplementary vitamin E is associated significantly with slower progression to AIDS in HIV-seropositive men.[42] Vitamin E has also been shown to increase the CD4+/CD8+ lymphocyte ratio in AIDS patients by enhancing CD4+ cell counts.[43]

α-Lipoic acid

Recently, α-lipoic acid was found to exert antioxidant action *in vivo* and *in vitro*.[44] In addition, α-lipoic acid has been shown to inhibit HIV-1 replication in infected cells.[45,46] This may be due to the inhibition of NF-κB activation imposed by the antioxidant properties of dihydrolipoic acid (DHLA) generated from α-lipoate.[14] DHLA can cause a complete inhibition of NF-κB activation induced by TNF-α by scavenging free radicals and recycling vitamin E.[14] The inhibitory action of α-lipoic acid was found to be very potent — only 4 mM was needed for a complete inhibition, whereas 20 mM was required for NAC,[45] which indicates that α-lipoic acid may be effective in AIDS therapeutics.

Vitamin C (ascorbic acid)

Vitamin C has a role in moderating the immune system, possibly by affecting natural killer cell, macrophage, and T cell activities.[47] Unfortunately, most of these studies have been done on mice, and mice can synthesize vitamin C internally. In humans, vitamin C properties seem to make it a potential anticancer treatment.[47] Vitamin C also appears to have direct effects on HIV, thus enhancing its importance in treating people with AIDS. *In vitro* vitamin C inhibits the replication of HIV by more than 90% at levels of no toxicity of vitamin C.[48,49] Vitamin C is apparently more efficient than GSH or NAC in reducing the HIV-1 replication in chronically infected T lymphocytes.[49] The effects of vitamin C on HIV can also be increased by the addition of NAC.[67]

Large amounts of vitamin C are consumed by HIV-infected patients.[50] No clinical benefit is associated with ingestion of vitamin C, in spite of the report that vitamin C can improve the clinical situation of patients suffering from different viral diseases and improve their CD4+ cell count with massive doses of vitamin C.[5] A survey of the nutritional status of HIV-seropositive patients[51] showed a nonsignificant decrease in serum vitamin C, and no significant difference in the prevalence of a low status even with an increase in vitamin C intake (10 times the RDA) due to supplementation.

Carotenoids

There is a severe deficit in plasma carotenoid including β-carotene levels in HIV-infected patients.[5] The degree of reduction in carotene levels is secondary to its depletion, given its ability to act as an antioxidant and scavenge the excess active oxygen.[52]

Other vitamins

In a study of micronutrients in HIV-infected patients, there was a decrease in vitamin A and vitamin B_2 (riboflavin) levels.[51] Vitamin B_2 deficiency results in a decreased activity of glutathione reductase, which regenerates oxidized GSH to reduced GSH, enabling it to rejuvenate its antioxidant functions. Mean serum levels of vitamin B_1 (thiamin), vitamin B_6 (pyridoxal), folate, and vitamin B_{12} were unchanged by HIV infection, whereas the prevalence of deficiencies in vitamin A, B_6, B_{12}, and E were significantly increased.[5]

Zinc

Zinc has a very interesting role in HIV infection. Zinc not only functions as an antioxidant, but it also has a more direct effect on the immune system. Zinc increases the secretion of IL-2, the activity of thymulin, and prevents apoptosis.[5] Zinc penetrates cells, enabling regulatory proteins to bind DNA, which results in expression of the IL-2 gene.[53] The addition of zinc to a serum-free culture medium increases the proliferation of T lymphocytes and the synthesis of IL-2 in response to stimulation.[54] In the presence of zinc, thymulin assumes an active cyclic form enabling zinc to be recognized by high affinity receptors on T lymphocytes. This results in the differentiation of T lymphocytes by the induction of antigen B and in response to concanavalin.[56] It is very important to note that Zn^{2+} inhibits the endogenous endonuclease activated by Ca^{2+} which is responsible for the apoptosis of CD4+ cells induced by TNF.[54] Additionally, zinc acts as an antiviral agent by inhibiting the reverse transcriptase.[5]

HIV-infected patients whose status remained stable for two years had normal plasma zinc levels,[56] whereas zinc levels of those who progressed towards AIDS were lower. Thymulin, which is also considered good marker of zinc status, was found to be extremely low in the blood of patients with AIDS.[57]

Faced with this decreased zinc status,[58] the effect of zinc supplementation was investigated in these patients. The most worrisome risk was that of an upsurge of viral activity due to the existence of several zinc-finger proteins in the structure of HIV-1.[59,60] It has been reported that the supplementation of zinc in AIDS patients can increase the CD4+/CD8+ lymphocyte ratio,[61] however, very few studies can confirm these results.

Selenium

Selenium is a cofactor of glutathione peroxidase (GPx). Due to its antiviral effects and its importance in all immunological functions, the administration of selenium is suggested as a supportive therapy in early as well as in advanced stages of HIV infection.[62] A characteristic of the protective effects of selenium against viral pathogens is that its benefits occur at supplemental levels above physiological requirements. This suggests that it may not be associated solely with its function in GPx.[62] Selenium inhibits reverse transcriptase activity in RNA-virus-infected animals, therefore supplemental selenium could also prevent the replication of HIV and retard the development of AIDS in newly HIV-infected subjects. Selenium is required for lymphocyte proliferation, macrophage-initiated tumor cytodestruction, and natural killer-cell activity.[63]

Subnormal serum or plasma selenium levels and erythrocyte GPx activities have been observed in patients with AIDS and AIDS-related complex (ARC).[64] Selenium levels and GPx activity were correlated to the total number of lymphocytes in HIV-infected patients.[64,65]

Selenium supplementation in HIV-infected patients causes symptomatic improvements, especially in appetite and intestinal functions,[66] and possibly slows the course of the disease. During the period of supplementation, CD4 cell numbers still tended to decline; however, this decline was often only slight, or not observed at all. CD8+ cells counts tended to decrease more often than to increase, causing the CD4+/CD8+ lymphocyte ratio to increase.[66]

Copper

It is extremely difficult to study the copper status in patients with inflammations. Cytokines, IL-1, and TNF, cause serum copper to undergo a clear-cut increase, due to the increase in ceruloplasmin, an "acute phase protein", even in copper-deficient subjects.[67]

Serum copper increased in AIDS patients after a decrease in the asymptomatic stage. Low serum zinc levels with high copper levels are predictive of progression towards AIDS, independent of the basal level of CD4+ cell counts.[51,58,68]

The measurement of copper-zinc superoxide dismutase (Cu-Zn SOD) in red cells is a more reliable marker of the zinc status with no variation in the enzyme, regardless of the stage of the disease.[67]

Antioxidant enzymes

The study of antioxidant enzyme activities, in addition to the changes in GPx described above, has shown a progressive and considerable increase in serum catalase,[69] while red cell SOD remains normal.[67]

Serum catalase activity increased progressively with advancing HIV infection (i.e., AIDS > symptomatic infection > asymptomatic infection > controls).[69] This correlates with increases in serum hydrogen peroxide (H_2O_2) scavenging ability, and may reflect or compensate for systemic GSH and other antioxidant deficiencies in HIV-infected individuals.[69]

Manganese-containing superoxide dismutase (Mn-SOD) is the key enzyme in cellular protection from apoptosis induced by TNF[70] via expression of the gene for Mn-SOD and for metallothioneins.[5] A decreased production of Mn-SOD was seen, while mRNA of this enzyme was overproduced in HIV-infected patients.[71] This results from the inhibition of translation of SOD mRNA caused by the binding of HIV tat protein to an RNA hairpin.[5] The sequence on which tat binds presents a sequence homology with a part of viral RNA, which is the biological target of tat, permitting the regulation of viral expression. The anomaly of Mn-SOD production is accompanied by signs of oxidizing stress in cells.[5]

Diethyldithiocarbamate (DDTC)

DDTC has a GPx-like activity. It is the only antioxidant drug that has been extensively studied in clinical trials, although it has not shown any *in vitro* antiviral activity.[72,73] In animals, DDTC increased GSH levels in a variety of tissues.[13] A significant reduction in these rates of new opportunistic infections was reported in AIDS patients receiving DDTC as compared to placebo.[73] However, a subsequent study apparently failed to demonstrate the similar benefit in a cohort study of HIV-infected asymptomatic patients.[13]

Desferrioxamine (DFX)

DFX is an iron chelator with strong antioxidant properties. DFX can inhibit *in vitro* HIV-1 replication in the H-9 T lymphocyte cell line. The rationale for this work is to explain the low rate of symptomatic HIV-1 infection in multiply transfused thalassaemic patients who have been intensively chelated with DFX.[76]

Plant-derived metabolites with synergistic antioxidant activity

Plants experience death due to oxidative stress, which closely parallels the process of apoptosis in humans, particularly as related to the destructive phenomena seen in HIV infection and AIDS. Primary and secondary metabolites found in plants act as synergistic antioxidants and can protect plants from oxidation-induced cell death. Some of these same metabolites can inhibit cell killing by HIV.[3] These metabolites are exemplified by phenolic compounds, nitrogen-containing compounds, enzyme systems and polypeptides, and vitamins. Therefore, use of these antioxidants in patients with HIV/AIDS is proposed as a mechanism by which viral replication and cell killing in HIV infection can be inhibited.[3]

Phenolic compounds (hydroxyl derivatives of aromatic hydrocarbons)

Ubiquinone.   Although ubiquinone (coenzyme Q_{10}, CoQ$_{10}$) is known for its activity as a redox component of transmembrane electron transport in mitochondria, its reduced form, ubiquinol, is an active antioxidant. Ubiquinol scavenges products from the peroxidation of membrane lipids even after the peroxidation process has been initiated. Lipid peroxidation will not occur, in fact, until all ubiquinol is consumed, which spares vitamin E in the process.[75]

Patients with AIDS had significantly lower blood CoQ$_{10}$ levels than healthy controls, while patients with ARC and asymptomatic HIV-seropositive infection had decreased blood levels of CoQ$_{10}$, but not to the extent of those of AIDS patients.[76] Supplementation with CoQ$_{10}$ retarded the progression from ARC to AIDS and has a positive effect on the T4+/T8+ lymphocyte ratio.[66] However, CoQ$_{10}$ may actually increase the level of free radicals thereby increasing oxidative stress.[66]

Flavonoids.   Flavonoids (plant phenolic pigment products, particularly the catechins and quercitin), scavenge peroxyl and hydroxyl free radial.[77] They are protective against lipid peroxidation probably by donating H+ atoms to peroxyl radicals and terminating the chain radical reaction.[78] They can also control the release of reactive oxygen products from macrophages and neutrophils by regulation enzymes such as NADPH oxidase.[79] Quercitin, in particular, can inhibit the PKC-induced phosphorylation of I-κB that can liberate NF-κB to play a role in activation of viral replication.[21,80]

Coumarins (benzopyrones).   Coumarins are effective against oxidative stress by acting in a similar manner to flavonoids.[81]

Nitrogen-containing compounds: di- and poly-amines (e.g., spermine, putrescine, cadaverine)

Nitrogen-containing compounds effectively inhibit lipid peroxidation and impede the release of superoxide radicals from senescing membranes. They exert their stabilizing effects by binding with negative charges of both nucleic acids and phospholipids.[82] They inhibit protease and RNAase activity, which is observed as a consequence of oxidative stress in plants.[82] Similar actions of polyamines in humans have been shown to help maintain intracellular Ca^{2+} homeostasis.[3]

Polyamines decline during oxidative stress, particularly when their necessary precursor, arginine, is either deficient or diverted. Arginine is consumed during nitric oxide production in HIV infection.[3]

Enzyme systems and polypeptides

Dismutase, catalases, and peroxidases all exist in plants, and their enhancement can increase resistance to oxidative stress.[85] The reduced form of GSH (a tri-peptide), so integral to the discussion of oxidative stress in HIV infection, is a scavenger of peroxides in plants and arrests senescence.[86]

Vitamins

Vitamin C and E and the various carotenoids are ubiquitous in plants. As in humans, they do not suffice as protection from superoxidative stress. This is confirmed by the multiplicity of the antioxidant systems that are necessary to synergize with vitamins and provide adequate protection.[85,86]

Conclusion

Oxidizing stress is not merely an epiphenomenon, but is at the heart of the pathogenesis of HIV disease. This has incited researchers to test the effect of antioxidants in cell models, showing the high efficacy of certain micronutrients, but also of some other antioxidants. It is indispensable to combine the return of a deficient antioxidant nutritional status to normal (zine, selenium, carotene, and vitamins C and E) with the supply of high doses of synthetic antioxidant-generating glutathione as N-acetyl cysteins.

Generally, supplementation with antioxidants appears to offer some hope in slowing the progression of HIV infection. Currently there is considerable debate over the use of antioxidant therapies in many illnesses, although more and more mainstream practitioners are considering the potential benefits of such therapies.[87] While the substances discussed here are largely free of toxic effects, caution still must be taken, and the development of adverse effects should be carefully monitored. It is also important for practitioners to stress to their patients the importance of a basic balanced diet as the essential groundwork underlying any additional supplementation or drug treatment. The research into antioxidants is still at an early stage of development, but future studies will likely resolve which of these substances can be used effectively in treating HIV infection.[67]

References

1. Yuichiro, J.S., Bharat B.A., and Lester P., Inhibition of NF-κB activation by vitamin E derivatives, *Biochem. Biophys. Res. Commun.*, 193, 277, 1993.
2. Buttke, T.M. and Sandstron P.A., Oxidative stress as a mediator of apoptosis, *Immunol. Today*, 15, 7, 1994.
3. Greenspan, H.C. and Arouma, O., Could oxidative stress initiate programmed cell death in HIV infection? A role for plant derived metabolites having synergistic antioxidant activity, *Chem. Biol. Interact.*, 91, 187, 1994.
4. Paul, A.R., Leonore, A.H., Leonard, A.H., and Mario, R., Glutathione precursor and antioxidant activities of N-acetylcysteine and oxothiazolidine carboxylate compared in *in vitro* studies of HIV replication, *AIDS Res. Hum. Retrovir.*, 10, 961, 1994.
5. Favier, A., Sappey, C., Leclerc, P., Faure, P., and Micoud, M., Antioxidant status and lipid peroxidation in patients infected with HIV, *Chem. Biol. Interact.*, 91, 165, 1994.

6. Braun, D.P., Kessler, H., Falk, L., Paul, D., Harris, J.E., Blauw, B., and Landay, A., Monocyte functional studies in asymptomatic human immunodeficiency disease virus (HIV) infected individuals, *J. Clin. Immunol.*, 8, 486, 1988

7. Folks, T., Justement, J., Kinter, A., Dinarello, C., and Fauci, A., Cytokine induced expression of HIV-1 in a chronically infected promonocyte cell line, *Science*, 238, 800, 1987.

8. Poli, G., Kinter, A., Justement, J., Kehrl, J., Bressler, P., Stanley, S., and Fauci, A., Tumor necrosis factor a function in an autocrine manner in the induction of human immunodeficiency virus expression, *Proc. Natl. Acad. Sci. U.S.A.*, 87, 782, 1990.

9. Greenspan H.C. and Arouma, O., Oxidative stress and apoptosis in HIV infection: a role for plant-derived metabolites with synergistic antioxidant activity, *Immunol. Today*, 15, 209, 1994.

10. Greenspan, H.C., The role of reactive oxygen species, antioxidants and phytopharmaceuticals in human immunodeficiency virus activity, *Med. Hypotheses*, 40, 85, 1993.

11. Scott-algara D., Vuillier F., Marasescu M., de Saint Martin, J., and Dighiero, G., Serum levels of IL-2, IL-1 alpha, TNF-alpha, and soluble receptor of IL-2 in HIV-infected patients, *AIDS Res. Hum. Retrovir.*, 7, 381, 1991.

12. Floyd, R.A. and Schneider, J.E., Hydroxyl free radicals damage to DNA, in *Membrane Lipid Oxidation*, Vol. I., Vigo-pelfrey, C., Ed., CRC Press, Boca Raton, FL, 1990,

13. Salvain, B. and Mark A.W., The role of oxidative stress in disease progression in individuals infected by the human immunodeficiency virus, *J. Leukocyte Biol.*, 52, 111, 1992.

14. Lester, P. and Yuichire, J.S., Vitamin E and alpha-lipoate: role in antioxidant recycling and activation of the NF-κB transcription factor, *Mol. Aspects Med.*, 14, 229, 1993.

15. Kelleher J., Vitamin E and the immune response, Proc. Nutr. Soc. 50, 245, 1991.

16. Droge, W., Eck, H.P., Peckar, U., and Caniel, V., Glutathione augments the activation of cytotoxic T lymphocytes *in vivo*, *Immunol.*, 172, 151, 1986.

17. Gougerot-Poccidalo, M.A., Fay, M., Roche, Y., Chollet, M., and Martin, S., Mechanism by which oxidative injury inhibits the proliferative response for human lymphocytes to PHA. Effect of the thiol compound 2-mercaptoethanol, *Immunol.*, 164, 281, 1989.

18. Roederer, M., Staal, F.J., Osada, H., and Herzenberg, L.A., CD4 and CD8 T cells with high intracellular glutathione levels are selectively lost as the HIV infection progresses, *Int. Immunol.*, 199, 933, 1990

19. Staal, F.J.T., Roederer, M., and Herzenberg, L.A., Intracellular thiols regulate activation of nuclear factor kappa B and transcription of human immunodeficiency virus, *Proc. Natl. Acad. Sci., U.S.A.*, 87, 9943, 1990.

20. Mihm, S., Ennen, J., Pessare, U., Kurth, R., and Droge, W., Inhibition of HIV-1 replication and NF-kappa B activity by cysteine and cysteine derivatives, *AIDS*, 5, 497, 1991.

21. Schreck, R., Meier, B., Mannel, D.N., Droge, W., and Vaeuerle, P.A., Dithiocarbamates as potent inhibitors of nuclear factor kappa B activation in intact cells, *J. Exp. Med.*, 175, 1181, 1992.

22. Schreck, R., Rieber, P., and Baeuerle, P.A., Reactive oxygen intermediates as apparently widely used messengers in the activation of the NF-kappa B transcription factor and HIV-1, *EMBO. J.*, 10, 2247, 1991.

23. Schreck, R., Albermann, K., and Baeuerle, P.A., Nuclear factor kappa B: an oxidative stress-responsive transcription factor of eukaryotic cells, *Free Radic. Res. Commun.*, 17, 221, 1992.
24. Quey, B., Malinverni, R., and Lauterburg, B.H., Glutathione depletion in HIV-infected patients: role of cysteine deficiency and effect of oral N-acetyl-cysteine, *AIDS*, 5, 814, 1992.
25. Fidelus, R.K. and Tsan, M., Enhancement of intracellular glutathione promotes lymphocyte activation by mitogen, *Cell Immunol.*, 97, 155, 1986.
26. Fidelus, R.K., Ginouves, P., Lawrence, D., and Tsan, M., Modulation of intra-cellular glutathione concentrations alters lymphocyte activation and prolifer-ation, *Exp. Cell Res.*, 170, 269, 1987.
27. Suthanthiran, M., Anderson, M.E., Sharma, V.K., and Meister, A., Glutathione regulates activation-dependent DNA synthesis in highly purified normal hu-man T lymphocytes stimulated via the CD2 and CD3 antigens, *Proc. Natl. Acad. Sci. U.S.A.*, 87, 3343, 1990.
28. Liang, S.M., Lee, N., Finbloom, D.S., and Liang, C.M., Regulation by glu-tathione of interleukin-4 activity on cytotoxic T cells, *Immunol.*, 75, 435, 1992.
29. Droge, W., Eck, H.P., Gmunder, H., and Mihm, S., Modulation of lymphocyte functions and immune responses by cysteine and cysteine derivatives, *Am. J. Med.*, 91 (suppl.), 140, 1991.
30. Levy, D.M., Wu, J., Salibian, M., and Black, P.H., The effect of changes in thiol subcompartments on T-cell colony formation and cell cycle progression: rel-evance of AIDS, *Cell Immunol.*, 140, 370, 1992.
31. Kalebic, T., Kinter, A., Poli, G., Anderson, M.E., Meister, A., and Fauci, A.S., Suppression of human immunodeficiency virus expression in chronically in-fected monocytic cells by glutathione, glutathione ester, and N-acetyl-cys-teine, *Proc. Natl. Acad. Sci. U.S.A.*, 88, 986, 1991.
32. Papadopulos-Eleopulos, E., Turner, V.F., and Papadimitriou, J.M., Oxidative stress, HIV, and AIDS, *Res. Immunol.*, 143, 145, 1992.
33. Droge, W., Eck, H.P., and Mihm, S., HIV-induced cysteine deficiency and T-cell dysfunction — a rationale for treatment with N-acetylcysteine, *Immunol. Today*, 13, 211, 1992.
34. Gilden, D., Nutritional intervention in HIV disease, *BETA*, March, 3-11, 1994.
35. Rortert, L.R., Vanita, R.A., and Bonnie, J.A., N-acetylcysteine enhances anti-body-dependent cellular cytotoxicity in neutrophils and mononuclear cells from healthy adults and human immunodeficiency virus-infected patients, *J. Infect. Dis.*, 172, 1492, 1995.
36. Angela, K.T., Stephen, D., Seth, W.P., Sheila, C.D., Suryaram, G., Steven, M.F., Deborah, N., Leon, G.E., Howard, E.G., and Harris, A.G., Tumor necrosis factors alpha-induced apoptosis in human neuronal cells: protection by the antioxidant N-acetylcysteine and the genes *bcl*-2 and *crm*A, *Mol. Cell. Biol.*, 15, 2359, 1995.
37. Kinscherf, R., Fishbach, T., and Mihm, S., Effect of glutathione depletion and oral N-acetyl-cysteine treatment of CD4+ and CD8+ cells, *FASEB J.*, 8, 448, 1994.
38. Salbemini, D. and Botting, R., Modulation of platelet function by free radicals and free-radical scavengers, *TIPS*, 14, 36, 1993.
39. Shug, A.L. and Madsen, D.C., Protection of the ischemic rat heart by procys-teine and amino acids, *J. Nutr. Biochem.*, 5, 356, 1994.
40. Combs, G.F., Jr., *The Vitamins: Fundamental Aspects in Nutrition and Health*, Academic Press, San Diego, 1992.

41. Passi, S., Picardo, D.M., Morrone, A., and Ippolito, F., I valori ematici deficitari degli acidi grassi poliinsaturi dei fosfolipidi, della vitamin E e della glutathione peossidasi come possibili fattori di rischio nell' insorgenza e nello sviluppo della sindrome da immunodeficienza acquisita, *G. Ital. Dermatol. Venereol.*, 125, 125, 1990.

42. Abrams, B., Duncan, D., and Hertz-Picciotto I., A prospective study of dietary intake and acquired immune deficiency syndrome in HIV-seropositive homosexual men, *J. AIDS*, 6, 949, 1993.

43. Myrvik, Q.N., Immunology and nutrition, in *Modern Nutrition in Health and Disease*, 8th ed., Shils, M.E., Olson, J.A., and Shike, M., Eds., Lea & Febiger, Philadephia, 1994, 623.

44. Peinado, J., Sies, H., and Akerboom, T.P., Hepatic lipoate uptake, *Arch. Biochem. Biophys.*, 273, 389, 1989.

45. Yuichiro, J., Suzuki, B.B.A., and Lester, P., α-Lipoic acid is a potent inhibitor of NF-κB activation in human T cells, *Biochem. Biophys. Res. Commun.*, 189, 1709, 1992.

46. Baur, A., Harrer, T., Peukert, M., Jahn, G., Kalden, J.R., and Fleckenstien, B., Alpha-lipoic acid is an effective inhibitor of human immuno-deficiency virus replication, *Klin. Wochenschr.*, 69, 722, 1991.

47. Siegel, B.V., Vitamin C and the immune response in health and disease, in *Human Nutrition: A Comprehensive Treatise, Vol. 8: Nutrition and Immunology*, Plenum Press, New York, 1993, 167.

48. Harakeh, S., Jariwalla, R.J., and Pauling, L., Suppression of human immuno-deficiency virus replication by ascorbate in chronically and acutely infected cells, *Proc. Natl. Acad. U.S.A.*, 87, 7245, 1990.

49. Harakeh, S. and Jariwalla, R.J., Comparative study of the anti-HIV activities of ascorbate and thiol-containing reducing agents in chronically HIV-infected cells, *Am. J. Clin. Nutr.*, 54, 1231s, 1991.

50. Cathart, R., Vitamin C in the treatment of acquired immune deficiency syndrome (AIDS)., *Med. Hypotheses*, 14, 423, 1984.

51. Beach, R., Mantero-Antienza, E., and Shor-Posner, G., Specific nutrient abnormalities in asymptomatic HIV-1 infection, *AIDS*, 6, 701, 1992.

52. Bendich, A. and Olson, J.A., Biological actions of carotenoids, *FASEB J.*, 3, 1927, 1989.

53. Schwabe, J. and Rhodes, D., Beyond zinc fingers: a steroid hormone receptors have a novel structural motif for DNA recognition, *Tibs*, 16, 291, 1991.

54. Tanala, Y., Shiozawa, S., Morito, I., and Fujita, T., Role of zinc in interleukin 2 mediated T-cell activation, *Scand. J. Immunol.*, 31, 547, 1990.

55. Dardenne, M., Savino, W., Berrih, S., and Bach, J.F., A zinc dependent epitope in the molecule of thymulin athymic hormone, *Proc. Natl. Acad. Sci. U.S.A.*, 82, 7035, 1985.

56. Graham, N., Sorensen, D., Odaka, N., Brookmeyer, R., Chan, D., Willett, W., Morris, J., and Saah, A., Relationship of serum copper and zinc levels to HIV-1 seropositivity and progression to AIDS, *J. AIDS*, 4, 976, 1991.

57. Fabris, N., Mocchegiani, E., Galli, M., Irato, L., Lazzarin, A., and Moroni, M., AIDS, zinc deficiency and thymic hormone failure, *JAMA*, 259, 839, 1988.

58. Sergio, W., Zinc salts that may be defective against the AIDS virus HIV, *Med. Hypotheses*, 26, 251, 1988.

59. Maekawa, T., Sakura, H., Sudo, T., and Ishii, S., Putative metal finger structure of the human immuno-deficiency virus type 1 enhancer binding protein HIV-EP1, *J. Biol. Chem.*, 64, 14591, 1989.
60. South, T., Kim, B., Hare, D., and Summers, M., Zinc fingers and molecular recognition, structure and nucleic acid binding studies of an HIV zinc finger-like domain, *Biochem. Pharmacol.*, 40, 123, 1990.
61. Zazzo, J.F., Rouveix, B., Rajagopolan, P., Leracher, M., and Girard, P.M., Effect of zinc on immune status of zinc depleted ARC patients, *Clin. Nutr.*, 8, 259, 1989.
62. Schrauzer, G.N. and Sacher, J., Selenium in the maintenance and therapy of HIV-infected patients, *Chem. Biol. Interact.*, 91, 199, 1994.
63. Kiremidjian-Schumacher, L. and Stotzky, G., Selenium and immune responses, *Environ. Res.*, 42, 277, 1987.
64. Dwodkin, B.M., Rosenthal, W.S., Wormser, G.P., Weiss, L., Numez, M., Coline, C., and Herp, A., Abnormalities of blood selenium and glutathione peroxidase in patients with acquired immunodeficiency syndrome and AIDS-related complex, *Biol. Trace Elem. Res.*, 20, 86, 1988.
65. Dworkin, B., Rosenthal, W., Wormser, G., and Weiss, L., Selenium deficiency in the acquired immuno-deficiency syndrome, *JPEN. Parenter. Enteral. Nutr.*, 10, 405, 1986.
66. Adam, E.S., Antioxidant supplementation in HIV/AIDS, *Nurse Pract.*, 20, 8, 1995.
67. Walter, R., Oster, M., Lee, T., Flynn, N., and Keen, C., Zinc status in human immunodeficiency virus infection, *Life Sci.*, 47, 1579, 1990.
68. Beck, K., Scramel, P., Hedl, A., Jaeger, H., and Kaboth, W., Serum trace element levels in HIV-infected subjects, *Biol. Trace Elem. Res.*, 25, 89, 1990.
69. Leff, J., Oppegard, M., Curiel, T., Brown, K., Schooley, R., and Repine, J., Progressive increases in serum catalase activity in advancing human immunodeficiency virus infection, *Free Rad. Biol. Med.*, 13, 143, 1992.
70. Wong, G.H., Elwell, J., Oberley, L., and Goeddel, D., Manganous superoxide dismutase is essential for cellular resistance to cytotoxicity of tumor necrosis factor, *Cell*, 58, 923, 1989.
71. Flores, S.C., Marecki, J.C., Harper, Kp., Bose, S.K., Nelson, S.K., and McCoed, J, M., Tat protein of human immunodeficiency virus type 1 represses expression of manganese superoxide dismutase in Hela cells, *Proc. Natl. Acad. Sci. U.S.A.*, 90, 7632, 1993.
72. Reisinger, E.C., Kern, P., Ernst, M., Bock, P., Flad, H.D., and Dietrich, M., Inhibition of HIV progression by dithiocarb, *Lancet*, 335, 679, 1990.
73. Hersh, E.M., Brewton, G., Abrams, D., Bartlett, J., Galpin, J., Parkash, G., Gorter, R., Gottlieb, M., Jonikas, J.J., Landesman, S., Levine, A., Marcel, A., Petersin, E.A., Whiteside, M., Zahradnik, J., Negron, C., Boutitie, F., Caraux, J., Dupuy, J-M., and Salmi, L.R., Dithiocarb sodium (diethyldithiocarbamate) therapy in patients with symptomatic HIV infection and AIDS. A randomized double blind, placebo-controlled multicenter study, *JAMA*, 265, 1538, 1991.
74. Baruchel, S., Gao, Q., and Wainberg, M.A., Desferrioxamine and HIV, *Lancet*, 337, 1356, 1991.
75. Feid, B., Kim, M.C., and Ames, B.N., Ubiquinol-10 is an effective lipid-soluble antioxidant at physiological concentrations, *Proc. Natl. Acad. Sci. U.S.A.*, 87, 4879, 1990.

76. Langsjoen, P.H., Folkers. K., and Richardson, P., Treatment of patients with human immunodeficiency virus infection with coenzyme Q_{10}, in *Biomedical and Clinical Aspects of Coenzyme Q*, Vol. 6, Folkers, K., Litatarru, G.P., and Yamagami, T., Eds., Elsevier, Amsterdam, 1991, 40916.
77. Afanas'ev, I.B. and Dorozhko, A.I., Chelating and free radical scavenging mechanisms of inhibitory action of rutin and quercitin in lipid peroxidation, *Biochem. Pharmacol.*, 38, 1763, 1989.
78. Laughton, M.J., Evans, P.J., Moroney, M.A., Hoult, J.R.S., and Halliwell, F., Inhibition of mammalian 5-lipoxygenase and cyclo-oxygenase by flavonoids and phenolic dietary additives, *Biochem. Pharmacol.*, 42, 1673, 1993.
79. Torel, J., Cillard, J., and Dillard, P., Antioxidant activity of flavonoids and reactivity with peroxy radical, *Phytochemistry*, 25, 383, 1986.
80. Greenspan, H.C., The role of reactive oxygen species, antioxidants and phytopharmaceuticals in human immunodeficiency virus activtity, *Med. Hypotheses*, 40, 85, 1993.
81. Paya, M., Halliwell. B., and Hoult, J.R.S., Interactions of a series of coumarins with reactive oxygen species, *Biochem. Pharmacol.*, 44, 205, 1992.
82. Drolet, G., Dumbroff, E.B., Legge, R.L., and Thompson, J.E., Radical scavenging properties of polyamines, *Phytochemistry*, 25, 367, 1986.
83. Bowler, C. and Slooten, L., Manganese superoxide dismutase can reduce cellular damage mediated by oxygen radicals in transgenic plants, *EMBO J.*, 10, 1732, 1991.
84. Alscher, R.G., Biosynthesis and antioxidant function of glutathione in plants, *Physiol. Plant*, 77, 457, 1989.
85. Garewal, H.S., Ampel, N.M., Watson, R.R., Prabhala, R.H., and Dols, C.L., A preliminary trial of beta-carotene in subjects infected with the human immunodeficiency virus, *J. Nutr.*, 22, 728, 1992.
86. Watson, R.R., Prabhala, R.H., Plezia, P.M., and Alberts, D.S., Effect of beta-carotene on lymphocyte subpopulations in elderly humans; evidence for a dose-response relationship, *Am. J. Clin. Nutr.*, 53, 90, 1991.
87. Voelker, R., Recommendations for antioxidants: how much evidence is enough? *JAMA*, 271, 1148, 1994.

chapter fourteen

Vitamin E supplementation retards the development of acquired immune deficiency syndrome

James Y. Wang and Bailin Liang

Introduction

Acquired immune deficiency syndrome (AIDS), caused by human immunodeficiency virus (HIV), is a clinical disorder representing the end point in a progression sequence of immune suppressive changes that render the body highly susceptible to life-threatening tumors and opportunistic infections. AIDS has been identified as a major public health priority in the U.S. with heavy social and economic impact. A recent analysis estimated that 700,000 to 900,000 U.S. residents (approximately 0.3% of the population) are infected with HIV, and about 40,000 persons are infected annually in the U.S.[1,2] Each year, around 60,000 are diagnosed with an AIDS-related opportunistic infection.[2] The Centers for Disease Control reported that 85,430 persons died from this condition.[3] Through 1994, more than 325,000 persons diagnosed with AIDS residing in the U.S. had died.[4] AIDS is the leading cause of death among all Americans aged 25 to 44.[4] The World Health Organization estimates that more than 10 million people throughout the world are infected with HIV.[5] Immune and other physiological defects induced by HIV infection appear to be progressive and irreversible with a high mortality rate that approaches 100%.[6]

Despite the recent optimism in the clinical care arena elicited by the finding that protease inhibitors can dramatically reduce viral load, we are still years or even a decade away from a cure or an effective vaccine. In view of the remarkable ability of HIV to mutate, avoid immune surveillance, and resist pharmacologic treatments, the development of effective treatments or vaccines against HIV will be difficult and expensive, especially in those at

0-8493-8561-X/98/$0.00+$.50
© 1998 by CRC Press LLC

the highest risk. Even when effective treatments or vaccines pass the rigors of clinical trials and become available for general use, they are unlikely to be 100% effective or to reach 100% of the at-risk population. Therefore, there is a pressing need for developing alternative or complementary approaches to prevention and treatment of AIDS.

One such possible approach is nutritional intervention. One of the most attractive nutrients in this respect is vitamin E, an antioxidant, free radical scavenger and immunoenhancer. Vitamin E is a widely distributed, fat-soluble vitamin composed of several tocopherols and tocotrienols, the most biologically active of which is α-tocopherol.[7] In this chapter, we summarize our current understanding as to immunological, nutritional, and oxidative stress caused by HIV infection, and properties of immunoenhancing, anti-oxidant, and undernutrition-improvement of vitamin E supplementation. Since there is a paucity of information available regarding the nutritional therapy in AIDS individuals, our purpose is to provide evidence from a murine AIDS model[8] for humans of the potential therapeutic role of vitamin E supplementation in the prevention and treatment of AIDS/HIV+ individuals.

AIDS and immune functions

HIV infection in humans progresses to significant immunosuppression.[9] The role of T cells is critical to AIDS development in humans. HIV causes abnormalities in the immune system by depleting the CD4+ T helper cells, and by changing their functions.[9,10] In addition, HIV activates B cells and infects macrophages which can be critical to antigen presentation.[10] HIV induces an early phase of B cell hyperactivity and polyclonal activation.[11] B cells and their production of immunoglobulin (Ig) show a significant number of alterations due to retroviral infection in men.[9] Activation of both T and B lymphocytes can be detected within one week of infection, as judged by flow cytometric analysis of size of T and B cells and measurements of the percentage of B cells secreting IgM. There is an absolute increase in the number of B cells in the spleen and lymph nodes, and a three-fold increase in the fraction of B cells in cell cycle.[12]

Cytokines mediate a variety of biological and physiological processes providing an interactive complexity of potentially immunomodulating agents which integrate cellular and humoral function within higher mammals. These pleiotropic cell regulators are secreted primarily from immunocompetent cells.[13] They play a crucial role in transmitting and regulating signals for proliferation, differentiation, and expression of cellular function in a variety of targets especially in relation to immune responses. Target cell functions are usually affected by the interactions of one or more of these regulatory molecules. Cytokine dysregulation may be a key component to induce AIDS in HIV-infected subjects. Interleukin 2 (IL-2) is a pivotal cytokine for the growth and differentiation of T and B cells, and for the enhancement of B cell growth and Ig production.[14] It is secreted mainly by the Th1 subset of activated T helper cells. In addition to T cell proliferation, subsequent studies have shown that B cells, NK cells, and LAK cells also respond to IL-2.[15] IL-4, IL-5, and IL-6 are synthesized predominantly by stimulated T cells.[16,17] IL-4, IL-5, and IL-6, respectively, promote the activation, growth, and differentiation of B lymphocytes into antibody-secreting cells, but have also been found to have various effects on T cell activation and growth.[15,18-25] IL-10 is produced during a variety of immune-activated conditions by Th0 and Th2 cell subsets as well as by monocytes, macrophages, and B cells.[26] It suppresses Th1 cytokine production (IL-2, IFN-γ, and lymphotoxin) and antigen-specific proliferation of Th1 cell subsets after activation in an accessory cell-dependent manner. It also diminishes delayed-type hypersensitivity reactions and other Th1 cell-mediated responses. Acting indirectly, IL-10 suppresses the capacity of certain accessory cells to promote Th1 cell development.[22] Furthermore, it suppresses murine macrophage functions such as the inhibition of macrophage-mediated immunity and the production of reactive nitrogen oxides which are involved in the elimination of intra- and extra-cellular parasites. Interferon-gamma (IFN-γ) is a multiple immunoregulatory cytokine that is secreted primarily by activated T lymphocytes (CD4+, CD8+, and CD4-8-), cells of the monocyte lineage, and NK cells.[27-30] The production of IFN-γ is modulated by the simultaneous production of IL-1, IL-2, IL-4, and tumor necrosis factor-α (TNF). IFN-γ primes macrophages for microbicidal and tumoricidal activity and enhances NK cytotoxicity.[31,32] Moreover, its functions include the inhibition of some IL-4-induced B cell activations, the modulation of B cell differentiation, the augmentation of Ig secretion in B lymphocytes,[33-35] and the up-regulation of expression of the secretory component required for binding and transport of secreted IgA and IgM.[36] Furthermore, it down-regulates Th2 cytokine production (IL-4, IL-6, and IL-10) and cell proliferation of Th2 cell clone. Finally, TNF is a cytokine that expresses activities including inflammation and anti-tumor activity.[32,37,38] Activated monocytes/macrophages are the primary source of TNF-α.[39,40] The production of TNF is regulated by IFN-γ released from stimulated T cells.[41]

AIDS and nutrition

The estimated median incubation time from infection with HIV to development of AIDS is 8 to 10 years.[42] Because some individuals infected with HIV develop AIDS quickly, while others do not, additional factors may modify the course of HIV infection and development of AIDS. It has been proposed that nutritional status is one of these factors.[43,44] An association between nutrition and AIDS development is suggested by evidence that certain nutrients influence immune responses[45] and by the observation that many of the physical manifestations of AIDS, for example, opportunistic infections and wasting, are also associated with protein energy malnutrition.[46]

Since progression to AIDS is often complicated by various nutritional disorders, the additional immune dysfunction due to undernutrition can have precluded recovery from infectious events which earlier represented survivable episodes. This hypothesis is based on findings that malnutrition has been associated with immunological dysfunction,[47,48] development of infectious processes,[49] and vital organ dysfunction.[50] Thus, the severe malnutrition seen in patients with AIDS may set up a vicious cycle in which the underlying immunological defects related to HIV infection are aggravated by the malnutrition-induced immune dysfunction.

Although the roles of vitamins and minerals in the clinical manifestation of HIV infection has not been well defined,[51] a growing number of studies have suggested important links between vitamins or minerals and HIV infection.[52] Vitamin B_{12} and B_6 deficiencies are common in patients with HIV infection.[53-56] Patients at various stages of HIV disease have serum vitamin A and E deficiencies.[57-59] Malabsorption secondary to HIV-induced intestinal dysfunction appears to be the likely cause of vitamin A deficiency, but no further study about pathogenesis has been reported. The cause of vitamin E deficiency is unclear, although it may relate to the malabsorption associated with worsening HIV infection. A recent study found that a major percentage of patients with AIDS (50%), ARC (58%), and HIV (38%) had a vitamin E intake of less than 50% the Recommended Daily Allowance.[51] Zinc deficiency in HIV infection has been identified consistently.[59-62] One study reported marginal copper deficiency in 22% of their AIDS patients.[63] Selenium deficiency also occurs in AIDS-related malnutrition, though its mechanism has not been determined.[63,64] A recent study indicated significant lower levels of lycopene, retinol, tocopherol, transthyretin, and serum albumin in HIV-infected children compared to controls. Thus, patients with HIV infection can be increasingly compromised nutritionally as the disease progresses. Indeed, it has been suggested that HIV infection might play a pathogenic role in gastrointestinal cells. *In situ* hybridization studies have localized HIV infection in various types of epithelial cells of the bowel mucosa.[65,66] HIV infection of gastrointestinal cell lines has been documented *in vitro*.[67-69] Since the lymphoid tissue, the main target of HIV, is present throughout the gastrointestinal tract, and CD4-related receptors on the epithelial cells have been demonstrated,[70] it is conceivable that AIDS patients have dysfunction of some portion of gastrointestinal tract due to retrovirus infection, thereby leading to nutrient malabsorption and then malnutrition.

AIDS and oxidative stress

Highly reactive oxygen-containing molecules, superoxide radicals, hydrogen peroxides, hydroxyl radicals, and their products lipid peroxides are being shown to play an important role in human diseases.[71] Oxidative stress may be a cofactor of disease progression from asymptomatic HIV infection to AIDS based on a recent review.[72] Reduced levels of potent antioxidants such as glutathione and other acid-soluble thiols correlated well with the progression to AIDS.[71] As two thiols inhibited HIV replication *in vitro*,[73,74] oxidative stress may be a potent inducer of viral activation as well as DNA damage in infected cells, producing one of the long-term consequences of HIV infection, immunosuppression.[75,76] In addition to antioxidant function, glutathione is also involved in synthesis of proteins and DNA precursors; in acting as a cofactor for a variety of enzymes; in the initiation and progression of lymphocyte activation;[77] and in natural killer activity and lymphokine-mediated cytotoxicity.[78] Another important function of glutathione is that of regeneration of vitamin E,[79,80] the body's principal antioxidant. *In vitro* and *in vivo* vitamin E can compensate for glutathione deficiency, maintain cellular levels of glutathione by diminishing the oxidant load, and contribute to regeneration of oxidized glutathione to reduced glutathione.[81-84] Therefore, vitamin E supplementation in humans with genetic glutathione deficiencies exerts a compensatory effect,[85,86] increasing serum glutathione peroxidase activity.[87]

Cytokine-induced oxidative stress is an important factor for replication of HIV.[88] TNF-α generates reactive oxygen species through neutrophils at concentration as low as 0.5 ng/ml.[89] Since reactive oxygen species induce the expression of HIV in human T cell lines by activating transcription of NF-κB,[90,91] TNF-α levels are elevated in the serum of HIV patients and murine AIDS,[92,93] and thus TNF-α, produced by retrovirus-infected macrophages/monocytes, can use oxidative stress as a second messenger to stimulate HIV replication.

Vitamin E and AIDS therapy

High doses of vitamin E decrease CD8+ T cells and increase CD4+/CD8+ ratio, increase total lymphocyte count, stimulate activity of cytotoxic cells and natural killer (NK) cells, and increase phagocytosis of macrophages and mitogen responsiveness.[94] The immunostimulatory nature of vitamin E does provide a basis for its use in the modulation of the various cell components and immune functions in humans and the consequent therapeutic use during AIDS. Furthermore, high doses of vitamin E supplementation provide essentially no toxicity.[95-97] Thus, the combination of existing medical therapy with vitamin E supplementation may provide a more successful and novel therapeutic approach for treatment of HIV-infected individuals.

Vitamin E supplementation exerts a positive effect on the immune system while its deficiency compromises the immune system.[94,98,99] Vitamin E has been found to stimulate Th cells, antibody response, delayed cutaneous hypersensitivity reaction, phagocytosis, mitogen responsiveness, the reticuloendothelial system, and host resistance in animal models.[100-102] In hemodialysis patients with low concentrations of vitamin E in the mononuclear cells, parenteral administration of physiological doses of vitamin E, repleting body stores, decreases the number of CD8+ T cells and increases the CD4+/CD8+ ratio.[103] Prasad demonstrated a significant increase in bactericidal activity in human leukocytes after ingestion of 300 mg of vitamin E daily for 3 weeks.[104] Vitamin E deficiency in dogs leads to depression of lymphocyte activation by mitogens.[105] Vitamin E supplementation has also been shown to be beneficial in reducing the incidence or severity of infectious diseases in elderly persons and in rats.[106] In elder human subjects, vitamin E has been shown to increase IL-2 production while decreasing that of prostaglandin E2 (PG), to increase the response to delayed hypersensitivity skin testing, and to enhance lymphocyte proliferating in response to mitogens.[107] In patients with SLE, supplementation with vitamin E decreases the severity of this autoimmune disease with the plasma globulin level decreased and the plasma albumin level increased.[108] Therefore, vitamin E supplementation may decrease the heightened levels of gamma globulin from polyclonal B cell activation that occur in AIDS patients. The notion that vitamin E supplementation can enhance suppressed immune responses induced by retrovirus infection is strongly supported by our findings regarding the therapeutic role of vitamin E supplementation in murine AIDS.

Our results[109,110] in murine AIDS indicate that vitamin E supplementation with 15-fold increase significantly restores mitogen-induced splenic T and B cells proliferation, release of IL-2 and IFN-gamma produced by ConA-inducing splenocytes, and NK cell activity, which are suppressed during murine AIDS. Furthermore, vitamin E supplementation reduces the secretion of IL-6 and tumor necrosis factor-α (TNF), which are elevated in AIDS and may contribute to enhancement of HIV replication, oxidative stress, and other AIDS pathological symptoms.[111-113] It also reduces splenomegaly induced by retrovirus infection, and immunoglobulin G level, which are increased in AIDS.[110] Vitamin E supplementation in murine AIDS also modulates retrovirus-dysregulated cytokine secretion by thymocytes,[114] which play important roles in T cell maturation in the thymus.[115] Retrovirus infection may also target the thymus. This would damage T cell differentiation in the thymus by reducing CD4+CD8- thymocytes and dysregulating secretion of thymic cytokine and hormones.[116-119] Thus, the favorable effects of dietary vitamin E supplementation on T cell differentiation in the thymus with normalizing cytokine secretion during murine AIDS[114] may provide new mature helper T cells and replace retrovirus-infected and damaged peripheral T helper cells, explaining its restoration of immune response in murine AIDS. We also found that vitamin E reduced tumor size and number, which are increased during murine AIDS.[120] Taken together, vitamin E supplementation, which normalizes immune responses, may retard the progression of AIDS and improve host resistance to tumors and opportunistic infections.

Since AIDS is a disease associated with malnutrition, vitamin E supplementation may improve the nutritional status. Vitamin E supplementation has been shown to increase hepatic level of vitamin A in the rat.[120] However, the role of vitamin E in the absorption or transportation of minerals is still unclear. The hypothesis is that vitamin E may protect gastrointestinal mucosa cells from damages of retrovirus infection, thereby decreasing the malnutrition occurring often in AIDS. The hypothesis is supported by our findings in murine AIDS.

In murine AIDS, we found[121] that retrovirus infection significantly reduces the levels of vitamin A, E, zinc, and copper in the liver, as well as the levels of vitamin A, E, and zinc in the spleen. These data strongly support that retrovirus infection can directly cause undernutrition. Zinc, copper, vitamin A, and vitamin E deficiencies have also been associated with suppression of immune responses and loss of disease resistance.[122-124] Therefore, undernutrition secondary to retrovirus infection may aggravate immune dysfunctions initiated by retrovirus infection, thereby partially explaining their increasing the susceptibility of mice to tumors[125] and opportunistic infections[126,127] observed in murine AIDS. The 15-fold increase of vitamin E supplementation in murine AIDS[109] significantly normalizes levels of vitamin A, E, and zinc in the liver as well as their levels in the spleen. Therefore, vitamin E supplementation can improve some nutrient deficiencies initiated by retrovirus infection in the tissues including immune organs, concomitantly with enhanced immune response in AIDS.[110] In conclusion, undernutrition induced by retrovirus infection could facilitate the progression to AIDS and suppress immune responses as well as speed the onset of tumors and opportunistic infections. Vitamin E supplementation may reverse the progression of malnutrition initiated by retrovirus infection in AIDS/HIV subjects.

In addition, vitamin E may block activation of NF-κB by reducing oxidative stress,[128] thereby retarding the progression of AIDS. The reduction by vitamin E supplementation level of TNF-α, elevated in AIDS, could lower the oxidative burden initiated by the retrovirus infection.[109,110] The physiological effects of TNF-α in the body include increasing phospholipase A_2 activity, a potent inducer of HIV replication in monocytes,[129,130] and stimulating synthesis of PGE_2, an immunosuppressive substance produced by macrophages/monocytes in human and murine AIDS.[131] These effects of TNF-α on generation of reactive oxygen species could also be directly lessened by vitamin E supplementation, because vitamin E inhibits phospholipase A_2 and PGE_2 production.[132] Vitamin E may also inhibit viral replication through inhibition of protein kinase C. The HIV coat protein gp120 induces protein kinase C activity in lymphocytes and in the brain.[133] In turn, protein kinase C activation results in the transition of HIV from a state of latency to active replication in lymphocytes, and leads to upregulation of HIV replication in cells with nondormant HIV.[134-136] The antiretroviral compounds hypericin, pseudohypericin, and glycyrrhizin are effective against HIV *in vitro* and inhibit the activity of protein kinase C.[137,138] A unique feature of the retroviral life cycle is that virus can persist in a quiescent state, prior to activation, without production of either viral mRNA or proteins. Thus, antioxidant agents such as vitamin E may slow the retrovirus replication, thereby reducing the viral burden and retarding the progression to AIDS. Indeed, α-tocopherol succinate increased the anti-HIV activity of AZT in the MT-4 cell line of cultured lymphocytes.[136]

Our results[125] demonstrated that oxygen-free radicals, represented by ethane exhalation are markedly increased during the development of murine AIDS. This may partly explain the greater susceptibility to cancer and infectious diseases during AIDS, because oxygen radicals have a carcinogenic potential and impair ability of lymphoid cell membrane and cytokine secretion. Vitamin E supplementation significantly reduces this increased free radical in murine AIDS. Hepatic lipid peroxidation is also significantly elevated in murine AIDS, whereas vitamin E supplementation significantly reduces it.[125] Thus, vitamin E supplementation could protect immune cells from the disturbance of free radicals and lipid peroxidation, intensifying immune responses during the development of AIDS. In conclusion, the possible importance of antioxidant nutrient as an adjunct therapy in AIDS patients as highlighted by vitamin E deficiency could be a predisposing factor for the pathological conditions occurring from AIDS or from AIDS chemotherapy, and possibly a factor influencing the progression of the disease.

AIDS therapies involve pharmacological interventions (e.g., Ganciclovir and Zidovudine, AZT) to inhibit HIV replication.[140] However, these drugs are accompanied by deleterious toxic side effects. For example, Ganciclovir toxicities include bone marrow suppression, atrophy of the gastrointestinal tract mucosa, inhibition of spermatogenesis, nausea, vomiting, reduced white blood cell count, and headaches. In addition, these anti-HIV drugs do not repair damaged immune functions or improve nutritional deficiencies and other pathological symptoms caused by retrovirus infection in AIDS individuals. Furthermore, a strain of AZT-resistant HIV was reported in a human individual possibly due to high dose and prolonged use of AZT.[141] Thus, new strategies including specific dietary nutrient supplementation could provide additional approaches to ameliorate malnutrition and thereby immune dysfunctions in infected individuals, eventually slowing the progression of disease to AIDS.

Vitamin E and toxicity

Vitamin E has unique therapeutic potential in that it has little, if any, toxicity when taken orally.[95,96] In several species the oral LD-50 was found to be ≥2,000 I.U./kg body weight.[142] Frogs, rabbits, cats, dogs, and monkeys can tolerate 200 I.U. vitamin E/Kg body weight without apparent toxic signs.[142] In general, deleterious effects have been observed in animals only when daily doses were ≥1,000 I.U./kg body weight.[143] No adverse effects are noted from vitamin E supplementation in doses of 800 I.U./d and 2,000 I.U./d (RDA: 30 I.U./d for adult humans) given to elderly patients to assess its effect on immunity and on the development of Parkinson's disease.[144-146] In six double-blind placebo-controlled studies involving oral intake of 600–3,200 I.U. vitamin E/d for 3 weeks to 6 months conducted since 1974, very few adverse side effects are noted and no specific side effect is consistently observed in all the studies.[142] In case of vitamin K deficiency, vitamin E can exacerbate the defect in coagulation; however, vitamin K deficiency is not common in AIDS patients.[147] While there could be concern that intake of an antioxidant could inhibit the superoxide mechanism of bacterial killing by neutrophil, this would not be a problem since oral supplementation does not allow the attainment of plasma levels of vitamin E sufficient to exert this side effect.[148]

Our study,[149,150] investigating the effects of different supplemental vitamin E levels during murine AIDS on cytokine secretion and immune functions, suggests that vitamin E supplementation at 150- and 450-fold (higher than mouse RDA) is not immunotoxic, even though in some cases this extremely high vitamin E supplementation appears to further normalize immune dysfunction and cytokine dysregulation only marginally compared to that normalized by 15-fold increase of vitamin E. Our results also indicate that higher levels of vitamin E supplementation appear more effective in normalizing the same clinical disorders during murine AIDS. These results suggest a possible role for a higher vitamin E dosage as a potential therapeutic nutrient to help normalize immune dysfunction and nutrient deficiency caused by HIV infection, thereby retarding the development of AIDS. In addition, animal studies show that vitamin E is not mutagenic, carcinogenic, or teratogenic.[144,148] In conclusion, oral intakes of vitamin E are safe. Thus, vitamin E nutritional supplementation may provide an additional therapeutic approach for treatment of HIV+/AIDS patients without additional toxicity.

Conclusions

Vitamin E should not be considered as a direct antiretroviral drug, but rather as a potentially immunomodulating and antioxidant agent that achieves its antiretroviral effect through indirect mechanisms, possibly through immunoenhancing, modulation of signal transduction, improvement of undernutrition, and anti-oxidative stress. Its use as combination therapy with other pharmacologic agents such as AZT could have several advantages. First, it could lead to more complete viral suppression than any single drug used alone by decreasing oxidative stress and enhancing immunity, associated with this retrovirus infection. Second, it may allow each drug to be used in lower doses, thus limiting drug toxicities and decreasing frequency of production of drug-resistant HIV strains. Third, such immunorestorative treatment may be given during maintenance therapy of the AIDS patient following the control of tumors and immune dysfunction by chemotherapy. Fourth, the use of vitamin E may be important in forestalling initial episodes of general immune disorders in some patients by extending the period between HIV infection and the appearance of clinical symptoms of AIDS.

Experimental results from animal studies have implied that vitamin E supplementation may act on various immune components to repair immune defects and lessen malnutrition status induced by retrovirus infection. Although the animal data may not be totally extrapolated to HIV-infected individuals, information obtained from murine model may potentially serve as a basis for the study of therapeutic roles of vitamin E in AIDS/HIV individuals.

References

1. Karon, J.M., Rosenberg, P.S., McQuillan, G., Khare, M., Gwinn, M., and Persen, L.P. Prevalence of HIV infection in the United States, 1984 to 1992, *JAMA*, 276, 126, 1996.
2. Holmberg, S.D., Estimated HIV prevalence and incidence in 96 large metropolitan areas in the United States, *Am. J. Public Health*, 86, 642, 1996.
3. Berkelman, R.L., Heyward, W.L., Stehr-Green, J.K., and Curran, J.W., Epidemiology of human immunodeficiency virus infection and acquired immunodeficiency syndrome, *Am. J. Med.*, 86, 761, 1989.
4. AIDS leading cause among men 25 to 44 (News), *Oncology*, 8, 94, 1994.
5. World Health Organization, The HIV-AIDS pandemic: 1993 overview, WHO/GPA/GNP/93.1, Geneva, 1993.
6. U.S. Public Health Service, Public Health Report Mortality and AIDS, 101, 341, 1986.
7. Burton, G.W. and Traber, M.G., Vitamin E: antioxidant activity, biokinetics, and bioavailability, *Ann. Rev. Nutr.*, 10, 357, 1990.
8. Liang, B., Wang, J.Y., and Watson, R.R., Murine AIDS: a key to understand pathogenesis of retrovirus, *Viral Immunol.*, 9, 225, 1996.
9. Koenig, S. and Fauci, A.S., AIDS: Etiology, diagnosis, treatment and prevention, Devita, V.T., Hellman, S., and Rosenberg, S.A., Eds. J.B., Lippincott, New York, p. 61, 1990.
10. Bowen, D.L., Lane, H.C., and Fauci, A.S., Immunopathogenesis of the acquired immunodeficiency syndrome, *Ann. Intern. Med.*, 103, 704, 1985.
11. Fauci, A.S., The human immunodeficiency virus: infectivity and mechanisms of pathogenesis, *Science*, 239, 617, 1988.
12. Mosier, D.E., Animal models for retrovirus-induced immunodeficiency disease, *Immunol. Invest.*, 15, 233, 1986.
13. Balkwill, F.R. and Burke, F., The cytokine network, *Immunol. Today*, 10, 299, 1989.
14. Mitl, B.S., The interleukins, *FASEB J.*, 3, 2379, 1989.
15. Hamblin, A.S., Lymphokines and interleukins, *Immunol.* (suppl.), 1, 39, 1989.
16. Yokota, T., Coffman, R.L., and Hagiwara, H., Isolation and characterization of lymphokine (IL-5), *Proc. Natl. Acad. Sci. U.S.A.*, 84, 7388, 1987.
17. Yokota, T., Otsuka, T., and Mosmann, T., Isolation and characterization of a human interleukin cDNA clone that expresses B-cell and T-cell stimulating activation, *Proc. Natl. Acad. Sci. U.S.A.*, 83, 5894, 1986.
18. Snapper, C., Finkelman, F.D., and Paul, W.E., Regulation of IgG1 and IgE production by interleukin 4, *Immun. Rev.*, 102, 51, 1988.
19. Tonkonogy, S.L., Mckenzie, D.T., and Swain, S.L., Regulation of isotype production by IL-4 and IL-5: effects of lymphokines on Ig production depend on the state of activation of the responding B cells, *J. Immunol.*, 142, 4351, 1989.
20. Van Vlasselaer, P., Gascan, H., De Wall Malefyt, R., and Devries, J.E., IL-2 and a contact-mediated signal provided by TDR alpha beta+ or TCR gamma delta+ CD4+ T cells induce polyclonal Ig production by committed human B cells. Enhancement by IL-5, specific inhibition of IgA synthesis by IL-4, *J. Immunol.*, 148, 1674, 1992.
21. Hsieh, C.S., Macatonia, S.E., Tripp, C.S., Volf, S.F., O'Garra, A., and Murphy, K.M., Development of Th1 CD4+ T cells through IL-12 produced by *Listeria*-induced macrophages, *Science*, 260, 547, 1993.

22. Scott, P., IL-12: initiation cytokine for cell-mediated immunity, *Science*, 260, 496, 1993.
23. Harriman, G., Kunimoto, D.Y., Strober, S., Elliott, J.F., and Pactkau, V., The role of IL-5 in IgA B cell differentiation, *J. Immunol.*, 140, 3033, 1988.
24. Murakami, S., Ono, S., Havad, N., Hava, Y., Katoh, Y., Dobash, K., Takatsu, K., and Hamaka, T., T cell derived factor B151-TRF1/IL-5 activates blastoid cells among unprimed B cells to induce a polyclonal differentiation into immunoglobulin M secreting cells, *Immunol.*, 65, 221, 1988.
25. Taga, T., Kawanishi, Y., Hardy, R.R., Hirano, T., and Kishimato, T., Receptors for B cell stimulatory factor 2: quantitation, specificity, distribution, and regulation of their expression, *J. Exp. Med.*, 166, 967, 1987.
26. Howard, M. and O'Garra, A., Biological properties of interleukin 10, *Immunol. Today*, 13, 198, 1992.
27. Biondi, A., Roach, J.A., Schlossmann, S.F., and Todd, R.F., Phenotypic characterization of human T-lymphocyte populations producing macrophage activating factor lymphokines, *J. Immunol.*, 133, 281, 1984.
28. Kuwano, K., Kawashima, T., and Arai, S., Antiviral effect of TNF-α and IFN-γ secreted from a CD8+ influenza virus specific CTL clone, *Viral Immunol.*, 6, 1, 1993.
29. Michael, A., Hackett, J., Bennett, M., Kumar, V., and Yuan, D., Regulation of B lymphocytes by natural killer cells, *J. Immunol.*, 142, 1095, 1989.
30. Sandvig, S., Taskay, T., Andersson, J., and De Ley, M., Andersson U. Gamma-interferon is produced by CD3+ and CD3- lymphocytes, *Immunol. Rev.*, 97, 51, 1987.
31. Van Der Merwe, P.A., Tumor necrosis factor, *S. Afr. Med. J.*, 74, 411, 1988.
32. Pace, J.L., Russell, S.W., Torres, B.A., Johnson, H.M., and Gray, P.W., Recombinant mouse γ-interferon induces the priming step in macrophage activation for tumor cell killing, *J. Immunol.*, 130, 2011, 1983.
33. Leibson, H.J., Geftar, M., Zlotnik, A., Marrack, P., and Kappler, J.W., Role of gamma-interferon in antibody-producing responses, *Nature*, 309, 799, 1984.
34. Nakamura, M., Daky, M., Gafter, M., Manser, T., and Pearson, G., Effect of IFN-γ on the immune response *in vivo* and on gene expression *in vitro*, *Nature*, 307, 381, 1984.
35. Sidman, C., Marshall, J., Shultz, I., Gray, P., and Johnson, H.M., γ-interferon is one of several direct B cell-maturing lymphokines, *Nature*, 309, 801, 1984.
36. Sollid, I., Kvale, D., Brandtzaeg, P., Markussen, G., and Thorsby, E., Interferon-γ enhances expression of secretory component, the epithelial receptor for polymeric immunoglobulins, *J. Immunol.*, 138, 4303, 1987.
37. Grunfeld, C., Palladino, M.A., Jr., Tumor necrosis factor: Immunologic, antitumor, metabolic, and cardiovascular activities, *Adv. Int. Med.*, 35, 45, 1990.
38. Feinmau, R., Henriksen-Destefazno, D., Tsujimoto, M., and Vilcek, J., Tumor necrosis factor is an important mediator of tumor cell killing by human monocytes, *J. Immunol.*, 138, 635, 1987.
39. Cuturi, M.C., Murphy, M., Costa Giomi, M.P., Weinmann, R., Perussia, B., and Trinchieri, G., Independent regulation of tumor necrosis factor and lymphotoxin production by human peripheral blood lymphocytes, *J. Exp. Med.*, 165, 1581, 1987.
40. Beutler, B., The tumor necrosis factors: cachectin and lymphotoxin, *Hosp. Pract.*, 15, 45, Feb. 1990.

41. Paya, C.V., Kenmotsu, N., Schoon, R.A., and Leibson, P.J., Tumor necrosis factor and lymphotoxin secretion by human natural killer cells leads to antiviral cytotoxicity, *J. Immunol.*, 141, 1989, 1988.
42. Biggar, R.J., International Registry of Seroconverters. AIDS incubation in 1991 seroconverters from different exposure groups, *AIDS*, 4, 1059, 1990.
43. Moseson, M. and Zeleniuch-Jacquotte, A., The potential role of nutritional factors in the induction of immunologic abnormalities in HIV-positive homosexual men, *J. AIDS*, 2, 235, 1989.
44. Chandra, R.K., 1990 McCollum Award Lecture. Nutrition and immunity: lessons from the past and new insights into the future, *Am. J. Clin. Nutr.*, 53, 1087, 1991.
45. Tomkins, A. and Watson, F., Malnutrition and infection: a review, United Nations Administrative Committee on Coordination — Subcommittee on Nutrition, Geneva, WHO, 1989.
46. Jain, V. and Chandra, R., Does nutritional deficiency predispose to acquired immune deficiency syndrome? *Nutr. Res.*, 4, 537, 1984.
47. Chandra, R.K. and Scrimahaw, W.S., Immunocompetence in nutritional assessment. *Am. J. Clin. Nutr.*, 33, 2694, 1980.
48. Chandra, R.K., Nutrition, immunity and infections: present knowledge and future directions, *Lancet*, i, 688, 1983.
49. Dorsetor, J., Whittle, H.C., and Granwood, B.M., Persistent measles infection in malnourished children, *Br. Med. J.*, 2, 1633, 1977.
50. Grunt, J.P., Clinical impact of protein malnutrition on organ mass and functions, in *Amino Acid Metabolism and Medical Applications*, Blackhur, G.L., Grant, J.P., and Young, V.P., Eds., Wright, Boston, 347, 1977.
51. Dworkin, B.M., Wormser, G.P., and Axelrod, R., Dietary intake in patients with acquired immunodeficiency syndrome (AIDS), patients with AIDS-related complex, and serologically positive human immunodeficiency virus patients: correlations with nutritional status, *J. Parent. Enter. Nutr.*, 14, 605, 1990.
52. Coodley, G. and Girard, D.E., Vitamins and minerals in HIV infection, *J. Gen. Intern. Med.*, 6, 472, 1991.
53. Beach, R.S., Mantero-Atienza, E., and Eisdorfer, C., Altered folate metabolism in early HIV infection, *JAMA*, 259, 3129, 1988.
54. Harriman, G., Smith, P.D., and Horne, M.K., Vitamin B_{12} malabsorption in patients with acquired immunodeficiency syndrome, *Arch. Intern. Med.*, 149, 2039, 1989.
55. Herbert, V., B_{12} deficiency in AIDS, *JAMA*, 260, 2837, 1988.
56. Remacha, A., Acquired immune deficiency syndrome and vitamin B_{12}, *Eur. J. Haematol.*, 42, 506, 1989.
57. Bogden, J.D., Baker, H., and Frank, O., Micronutrient status and human immunodeficiency virus (HIV) infection, *Ann. N.Y. Acad. Sci.*, 587, 189, 1990.
58. Malcolm, J.A., Tynn, D.F., Sutherland, D.C., Dobsm, P., Kelson, W., and Carlton, J., *Proceedings of the 6th International Conference on AIDS*, Abst. Th.B., p. 206, 1990.
59. Passi, S., De Luca, C., Oicardo, M., Morrone, A., and Lppolito, F., Blood deficiency values of polyunsaturated fatty acids of phospholipids, vitamin E and glutathione peroxidase as possible risk factors in the onset and development of acquired immunodeficiency syndrome, *G. Ital. Dermoatol. Venereol.*, 125, 125, 1990.

60. Falut, J., Tsoukas, C., and Gold, P., Zinc as a cofactor in human immunodeficiency virus-induced immunosuppression, *JAMA*, 259, 2850, 1988.
61. Fordycc-Baum, M.K., Mantero-Atinza, E., Van Riel, P., Morgan, R., and Beach, R.S., *Proceedings of the 5th International Conference on AIDS*, Abstr. Th.B., p. 310, 1989.
62. Coulston, A., Mccorkindale, C., Dyhevik, W., and Menigun, T., *Proceedings of the 5th International Conference on AIDS*, Abstr. Th.B., pp. 200, 1990.
63. Dworkin, B.D., Rosenthal, W.A., Wormser, G.P., and Weiss, I., Selenium deficiency in AIDS, *J. Parent. Enter. Nutr.*, 10, 405, 1986.
64. Colman, N. and Grossman, F., Nutritional factors in epidemic Kaposi's sarcoma, *Semin. Oncol.*, 14(suppl), 54, 1987.
65. Nelson, T.A., Wiley, C.A., Reynolds-Kohler, C., Neese, L.E., Margaretten, W., and Levy, J.A., Human immunodeficiency virus detected in bowel epithelium from patients with gastrointestinal symptoms, *Lancet*, i, 259, 1988.
66. Levy, J.A., Margaretten, W., and Nelson, J., Detection of HIV in enterochromaffin cells in the rectal mucosa of an AIDS patient, *Am. J. Gastroenterol.*, 84, 787, 1989.
67. Adachi, A., Koenig, S., Gendelman, H.E., Dauherty, D., Gattoni-Celli, S., Fauci, A.S., and Martin, M.A., Productive, persistent infection of human colorectal cell lines with human immunodeficiency virus, *J. Virol.*, 61, 209, 1987.
68. Moyer, M.D., Hout, R.I., Tamirez, A., Jol, S., Meltzer, M.S., and Gendelman, H.E., Infection of human gastrointestinal cells by HIV-1, *Res. Hum. Retrovir.*, 6, 1409, 1990.
69. Barnett, S.W., Barboza, A., Wilcox, C.M., Forsmark, L.E., and Levy, J.A., Characterization of human immunodeficiency virus type 1 strains recovered from bowel of infected individuals, *Virology*, 182, 802, 1991.
70. Moyer, M.P., Hout, R., Wideman, D., and Martin, D., Expression of a potential HIV receptor on human gastrointestinal epithelial cells (giecs), *International Conference on AIDS*, Montreal, Abstr. WCP 607, 1989.
71. Staltman, P., Oxidative stress: a radical view, *Semin. Hematol.*, 26, 249, 1989.
72. Baruchel, S. and Xainberg, M.A., The role of oxidative stress in disease progression in individuals infected by the human immunodeficiency virus, *J. Leuko. Biol.*, 52, 111, 1992.
73. Kalebic, T., Kinter, A., Poli, G., Anderson, M.E., Mester, A., and Fauci, A.S., Suppression of human immunodeficiency virus expression in chronically infected monocytic cells by glutathione, glutathione ester, and N-acetyl-L-cysteine, *Proc. Natl. Acad. Sci. U.S.A.*, 88, 986, 1990.
74. Staal, F.J.T., Roederer M, Herzenberg LA. Intracellular thiols regulate activation of nuclear factor κB and transcription of HIV, *Proc. Natl. Acad. Sci. U.S.A.*, 87, 9943, 1990.
75. Floyd, R.A. and Schneider, J.E., Hydroxy free radicals damage to DNA, in *Membrane Lipid Oxidation*, Vol. I., Vigo-Pelfrey, C., Ed., CRC Press, Boca Raton, FL, p. 245, 1989.
76. Halliwell, B. and Gutterbridge, J.M.C., The importance of free radicals and catalytic metal ions in human disease, *Mol. Aspects Med.*, 8, 89, 1985.
77. Suthanthiran, M., Anderson, M.E., Sharma, V.K., and Meister, A., Glutathione regulates activation-dependent DNA synthesis in highly purified normal human T lymphocytes stimulated via the CD2 and CD3 antigens, *Proc. Natl. Acad. Sci. U.S.A.*, 87, 3343, 1990.

78. Buhl, R., Jaffe, H.A., and Holroyd, K.J., Systemic glutathione deficiency in symptom-free HIV-seropositive individuals, *Lancet,* ii, 1294, 1989.
79. Niki, E., Tsuchiya, J., Tanimura, R., and Kamiya, Y., Regeneration of vitamin E from alpha-81 romanoxyl radical by glutathione and vitamin C, *Chem. Lett.,* 24, 789, 1982.
80. Reddy, R.C., Scholz, R.W., Thomas, C.E., and Mawsaro, E.J., Vitamin E dependent reduced glutathione inhibition of rat liver microsomal lipid peroxidation, *Life Sci.,* 31, 571, 1982.
81. Casini, A.F., Maellaro, E., Del Bello, B., and Comporti, M., The role of vitamin E in the patotoxicity by glutathione depleting agents, *Adv. Exp. Med. Biol.,* 264, 105, 1990.
82. Pascoe, G.A., Olafsdottir, K., and Reed, D.J., Vitamin E protection against chemical-induced cell injury. I. Maintenance of cellular protein thiols as a cryoprotective mechanisms, *Eur. J. Biochem.,* 166, 241, 1987.
83. Costagliola, C. and Menzione, M., Effect of vitamin E on the oxidative state of glutathione in plasma, *Clin. Physiol. Biochem.,* 8, 140, 1990.
84. Leedle, R.A. and Aust, S.D., The effect of glutathione on the vitamin E requirement for inhibition of liver microsomal lipid peroxidation, *Lipids,* 25, 241, 1990.
85. Boxer, L.A., Oliver, J.M., Spielberg, S.P., Allen, J.M., and Schulman, J.D., Protection of granulocytes by vitamin E in glutathione synthetase deficiency, *N. Engl. J. Med.,* 301, 901, 1979.
86. Corash, L.M., Sheetz, M., and Bieri, J.G., Chronic hemolytic anemia due to glucose-6-phosphate dehydrogenase deficiency or glutathione synthetase deficiency: the role of vitamin E in its treatment, *Ann. N.Y. Acad. Sci.,* 393, 348, 1982.
87. Sundstrom, H., Korpela, H., Sajanti, E., and Kaupplia, A., Supplementation with selenium, vitamin E and their combination in gynecological cancer during cytotoxic chemotherapy, *Carcinogenesis,* 10, 273, 1989.
88. Roederer, M., Stall, F.J., Raju, P.A., Ela, S.W., and Herzenberg, L.A., Cytokine-stimulated human immunodeficiency virus replication is inhibited by N-acetyl-L-cysteine, *Proc. Natl. Acad. Sci. U.S.A.,* 87, 4884, 1990.
89. Klebanoff, S.J., Vadas, M.A., and Harlan, J.M., Stimulation of neutrophils by tumor necrosis factor, *J. Immunol.,* 136, 4220, 1986.
90. Paeck, R., Rubin, P., and Bauerle, P.A., Reactive oxygen intermediates as apparently widely used messengers in the activation of the NF-κB transcription factor and HIV, *EMBO J.,* 10, 2247, 1991.
91. Toledano, M. and Leonard, W., Modulation of transcription factor NF-κB by oxidation-reduction *in vitro, Proc. Natl. Acad. Sci. U.S.A.,* 88, 4328, 1991.
92. Wang, Y., Huang, D.S., Giger, P.T., and Watson, R.R., Kinetics of cytokine production by T cells and macrophages during murine AIDS, *Adv. Biol. Sci.,* 86, 335, 1993.
93. Boue, F., Wallon, C., Goujard, C., Barresinouss, F., Galand, P., and Defraissy, J.F., HIV induced IL-6 production by human B lymphocytes: role of IL-4, *J. Immunol.,* 148, 3761, 1991.
94. Odeleye, O.E. and Watson, R.R., The potential role of vitamin E in the treatment of immunological abnormalities during acquired immune deficiency syndrome, *Prog. Food Nutr. Sci.,* 15, 1, 1991.
95. Bendich, A. and Machlin, L.J., Safety of oral intake of vitamin E, *Am. J. Clin. Nutr.,* 48, 612, 1988.

96. National Research Council (U.S.) Subcommittee on the 10th edition of the RDAS, Fat soluble vitamin, in *Subcommittee of the 10th edition of the RDAS*, (Recommended Dietary Allowances), Washington, D.C., National Academy Press, p. 78, 1989.

97. Mino, M., Use and safety of elevated dosages of vitamin E in infants and children, *Int. J. Vitam. Nutr. Res. Suppl.*, 30, 69, 1989.

98. Meydani, S.N., Meyani, M., and Blumberg, J.B., Antioxidants and the aging immune response, *Adv. Exp. Med. Biol.*, 262, 57, 1990.

99. Meydani, S.N., Barklund, M.P., and Liu, S., Vitamin E supplementation enhances cell-mediated immunity in healthy elderly subjects, *Am. J. Clin. Nutr.*, 52, 557, 1990.

100. Watson, R.R. and Leonard, T.K., Selenium and vitamin A, E and C, nutrients with cancer prevention properties, *J. Am. Diet. Assoc.*, 86, 505, 1986.

101. Watson, R.R., Moriguchi, S., Jackson, J., Werner, J., Wilmore, J., and Freund, B., Modification of cellular immune functions in humans by endurance excise training during β-adrenergic blockade with ateholol or propranolol, *Med. Sci. Sport Exercise*, 18, 95, 1986.

102. Shefty, B. and Schultz, R., Influence of vitamin E and selenium on immune response mechanisms, *Fed. Proc.*, 38, 2139, 1979.

103. Taccone-Galluci, M., Giardini, D., Piazza, A., Spagnoli, G.C., Bandino, D., Lubrand, R., Taggi, F., Evangeli, B., and Monaco, P., Vitamin E supplementation in hemodialysis patients: effects on peripheral blood mononuclear cell lipids peroxidation and immune response, *Clin. Nephrol.*, 25, 81, 1986.

104. Prasad, J.N., Effect of vitamin E supplementation on leukocyte function, *Am. J. Clin. Nutr.*, 33, 606, 1980.

105. Bendich, A., Antioxidant vitamins and their functions in immune responses, *Adv. Exp. Med. Biol.*, 262, 35, 1990.

106. Kline, K., Rao, A., Romach, E.H., Kidao, S., Morgan, T.J., and Snaders, B.G., Vitamin E modulation of disease resistance and immune responses, *Ann. N.Y. Acad. Sci.*, 587, 294, 1990.

107. Meydani, S.N., Meydani, M., Verdon, C.P., Shapiro, A.A., Blumberg, J.B., and Hayes, K.C., Vitamin E supplementation suppresses prostaglandin E2 synthesis and enhances the immune response of aged mice, *Mech. Aging Dev.*, 34, 191, 1986.

108. Welsh, A., Lupus erythematosus; Treatment by combined use of massive amounts of calcium pantothenate with synthetic vitamin E. SO-A.M.A. *Arch. Dermatol. Syph.*, 1952.

109. Wang, Y., Huang, D.S., Eskelson, C.D., and Watson, R.R., Normalization and restoration of nutritional status and immune functions by vitamin E supplementation in murine AIDS, *J. Nutr.*, 124, 2024, 1994.

110. Wang, Y., Huang, D.S., Liang, B., and Watson, R.R., Normalization of nutritional status by various levels of vitamin E supplementation during murine AIDS, *Nutr. Res.*, 14, 1375, 1994.

111. Larrick, J.M. and Wright, S., Cytotoxic mechanism of tumor necrosis factor alpha, *FASEB J.*, 4, 3215, 1990.

112. Gieger, T., Andus, T., Klapproh, J., Hirano, T., Kishimoto, T., and Heinrich, P.C., Induction of rat acute-phase proteins by interleukin-6 *in vivo*, *Eur. J. Immunol.*, 18, 717, 1988.

113. Van Snick, J., Interleukin-6: an overview, *Ann. Rev. Immunol.*, 8, 253, 1990.

114. Wang, Y., Huang, D.S., and Watson, R.R., Vitamin E supplementation modulates cytokine production by thymocytes during murine AIDS, *Immunol. Res.*, 12, 358, 1994.
115. Wang, Y., Huang, D.S., Wood, S., Giger, P.T., and Watson, R.R., Kinetics of cytokine production by thymocytes during murine AIDS caused by LP-BM5 retrovirus infection, *Immunol. Lett.*, 47, 187, 1995.
116. Schuurman, H.J., Krone, W.J.A., Broekhuizen, R., Van Baarien, J., Van Veen, P., Goldtein, A.L., Huber, J., and Goudsmit, J., The thymus in acquired immunodeficiency syndrome, comparison with other types of immunodeficiency disease, and presence of components of human immunodeficiency virus type I, *Am. J. Pathol.*, 134, 1329, 1989.
117. Schnittman, S.M., Singer, K.H., Greenhouse, J.J., Stanley, S.K., Whichard, L.P., Haynes, B.F., and Fausci, A.S., Thymic microenvironment induces HIV expression, *J. Immunol.*, 147, 2553, 1991.
118. Avino, W., Dardenne, M., Marche, C., Rophilme, D.T., Dupuy, J.M., Pekovic, D., Lapointe, N., and Bach, J.F., Thymic epithelium in AIDS, *Am. J. Pathol.*, 122, 302, 1986.
119. Lopez, M.C., Colombo, L.L., Huang, D.S., Wang, Y., and Watson, R.R., Modification of thymic cell subsets induced by long-term cocaine administration during a murine retroviral infection producing AIDS, *Clin. Immunol. Immunopathol.*, 65, 45, 1992.
120. Eskelson, C.D., Odeleye, O.E., Watson, R.R., Earnest, D.L., and Mufti, S.I., Modulation of cancer growth by vitamin E and alcohol, *Alcohol Alcoholism*, 28, 117, 1993.
121. Wang, Y., Liang, B., and Watson, R.R., Suppression of tissue levels of vitamin A, E, zinc and copper in murine AIDS caused by LP-BM5 retrovirus infection, *Nutr. Res.*, 14, 1031, 1994.
122. Keen, C.L. and Gershwin, M.E., Zinc deficiency and immune function, *Annu. Rev. Nutr.*, 10, 415, 1991.
123. Sherman, A.R. and Hallquist, N.A., in *Present Knowledge in Nutrition*, Brown, M.L., Ed., 6th ed., Nutrition Foundation, Washington, D.C., p. 463, 1990.
124. Ross, A., Vitamin A status: relationship to immunity and the antibody response, *Proc. Soc. Exp. Biol. Med.*, 200, 303, 1992.
125. Odeleye, O.E., Eskelson, C.D., Mufti, S.I., and Watson, R.R., Vitamin E protection against chemically-induced esophageal tumor growth in mice immunocompromised by retroviral infection, *Carcinogenesis*, 13, 1811, 1992.
126. Alak, J.I.B., Shahbazian, M., Huang, D.S., Wang, Y., Darban, H., Jenkins, E.M., and Watson, R.R., Alcohol and murine acquired immunodeficiency syndrome suppression of resistance to *Cryptosporidium parvum* infection during modulation of cytokine production, *Alcohol: Clin. Exp. Res.*, 17, 539, 1993.
127. Darban, H., Enriquez, J., Sterling, C.R., Lopez, M.C., Chen, G., and Watson, R.R., *Cryptosporidium* growth enhanced by retrovirally-induced immunosuppression in mice infected with LP-BM5 murine leukemia virus, *J. Infec. Dis.*, 164, 741, 1991.
128. Tappel, A.L., Vitamin E and free radical peroxidation of lipids, *Ann. N.Y. Acad. Sci.*, 203, 12, 1972.
129. Rabinovitch, A., Baquerizo, H., and Sumoski, W., Cytotoxic effects of cytokines on islet beta-cells: evidence for involvement of eicosanoids, *Endocrinology*, 126, 67, 1990.

130. Spriggs, D.R., Sherman, M.L., and Imamura, K., Phospholipase A₂ activation and autoinduction of tumor necrosis factor gene expression by tumor necrosis factor, *Cancer Res.*, 50, 7101, 1990.

131. Akama, H., Ichikawa, Y., Matsushita, Y., Shinozawa, T., and Homma, M., Mononuclear cells enhance prostaglandin E2 production of polymorphonuclear leukocytes via tumor necrosis factor-a, *Biochem. Biophys. Res. Commun.*, 168, 857, 1990.

132. Cao, Y.Z., Choy, P.C., and Chan, A.C., Regulation by vitamin E of phosphatidylcholine metabolism in rat heart, *Biochem. J.*, 247, 135, 1987.

133. Zorn, N.E., Weill, C.L., and Russell, D.H., The HIV protein, GP120, activates nuclear protein kinase C in nuclei from lymphocytes and brain, *Biochem. Biophys. Res. Commun.*, 166, 1133, 1990.

134. Jakobovits, A., Rosenthal, A., and Capton, D.J., Trans-activation of HIV-1 LTR-directed gene expression by tat requires protein kinase C, *EMBO J.*, 9, 1165, 1990.

135. Kinter, A.L., Poli, G., Maury, W., Folks, T.M., and Fauci, A.S., Direct and cytokine-mediated activation of protein kinase C induces human immunodeficiency virus expression in chronically infected promonocytic cells, *J. Virol.*, 64, 4306, 1990.

136. Matthes, E., Langen, P., and Brachwitz, H., Alteration of DNA topoisomerase II activity during infection of H9 cells by human immunodeficiency virus type 1 *in vitro*: a target for potential therapeutic agents, *Antiviral Res.*, 13, 273, 1990.

137. Takahashi, I., Nakanishi, S., Kobayashi, E., Nakano, H., Suzuki, K., and Tamaoki, T., Hypericin and pseudohypericin specifically inhibit protein kinase C: possible relation to their antiretroviral activity, *Biochem. Biophys. Res. Commun.*, 165, 1207, 1989.

138. Ito, M., Sato, A., and Hirabayashi, K., Mechanism of inhibitory effect of glycyrrhizin on replication of human immunodeficiency virus, *Antiviral Res.*, 10, 289, 1988.

139. Gogu, S.R., Beckman, B.S., Rangan, S.K., and Argawal, K.C., Increased therapeutic efficacy of zidovudine in combination with vitamin E, *Biochem. Biophys. Res. Commun.*, 165, 401, 1989.

140. Gutmann, L., Shockcor, W., and Kien, C.L., Vitamin E-deficient spinocerebellar syndrome due to intestinal lymphangiectasia, *Neurology*, 36, 554, 1986.

141. Apfel, S.C., Lipton, R.B., Arezzo, J.C., and Kessler, J.A., Nerve growth factor prevents toxic neuropathy in mice, *Ann. Neurol.*, 29, 87, 1991.

142. Machlin, L.J., Vitamin E. in *Handbook of Vitamins: Nutritional, Biochemical, and Clinical Aspects*, Machlin, L.J., Ed., Marcel Dekker, New York, p. 100, 1984.

143. Federation of American Societies for Experimental Biology (FASEB), Evaluation of the *Health Aspects of Tocopherols and α-Tocopherol Acetate as Food Ingredients*, FASEB, Washington, D.C., 1975.

144. Committee on Dietary Allowances, Food and Nutrition Board, National Research Council. *Recommended Dietary Allowances*, 10th ed. National Academy Press, Washington, D.C., 1989.

145. Shoulson, I., Deprenyl and tocopherol antioxidative therapy of Parkinsonism (DATATOP), Parkinson Study Group, *Acta Neurol. Scand. Suppl.*, 126, 171, 1989.

146. The Parkinson Study Group, Effect of deprenyl on the progression of disability in early Parkinson's disease, *N. Engl. J. Med.*, 321, 1364, 1989.

147. Moseson, M., Zeleniuch-Jacquotte, A., and Belsito, D.V., The potential role of nutritional factors in the induction of immunological abnormalities in HIV-positive homosexual men, *J. AIDS*, 2, 235, 1989.

148. Mino, M., Use and safety of elevated dosages of vitamin E in infants and children, *Int. J. Vitam. Nutr. Res. Suppl.*, 30, 69, 1989.

149. Wang, Y., Huang, D.S., Wood, S., and Watson, R.R., Effects of very high intake of vitamin E on immune response and cytokine production in murine AIDS, *Immunopharmacol.*, 29, 225, 1995.

150. Wang, Y. and Watson, R.R., Effects of very high intake of vitamin E on cytokine production by thymocytes in murine AIDS, *Thymus*, 22, 153, 1994.

section four

Fruits and HIV progression

chapter fifteen

Pomegranate: a role in health promotion and AIDS?

Jeongmin Lee and Ronald R. Watson

People of classical times were conscious of plants or fruits as important producers of food, oils, fibers, woods, and medicine. The history of pomegranate as a natural medicine and food is shown in the paintings and mosaics of Pompeii, the city destroyed by an eruption of Vesuvius in 79 A.D.[1] The plants or fruits that appear in the paintings and mosaics of Pompeii are chiefly edible and medicinal. They include lemon, cherry, strawberry, grape, leaves of grape, olive, fig, apple, olive, flowers of corn cockle, and pomegranate. Some of these plants or fruits are mentioned to have diuretic properties in *Naturalis Historia* of Pliny the Elder.[2]

Pomegranate (*Punica granatum*) is the reddish-purple fruit of the pomegranate tree with juicy red seeds. It is a dicotyledon angiosperm plant of the *Punicaceae* family, originally from Persia, Khurdistan, and Afghanistan. It was brought to the Mediterranean countries by the Phoenicians, and spread from there by the Romans and Arabs.[3] Spain is a major pomegranate producer, particularly in the south. Approximately 10,400 to 22,000 tons are exported, mainly to the U.K., Italy, and France.[3] The pomegranate tree flowers in May and June, and its fruits mature in September and October. It is not botanically related to any other fruit for human consumption. Thus, it may have unique properties and constituents for health promotion.

One gram of pomegranate contains 0.003 g protein, 0.002 g fat, 0.09 g carbohydrate, 0.02 mg calcium, 0.045 mg phosphorus, 0.002 mg iron, 0.02 mg sodium, 1.5 mg potassium, small amounts of vitamin A, thiamin, riboflavin, niacin, and large quantities of vitamin C.[4] The pomegranate tree contains several alkaloids, mainly in the root cortex, in a proportion of 0.3 to 0.7% with up to 25% tannic compounds.[5] Cortex activity is preserved for many years and has important medicinal components, e.g., as a vermicide. The pomegranate seeds comprise water, glucose, citric acid, malic acid, and large quantities of vitamin C.[6] Pomegranate seeds also contain 1.09 mg estrogen/100 g.[7]

A possible role of crushed pomegranate seeds in the development of esophageal carcinoma has been suggested, due to its local erosive or irritant action.[8] Physical irritation, as well as a diet deficient in major nutrients, may promote the occurrence of esophageal cancer. In the high-risk region of the Turkoman Sahara, the main diet of pregnant women consists of a special mixture, known as *majoweh* or *majum*, composed of crushed sour pomegranate seeds, black pepper, raisins, and occasionally garlic.[9] The sharp, crushed pomegranate seeds could cause physical irritation and thus stimulate development of the esophageal cancer.

A recidivant tongue angioedema can be caused by a late adverse reaction (intolerance) to the ingestion of 40 g of crushed pomegranate seeds.[10] This was due to an allergic reaction to pomegranate seeds in which Ig-E mediated immunological mechanism had not been shown. Ingestion of several pomegranate seeds by a 7-year-old Ig-E dependent asthmatic child caused allergic reaction and bronchospasm which responded to treatment with inhaled salbutamol.[11]

Pomegranate seeds contain estrone (1.09 mg in 100 g) which is one of the main metabolites of 17 beta-estradiol. It is commonly found in urine, ovaries, and placenta with considerably less biological activity than 17 beta-estradiol.[7] Nonsteroidal estrogen, coemestrol, occurred at the concentration of 0.036 mg/100 g of pomegranate seeds.[7] However, its role in adverse reactions to pomegranate was not established.

Alkaloids and tannins extracted from pomegranate roots inhibited bacterial growth.[5] Two ml of aqueous extract containing alkaloids and tannins had higher activity on cultures from *E. histolytica* than *E. invadens* strains, producing growth inhibitions of about 100 and 40%, respectively. Alkaloid concentrations of 1 mg/ml had no bactericide activity, however tannins at concentration of 10 µg/ml for *E. histolytica*, and 100 µg/ml for *E. invadens* were sufficient to produce a growth inhibition of almost 100%.

Boiled-water extract of the pomegranate peel has genotoxic property on human cell lines, Raji and P3HR-1.[12] Cell growth and viability were dose dependently reduced without induction of chromosomal aberrations. Administration of pomegranate extract induced apoptotic DNA fragmentation.

A mixture of a ferrous salt and an extract of pomegranate rind completely inhibited the growth of fungus, *powdery mildew*, in the apple leaves within 24 h.[13] Through microscopic test, both spores and mycellium of *powdery mildew* treated with the mixture were destroyed after 1 h at room temperature. The 144 µg of the mixture was tested to identify the effect on the growth of poliovirus, herpes simplex virus type 1 (HSV-1), and human immunodeficiency virus type 1 (HIV-1).[13] In the cell culture assays using HT-29 cells for poliovirus, MRC-5 cells for HSV-1 and IIUT-78 cells for HIV-1, there was complete reduction of infectivity of these viruses, which indicated that the extract of pomegranate could be used to control the spread of herpes

and as protection against HIV-1. However, there was no ap
genic effect on MRC-5 cells or HT-29 cells.

In trying to understand the potential actions of por
promotion it is important to focus on it as a rich sourc
vanoids. They are a ubiquitous group of nontoxic plant cu..ֽ
impact on a variety of disease processes in humans. Their primary action ıs
oxygen free-radical scavenging. They also inhibit lipoxygenase, which converts arachidonic acid to leukotrienes. These actions should affect inflammation, cancer, and pathogen growth. The presence of pomegranate tannins,
polyphenolic compounds, should also promote inhibition of microbes,
including opportunistic pathogens present in AIDS patients.

In conclusion, pomegranate has both antibacterial and antiviral effects,
although it can have adverse effects on the human esophagus and tongue
due to physical irritation and allergic reaction. Alkaloids and tannic compounds extracted from pomegranate root cortex significantly inhibited the
growth of *E. histolyca* and *E. invadens* strains. An extract of pomegranate rind
showed the complete growth inhibition of the fungus, *powdery mildew*, indicating that it might be effective in controlling the growth of eukaryotic cells.
A mixture containing the extract of pomegranate exhibited complete reduction of infectivity of poliovirus, HSV-1, and HIV-1. Thus, the extracts of
pomegranate and its seeds might be useful for therapeutic purposes to
promote health in humans. However, the mode of action of pomegranate
extracts on bacteria and virus and its long-term effects on humans is not
established.

Reference

1. Melillo, L., Diuretic plants in the paintings of Pompeii, *Am. J. Nephrol.* 14, 423, 1994.
2. Penso, G., *Le Piante Medicinali nella Terapia Medica,* Org. Ed. Med. Farm, Milan, 1987.
3. Granada, S., Informe-resumen de la campana de exportacion, Ministerio de Agricultura, Madrid, 1972.
4. Adams, C.F., Nutritive value of American foods, *Agric. Handbook,* 456, 125, 1995.
5. Segura, J.J., Morales-Ramos, L.H., Verde-Star, J., and Guerra D., Growth inhi-bition of *Entamoeba histolytica* and *E. invadens* produced by pomegranate root, *Arch. Invest. Med.,* 21, 235, 1990.
6. Quer, P.F., Plants medicinals: el Dioscorides renovado, Editorial Labor, Barce-lona, 456, 1980.
7. Moneam, N.M., Sharaky, A.S., and Badreldin, M.M., Oestrogen content of pomegranate seeds, *J. Chromatogr.,* 438, 438, 1988.
8. Ghadirian, P., Ekoe, J.M., and Thouez, J.P., Food habits and esophageal cancer, *Cancer Detect. Prev.,* 16, 163, 1992.
9. Ghadirian, P., Food habits of the people of the Caspian Littoral of Iran in relation to esophageal cancer, *Nutr. Cancer,* 9, 147, 1987.

10. Igea, J.M., Cuesta, J., Cuevas, M., Elias, L.M., Marcos, C., Lazaro, M., and Compaired, J.A., Adverse reaction to pomegranate ingestion, *Allergy,* 46, 472, 1991.
11. Gaig, P., Botey, J., Gutierrez, V., Pena, M., Eseverri, J.L., and Marin, A., Allergy to pomegranate (*Punica granatum*), *J. Invest. Allergy Clin. Immunol.,* 2, 216, 1992.
12. Settheetham, W. and Ishida, T., Study of genotoxic effects of antidiarrheal medicinal herbs on human cells *in vitro, S. Asian J. Trop. Med. Public Health,* 26, 306, 1995.
13. Stewart, G., Antiviral and antifungal compositions comprise a mixture of a ferrous salt and a plant extract of pomegranate rind, *Viburnum plicaum,* leaves or flowers, tea leaves or maple leaves in aqueous solution, *Int. Search Rep.,* 1995, (patent pending).

chapter sixteen

Cranberry: a role in health promotion

Jeongmin Lee and Ronald R. Watson

Introduction

Cranberry is the fruit of several small creeping or trailing woody plants. The small-fruited or northern cranberry (*Vaccinium oxycoccos*) is found in marshy land in northern North America, northern Asia, and northern and central Europe. Its stems are wiry and creeping, cranberry flowers appear in June, and its fruit ripens in September. The American or mountain cranberry (*V. macrocarpon*) is found wild from Newfoundland to the Carolinas and westward to Minnesota and Arkansas. The cranberry is cultivated on acid soils of peat or vegetable mold that is free of loam and clay and cleared of turf, having a surface layer of sand. It is grown extensively in Massachusetts, New Jersey, and Wisconsin and near the coast in Washington and Oregon. Cranberries are used mostly as a sauce and as a relish for meats but are also used in pies and fresh fruit beverages. Cranberry consumption is highest in the U.S. and Canada.

Cranberries are a good source of ascorbic acid (vitamin C), potassium, and micronutrients. One gram of cranberry contains 0.004 g of protein, 0.007 g of fat, 0.1 g of carbohydrate, 0.13 mg of calcium, 0.1 mg of phosphorus, 0.005 mg of iron, 0.02 mg of sodium, 0.8 mg of potassium, 0.4 IU of vitamin A, 0.0003 mg of thiamin, 0.0002 mg of riboflavin, 0.009 mg of niacin, and 0.1 mg of ascorbic acid.[1] Cranberries also contain flavonoids — such as anthocyanin — flavonols, and proanthocyanidins, as well as other phenolic compounds which have anti-cancer properties.[2] Anthocyanin and proanthocyanidin have been recently recognized as antioxidants. Malic, quinic, and citric acids are constituents of major organic acids in cranberry juice or extract.[3] Cranberry juice is rich in benzoic acid, which is excreted as hippuric acid in the urine.

0-8493-8561-X/98/$0.00+$.50
© 1998 by CRC Press LLC

Antibacterial effects of cranberries

Significant variations in urinary pH can cause problems for all human beings, but these problems are magnified when an individual has a urostomy. Most significantly, stomal and peristomal complications are related to an alkaline urine including hyperleratosis, stoma bleeding, incrustation, ulceration, stoma stenosis, and urinary tract infection (UTI).[4] Cranberry juice has been increasingly recommended as a folk treatment to reduce or prevent urinary tract infection. Drinking cranberry juice to reduce UTI is very reasonable and effective.[5]

Cranberry juice or cocktail has bacteriostatic effects.[5] Regular intake of cranberry juice can reduce the frequency of bacteriuria and pyuria in older women.[5] Bacterial infection and influx of white cells into the urine were reduced by 50% with consumption of 300 ml of cranberry juice per day over 6 months. This indicates that the consumption of cranberry juice is more effective in treating than preventing bacteriuria and pyuria.[6] These findings suggest that prevalent beliefs about the effects of cranberry juice on the urinary tract may have microbiologic justification. There is an adverse effect with development of kidney stones if more than 2.5 l cartons of cranberry juice per day are drunk.[7] Cranberry juice improved vitamin B_{12} absorption, which had been decreased by omeprazole, a potent inhibitor of gastric acid secretion.[8] This activity was related to the ability of cranberry juice to change gastric and small intestine pH and to inhibit the overgrowth of pH-sensitive bacteria, which could bind with vitamin B_{12}.

Cranberry juice inactivates bacteria by inhibiting the bacterial adherence to uroepithelial cells, although this is not yet clearly proven. It was thought until the 1970s that the bacteriostatic effect of cranberry juice is caused by change in urinary pH[9,10] or increase in hippuric acid level.[11] However, there were conflicting results concerning urinary acidification and increased hippuric acid level in urine excretion.[12] Drinking cranberry juice did not acidify the urine. Improvements were seen in skin conditions of the study participants, suggesting that drinking cranberry juice positively impacts the incidence of skin complications of the patients.[27] Recent evidence suggested a different potential mechanism of cranberry juice's antipathogen activity. Both cranberry juice and the urine collected from mice fed cranberry cocktail inhibited adherence of *Escherichia coli* to uroepithelial cells by about 75 to 80%.[12] Similar activity was found in humans provided with 15 oz of cranberry cocktail. Thus, cranberry juice may affect urinary concentration of Tamm-Horsfall glycoprotein, which prevents adherence of *E.coli* strain to human kidney cells.[13] Cranberry juice also inhibited bacterial adherence and *E.coli* reproduction in the bowel.[14] Two active compounds, fructose and a nondialyzable polymer, were isolated from the cranberry cocktail that inhibited lectin-mediated adherence of *E.coli* to bladder cells. Cranberry cocktails inhibited a wide range of bacteria and the growth of yeast cells.[15]

Cranberries and AIDS

Infection is a common problem among the immunodeficient such as AIDS patients and the aged. Whereas a recent report suggested that pomegranates contained materials that inhibited HIV, nothing is known about cranberry's actions on viral growth. However, it does affect infections, which are more prevalent in the immunocompromised.

Cranberry: Role in Cancer Resistance

Cancer is one of the major causes of death in the U.S. Although the risk for cancer is multifunctional, a substantial portion of the cancer incidence rate is related to environmental factors including diet.[18] Thus, a large number of cancer-related deaths could be prevented by increased consumption of fruits and vegetables.[19] Members of *Vaccinium* species including *V. macrocarpon* Ait.(cranberry), *V. myrtillus* L.(bilberry), *V. angustifolium* Ait.(lowbush blueberry), and *V. vitis-idaea* L.(lingonberry) are rich resources of flavonoids and other phenolics which have anticancer properties.[20] Crude extracts of bilberry and lingonberry have anti-free-radical and anti-tumor activities.[21] However, there are few reports on the effects of cranberry juice or extracts on cancer resistance.

The extract of cranberry showed potential anticarcinogenic activity using an *in vitro* screening test.[18] Most research has been carried out with crude cranberry extracts, which can be subdivided into anthocyanin, proanthocyanidin, and ethyl acetate fractions. Cranberry extracts were tested for their ability to induce the phase II xenobiotic detoxification, quinone reductase (QR), and to inhibit the induction of ornithine decarboxylase (ODC), the rate-limiting enzyme in polyamine synthesis by the tumor promoter porbol 12-myristate 13-acetate (TPA). The crude extracts, anthocyanin and proanthocyanidin fractions, were not highly active in QR induction whereas the ethyl acetate fraction was. The concentration of ethyl acetate fraction required to double QR activity was 3.7 μg tannic acid equivalent (TAE). The study also showed that proanthocyanidin fraction of cranberry was an active inhibitor of ODC activity. The concentration needed to inhibit ODC activity by 50% was 7.0 μg TAE. The anthocyanin and ethyl acetate fractions were either inactive or relatively weak inhibitors of ODC activity. Thus, the proanthocyanidin of cranberry may play a role in exhibiting potential anticarcinogenic activity.

Anthocyanins extracted from cranberry had relatively less inhibitory activity in an *in vitro* test for anti-tumor promoting effect on Epstein-Barr virus early antigen (EBV-EA) induced by TPA than betanin extracted from *beta vulgaris* (beet) root, carotenoids from short red bell peppers, and anthocyanins from red onion skin.[19]

Unlike anthocyanin, cranberry proanthocyanidin may act as an anticarcinogen. Further study of proanthocyanidin *in vivo* as an anticarcinogen and strong antioxidant is recommended.

Antioxidants of Cranberry

There are few reports on proanthocyanidin and anthocyanin, which may be one of the active compounds of cranberry. Both proanthocyanidin and anthocyanin were recently defined as strong antioxidants. Proanthocyanidin has several functions concerning nutrition, metabolism, and enzyme, and antioxidant activities. Proanthocyanidin-A$_2$, a catechic dimer extracted from the bark of *Aesculus hippocastanum* L., has a tropic effect on reinnervated rat muscle.[23] It increased the contraction force and soleus muscle mass. Proanthocyanidin and proanthocyanidin-rich hulls prepared from beans (*Vicia faba* L.) depressed the digestibility of protein by 35 to 60%, starch by 5%, and lipid by 4%.[24] Proanthocyanidin also depressed digestive enzyme activities, trypsin by 60%, alpha-amylase by 76%, and lipase by 32%.[24]

Proanthocyanidin-A$_2$ prevents skin damage through two mechanisms of action that involve scavenging oxygen and carbon-center free radicals and inhibiting enzyme systems.[25] Proanthocyanidin inhibited all the enzyme systems including collagenase, elastas, hyaluronidase, and beta-glucuronidase noncompetitively, which indicates that proanthocyanidin interacts with the enzymes through a hydrogen-bonding mechanism, not substrate binding.[25] Proanthocyanidin inhibited all the phases of the lipid peroxidative cascade, the induction initiated by HO*, the propagation sustained by R* and ROO*.[25] In addition, proanthocyanidin was 10 times more active than the typical antioxidant vitamin E.[26]

Anthocyanin has also been classified as an antioxidant by nonenzymatic reaction. The antioxidant effect of anthocyanins on lipid peroxidation is partly due to its strong reactivity with hydroperoxides.[27]

Conclusion

In summary, bacteriuria is very common among elderly women. About 15% of older women suffer from repeated UTI. Cranberry juice or its extract is very effective in reducing urinary tract infection in older women.[16] The mechanisms by which cranberry juice prevent UTI include (1) urinary acidification due to increased hippuric acid, and (2) inhibition of bacterial adherence to uroepithelial cells. The former concept has recently yielded controversy among many researchers; the latter is much regarded as a possible mechanism of cranberry juice to prevent UTI. In addition, cranberry juice can reduce risk of UTI in sexually active young women.[17] However, the effect of cranberry juice on young women has not been established. Thus, further study will help treat UTI in young women by detecting the active compound in cranberry juice and defining clinical treatment with the active compound. Proanthocyanidin extracted from cranberry juice is an active inhibitor of ornithine decarboxylase (ODC) activity, indicating that the extract of cranberry may play a role in exhibiting potential anticarcinogenic activity. Proanthocyanidin is also ten times stronger than vitamin E as an antioxidant.

In trying to understand the potential actions of cranberry extracts in health promotion it is important to focus on it as a rich source of diverse bioflavanoids. They are a ubiquitous group of nontoxic plant compounds that impact on a variety of disease processes in humans.[14] Their primary action is oxygen free-radical scavenging. They also inhibit lipoxygenase which converts arachidonic acid to leukotrienes. These actions should affect inflammation, cancer, and pathogen growth.

Compared with its antibacterial effects, a role for cranberries in cancer and antiviral resistance has not been demonstrated. However, there is a recent report concerning the potential activity of cranberry against cancer. Thus, further studies are needed on the biochemical properties of the substances in cranberry juice to clarify its role in the prevention of UTI, and to help in understanding cancer resistance and antiviral effect.

References

1. Adams, C.F., Nutritive value of American foods, *Agric. Handbook*, 456, 125, 1995.
2. Bomser, J., Madhavi, D.L., Singletary, K., and Smith, M.A., *In vitro* anticancer activity of fruit extracts from *Vaccinium* species, *Planta Med.*, 62, 212, 1996.
3. Coppola, E.D., Conrad, E.C., and Cotter, R., High pressure liquid chromatographic determination of major organic acids in cranberry juice, *J. Assoc. Off. Anal. Chem.*, 61, 1490, 1978.
4. Walsh, B.A., Urostomy and urinary pH, *J. Nursing*, 19, 110, 1992.
5. Avorn, J., Monane, M., Gurwitz, J.H., Glynn, R.J., Choosnovskiv, I., and Lipsitz, L.A., Reduction of bacteriuria and pyuria after ingestion of cranberry juice, *JAMA*, 271, 751, 1994.
6. Fleet, J.C., New support for a folk remedy: cranberry juice reduces bacteriuria and pyuria in elderly women, *Nutr. Rev.*, 52, 168, 1994.
7. Kahn, H.D., Effect of cranberry juice on urine, *J. Am. Diet. Assoc.*, 51, 252, 1967.
8. Saltzman, J.R., Kemp, J.A., Golner, B.B., Pedrosa, M.C., Dallal, G.E., and Russel, R.M., Effect of hypochlorhydria due to omeprazole treatment of atrophic gastritis or protein-bound vitamin B_{12} absorption, *JACN*, 13, 584, 1994.
9. Schultz, A.S., Efficacy of cranberry juice and ascorbic acid in acidifying the urine in multiple sclerosis subjects, *J. Com. Health Nurs.*, 1, 159-169, 1984.
10. Kinney, A.B. and Blount, M., Effect of cranberry juice on urinary pH, *Nurs. Res.*, 29, 287, 1979.
11. Bode, P.T., Cranberry juice and the antibacterial action of hippuric acid, *J. Lab. Clin. Med.*, 54, 881, 1959.
12. Sobota, A.E., Inhibition of bacterial adherence by cranberry juice: potential use for the treatment of urinary tract infections, *J. Urol.*, 131, 1013, 1984.
13. Dulawa, J., Tamm-Horsfall glycoprotein interferes with bacterial adherence to human kidney cells, *Eur. J. Clin. Invest.*, 18, 87, 1998.
14. Sternlieb, P., Cranberry juice in renal disease, *N. Engl. J. Med.*, 268, 57, 1993.
15. Zafriri, D., Ofek, I., Adar, R., Pocino, M., and Sharon, N., Inhibitory activity of cranberry juice on adherence of type I and type P fimbriated *Escherichia coli* to eukaryotic cells, *Antimicrob. Agents Chemother.*, 33, 92, 1989.

16. Mollander, U., An epidemiological study of urinary incontinence and related urogenital symptoms in elderly women, *Maturitas*, 12, 51, 1990.
17. Betsy, F., Ann, M.G., Karen, P., Brenda, G., and James, S.K., First-time urinary tract infection and sexual behavior, *Epidemiology*, 6, 162, 1995.
18. Committee on Diet and Health: Implications for reducing chronic disease risk, *Natl. Acad. Press*, Washington, D.C., 593, 1989.
19. Block, G. and Patterson, B., Fruit, vegetables, and cancer prevention: a review of the epidemiological evidence, *A. Subar. Nutr. Cancer*, 18, 1, 1992.
20. Delong, M.J., Prochaska, H.J., and Talalay, P., Induction of NAD(P)H: quinone reductase in murine hepatoma cells by phenolic antioxidants, azo dyes, and other chemoprotectors — a model system for the study of anticarcinogens, *Proc. Natl. Acad. Sci.*, 83, 787,1986.
21. Seeger, P.G., The antocyans of *beta vulgaris var. rubra* (red beets), *Vaccinium myrtillis* (whortleberries), *vinum rubrum* (red wine) and their significance as cell respiratory activators for cancer prophylaxis and cancer therapy, *Arzneim.-Forsch.*, 21, 68, 1967.
22. Kapadia, G.J., Tokuda, H., Konoshima, T., and Nishino, H., Chemoprevention of lung and skin cancer by *beta vulgaris* (beet) root extract, *Cancer Lett.*, 100, 211, 1996.
23. Ambrogini, P., Cuppini, R., Bruno, C., and Bombrdelli, E., Effects of proanthocyanidin on normal and reinnervated rat muscle, *Boll.-Soc. Ital. Bio. Sper.*, 71, 227, 1995.
24. Yuste, P., Longstaff, M., and Mccorquodale, C., The effect of proanthocyanidin-rich hulls and proanthocyanidin extracts from bean (*Vincia faba* L.) hulls on nutrient digestibility and digestive enzyme activities in young chicks, *Brit. J. Nutr.*, 67, 57, 1992.
25. Facino, R.M., Carini, M., Brambilla, A., Bombardelli, E., and Morazzoni, P., Proanthocyanidin-A_2: a new polyphenol, *Cosmet. Toil.*, 111, 49, 1996.
26. Illou, J.P., Kinetics of photoperoxidation of arachidonic acid: molecular mechanism and effects of antioxidants, *Lipid*, 27, 959, 1992.
27. Yoshiki, Y., Okubo, K., and Igarashi, K., Chemiluminescence of anthocyanins in the presence of acetaldehyde and tert-butyl hydroperoxide, *J. Biol. Chem.*, 10, 335, 1995.

Index

Index